The Stenter's Notebook

Paul S. Phillips, MD
Director, Interventional Cardiology
Mercy Hospital
San Diego, California

Morton J. Kern, MD
Director, Cardiac Catheterization Laboratory
Saint Louis University Health Sciences Center
St. Louis, Missouri

Patrick W. Serruys, MD, PhD
Research Director, Cardiac Catheterization Laboratory
Thoraxcenter, Erasmus University
Rotterdam, the Netherlands

PHYSICIANS' PRESS

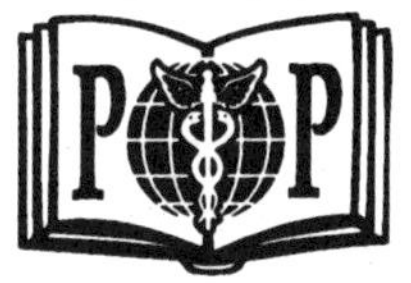

Birmingham, Michigan

ABOUT PHYSICIANS' PRESS

Physicians' Press is a unique entry into the medical publishing industry. Owned and operated by physicians, Physicians' Press specializes in innovative and user-friendly manuals, textbooks, and newsletters in the fields of Interventional Cardiology, Clinical Cardiology, and Internal Medicine. Physicians' Press stands apart from all other medical publishers in being able to produce completely current publications; literature references are ***less than 2 weeks old*** at the time of book release, compared to 18 months old for most other texts. We frequently receive comments such as "I am astounded at how current your information is," and, "The only books I bother reading are yours, the rest are outdated." Physicians' Press is committed to providing its readers with the most current, practical, and user-friendly information, as we continue to distinguish ourselves as the new gold-standard in medical publishing.

Be sure to visit us on the internet at **www.physicianspress.com**, where you'll find interventional cases, self-assessment questions and answers, information about upcoming meetings, and more.

If you are looking for a publisher or have comments and suggestions, please contact us at:

Physicians' Press
555 South Woodward Ave., Suite 1409
Birmingham, Michigan 48009
Tel: (248) 645-6443
Fax: (248) 642-4949
http://www.physicianspress.com

Printed in the United States of America ISBN 1-890114-06-5

DEDICATION

To Adrienne, Colin, Justin and Galen, to whom the time dedicated to this notebook properly belonged. Their support has provided personal meaning to the term "scaffolding."

— Paul Phillips

To Margaret and Anna Rose, my real-life stents.

— Morton Kern

To my wife, Danielle, and to my family.

— Patrick Serruys

PREFACE

"The Stenter's Notebook" was initiated as a result of a year's sabbatical with Dr. Carlos Macaya and the interventional team at the San Carlos University Hospital in Madrid, Spain. The majority of the cases presented were performed by Drs. Carlos Macaya, Javier Goicolea, Fernando Alfonso, Rosana Hernandez, Camino Banuclos, Javier Segovia, and Antonio Fernandez-Ortiz. In particular, Dr. Carlos Macaya's ability to make complex cases simple and dangerous interventions safe while maintaining a Spaniard's calm has left its indelible impression on me, and his thoughtful commentary and encouragement have been instrumental in the development of this book.

Paul S. Phillips, MD

The stent is one of the most important and unique devices to be introduced into the practice of cardiology since the advent of Gruntzig's angioplasty balloon catheter. "The Stenter's Notebook" is a lesion-specific approach to intracoronary stenting; case presentations and clinical discussions about technical pearls and pitfalls, device synergy, adjunctive imaging and pharmacotherapy, and recent trials provide a comprehensive and current overview of this important new technology. We have enjoyed working with Dr. Phillips in the presentation of his experience during the time spent with his colleagues at the San Carlos University Hospital in Madrid, Spain, and hope that you find "The Stenter's Notebook" a practical resource for patient care.

Morton J. Kern, MD
Patrick W. Serruys, MD, PhD

ACKNOWLEDGMENTS

We would like to acknowledge the dedicated and tireless efforts of Donna Sander in preparing this manuscript for publication, Casado for his patience in processing the numerous cineangiographic images into photographs for the case studies, Mark Snyder and Monica Crowder for typesetting and formatting, Norm Lyle of The Lyle Group for cover design, Dickinson Press for their printing expertise, to the stent manufacturers for providing photographs and technical specifications about their stents, and to Mark Freed, MD, and his staff at Physicians' Press, for their unique commitment to publishing excellence.

Paul S. Phillips, MD
Morton J. Kern, MD
Patrick W. Serruys, MD, PhD

NOTICE

The explosive growth of new equipment and drug therapy has resulted in the rapid evolution and acceptance of practice patterns often based on retrospective nonrandomized data and personal experience. Their ultimate role will require close inspection of prospective randomized trials. The clinical recommendations set forth in this book are those of the authors; they are offered as *general guidelines only and are not to be construed as absolute indications*. The cases in this book are purely illustrative, and are not intended to endorse one device over another, or one stent design over another. In addition, not all equipment or medications have been accepted by the U.S. Food and Drug Administration (USFDA) for usages described in this manual. The use of any device or drug should be preceded by a careful review of the package insert, which provides indications (and dosages) as approved by the USFDA. The reader is advised to consult the package insert before using any therapeutic agent. The authors and publisher disclaim responsibility for adverse effects resulting from omissions or undetected errors.

TABLE OF CONTENTS

INDEX OF CASES

CHAPTER 1

RESTENOSIS AND REMODELING WITHIN STENTS

CASE 1.1: Remodeling within Stents

A 75 year old man presented 14 years ago with unstable angina. He had an occluded right coronary artery and his angina was treated medically until four and a half years ago when he presented with unstable angina which failed medical therapy. Urgent catheterization demonstrated a new proximal left anterior descending stenosis in association with his chronically occluded right coronary artery (**Figure 1.1a**).

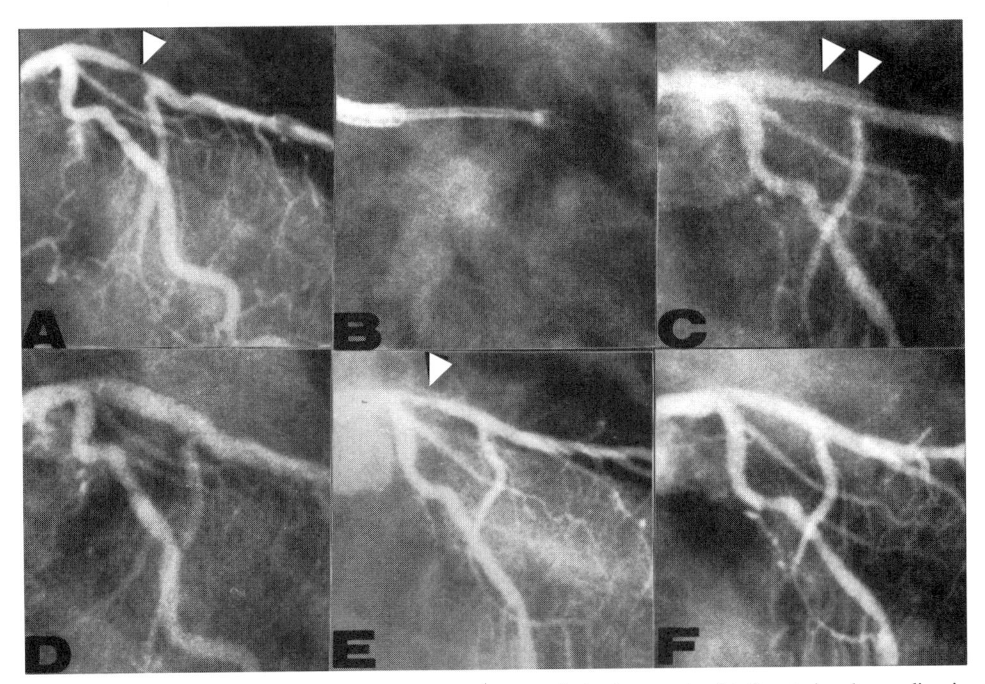

Figure 1.1 Remodeling within Stents. A severe stenosis in the proximal left anterior descending is noted (**a**; arrow). Because some projections suggested thrombus at the lesion, a transluminal extraction-endarterectomy catheter (TEC) was used to cross the lesion (**b**). A linear dissection resulted after the TEC procedure (**c**; arrows). After deployment of a Palmaz-Schatz I stent there is no residual lesion or dissection (**d**). Angiography 6 months after stent implantation revealed a 50% restenosis at the proximal stent segment (**e**; arrow). The patient was treated medically. Angiography four and a half years later revealed remarkable remodeling leaving no residual lesion at the restenotic site (**f**).

PROCEDURE 1.1

Because of the rapid progression of symptoms and the suggestion of thrombus on some angiographic projections, a staged transluminal extraction-endarterectomy (TEC) followed by angioplasty was planned. A TEC guidewire was easily passed through the lesion into the transapical left anterior descending artery (LAD). A 2.1mm TEC catheter was passed over the diseased area using a passage rate to maintain good return of aspirated matter (**Figure 1.1b**). Upon completion of the transluminal endarterectomy, a long Type C dissection without flow limitation was present (**Figure 1.1c**) and did not improve after a prolonged low pressure dilation with a 3mm balloon. Because of the very proximal location of the initial lesion and the occluded right coronary artery, a Palmaz-Schatz 15mm stent (**Figure 1.2**) was placed in the diseased segment and covered the dissection. There was no residual stenosis after stenting (**Figure 1.1d**).

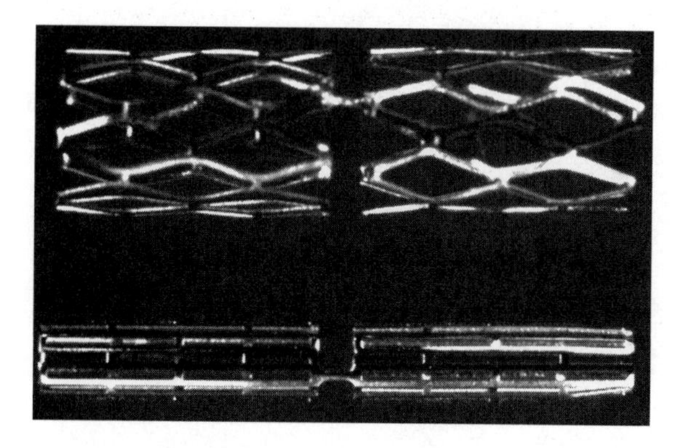

Figure 1.2 The Palmaz-Schatz stent. A slotted tube with central articulation

The patient was discharged and remained asymptomatic at follow-up evaluation six months later. At that time he exercised to 10 METS on a Bruce protocol stress test without symptoms nor electrocardiographic changes. However, an angiogram revealed a moderate (50% by QCA) restenosis (**Figure 1.1e**). As the patient was asymptomatic he was treated medically. He underwent angiography four and a half years after the original procedure because of atypical chest pains and was found to have remodeled his restenotic lesion to a remarkable extent leaving no residual stenosis (**Figure 1.1f**).

Materials 1.1

Guiding Catheter:	Interventional Technologies FL 3.5 TEC guiding catheter
Guidewires:	Interventional Technologies 0.014"x 300cm TEC guidewire
Atherotome:	Interventional Technologies TEC 2.1 mm coronary catheter
Balloons:	Schneider Speedy 3.0 x 20mm, ACS Low Profile II 3.5 x 20mm
Stents:	Johnson & Johnson P-S 153 (15mm)

DISCUSSION

Stents have become increasingly popular, overcoming the two major inadequacies of angioplasty: suboptimal results and restenosis. Compared to balloon angioplasty, a lower restenosis rate is the major rationale for an elective stent placement. Although various definitions of restenosis are used, review of available studies suggests that stent implantation provides an advantage over balloon angioplasty no matter which definition is employed.

The mechanisms of restenosis differ between balloon angioplasty and stent implantation as do the risk factors for restenosis after each treatment. This difference may provide support for one treatment over the other in certain defined clinical circumstances. The current case highlights the clinical importance of angiographic restenosis and the methods of treating intrastent restenosis.

Definitions of Restenosis

There has been little standardization of the definition of restenosis among different trials. Serruys et al.[1] in a survey of studies of restenosis report 13 different definitions in common use. In one comparison of restenosis trials, the most powerful single predictor of restenosis rate was the choice of definition.[2] Different definitions may identify different restenotic patient cohorts.[1] The most commonly used definition has been a percent diameter stenosis at follow-up of >50%. While this definition has some physiologic correlates with respect to coronary flow reserve,[3] it has been shown to be limited in two additional respects. Firstly, there is often progressive narrowing of the reference arterial segment after procedures which causes percent stenosis measurements at 6 months to underestimate the true amount of restenosis due to the fibroproliferative reaction at the lesion site.[4,5] Secondly, the change in minimal lumen diameter (MLD) at follow-up, when analyzed by quantitative angiographic (QCA) methods, distributes in a Gaussian fashion and not in a bimodal fashion. Artificially dividing this continuous biologic phenomenon into a dichotomy of groups with greater than and less than 50% stenosis does not adequately describe the process.[6] Consequently, the MLD has become the preferred measurement to assess restenosis after coronary interventions. The MLD can be examined as a continuous rather than a dichotomous display to demonstrate the restenosis spectrum for the intervention under study. The MLD does not incur the errors of choosing reference diameters which may themselves have significant atherosclerosis and variability.

Mechanisms of Stent Restenosis

The mechanisms of restenosis involve the following five processes, contributing to luminal narrowing to varying degrees:

1. Elastic recoil
2. Platelet deposition and arterial mural thrombus
3. Fibrocellular neointimal hyperplasia
4. Progression of the atherosclerotic plaque
5. Vascular remodeling: constriction and dilation

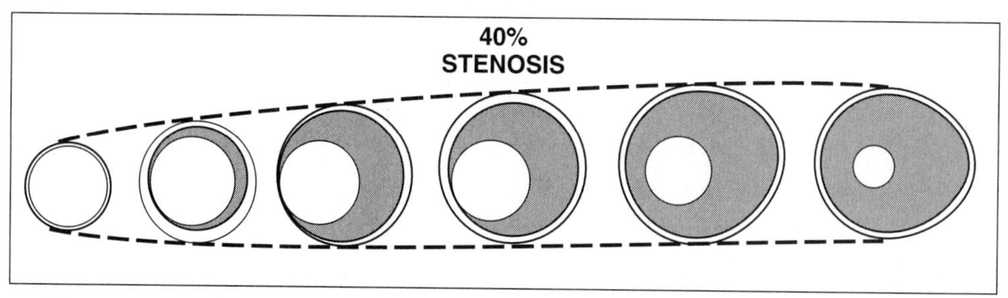

Figure 1.3 "Glagovian Remodeling" As atherosclerotic plaque accumulates within the arterial lumen, the artery enlarges or remodels to preserve the intraluminal area. This remodeling successfully maintains the lumenal area until the plaque causes 40% stenosis after which further plaque deposition results in progressive reduction of the lumen. Reprinted with permission from Dr. S Glagov and The New England Journal of Medicine. N Engl J Med 1987; 316:1374).

Restenosis may be viewed as the local vascular response to wound healing associated with the inevitable injury of balloon angioplasty.[7] The important steps in the model include platelet aggregation, the infiltration of inflammatory cells, growth factor mediated smooth muscle proliferation, and finally the remodeling of the extracellular matrix.[7] Thrombus now appears to contribute only minimally to the amount of intimal proliferation[8] while remodeling seems to play a larger role in the restenotic process.[9]

Vascular Remodeling

Remodeling refers to the changes in the arterial caliber in response to atherosclerotic plaque or after coronary interventions. Glagov[10] first described this phenomenon in left main coronary arteries where the vascular response to plaque caused vessels to dilate. This dilation maintained the lumen size until the plaque volume exceeded 30-40% of the lumen area (**Figure 1.3),** a finding confirmed in other arteries by monitoring the enlargement of their internal elastic lamina by intracoronary ultrasound.[11] In an animal model of angioplasty restenosis, the volume contained by the internal elastic lamina increased by 20% over the four weeks post procedure.[12] This compensatory enlargement accommodated almost 60% of the intimal proliferation which developed, and often maintained, the same lumen size. The intimal area was equal in restenotic and non-restenotic vessels and the difference in luminal areas between the groups was accounted for by differences in the area encompassed by the remodeled internal elastic lamina.[12] In humans after angioplasty, intravascular ultrasound (IVUS) data suggest that intimal hyperplasia comprises only 50% of the luminal narrowing leaving anti-Glagov remodeling or chronic constriction accountable for the remaining 50% of luminal loss.[13]

The ambiguity of the terms recoil, remodeling, and chronic constriction, often used imprecisely, leads to confusion. All three terms refer to changes in the luminal area which are not accounted for by intimal proliferation. Recoil, defined as the difference in the arterial dimensions within the first minutes of angioplasty, may be an artifact of the measurement technique. Recoil has been attributed to errors due to balloon-to-artery diameter inequities and varying amounts of vascular spasm or arterial paralysis. Recoil measured between 24 hours and six months after angioplasty is more likely to represent the restoration of vascular tone and is indistinguishable from adaptive remodeling or chronic constriction.[14-17]

Stent Restenosis

Remodeling may be used to describe both compensatory enlargement ("Glagovian") or constriction ("Anti-Glagovian") of an artery. When constriction is the predominant response, restenosis will occur with minimal intimal ingrowth.[9] While IVUS data suggest that differences in arterial remodeling after angioplasty have more impact on restenosis than differences in the quantity of intima formation,[12] the lumen response is precisely the opposite after stenting.

After stent placement, the intimal proliferative response, measured as late lumen loss, is significantly greater than after angioplasty.[18,19] The fixation of the arterial wall by the stent tends to prevent both vascular recoil and remodeling-induced changes in the arterial diameter. After placement of stainless steel mesh Wallstents, remodeling or vascular constriction was reduced to less than 20%.[20,21] Elastic recoil is reduced to 4-18% for Palmaz-Schatz stents,[22] 20% after Gianturco-Roubin stents,[23] and 8-22% after Wiktor stents.[24]

In the coronary circulation, late stent compression by external plaque or vascular recoil has been disproved as a mechanism of stent restenosis.[25,26] Thus, stents replace the problems of recoil and remodeling with a greater degree of intimal hyperplasia. The increased intimal reaction is attributable to the greater degree of vascular damage by stent placement and is consistent with Schwartz's concept of proportional injury (the greater the injury, the greater the injury response; see Chapter 8 and Figure 8.3).[28] Stents reduce restenosis despite the increase in intimal reaction because the initial lumen gain more than accommodates the increase in late lumen loss.

Findings in both the Benestent and STRESS trials indicated that stents offered, on average, a 30% reduction in restenosis in de novo lesions compared to balloon angioplasty. These results have been supported by other restenosis trials. In the REST study using Palmaz-Schatz stents to treat restenotic lesions, angiographic restenosis was 18% in the stented group compared to 38% in the repeat angioplasty group.[29] The START trial was similarly designed and demonstrated a 22% restenosis rate in the stent group compared to 37% restenosis rate in the repeat angioplasty group.[30] The preliminary data from the Benestent-II trial using higher pressure inflations to insure optimal stent deployment, reduced restenosis rates to 17%.[31]

The differences in the mechanisms of restenosis between angioplasty and stents may also involve differences in the risk factors for restenosis after treatment. **Table 1.1** profiles these differences.

Table 1.1 Risk Factors for Restenosis after Angioplasty and Stent Implantation

RISK FACTOR	PTCA RESTENOSIS	STENT RESTENOSIS
DIABETES	↑[32] 4-fold on insulin[33]	↑[34, 35]
UNSTABLE ANGINA or MI	↑[36]	-[37]
LONG LESIONS	↑[32,38]	↑[35, 40]
LESIONS ON CURVES	↑for angle > 45%[41]	-[57]
RELATIVE GAIN	↑[39]	↑[42]
CHRONIC OCCLUSIONS	↑[43]	↑[44, 45]
VESSELS < 2.5mm	-	↑[35]
PROXIMAL LAD	↑[41, 46, 47, 48, 49]	-[50,74]
RESTENOTIC LESIONS	↑[51]	↑[35, 52, 53]
OSTIAL LOCATION	↑[54]	↑[35]
SMALL POST PROCEDURE MLD	↑[39]	↑[35]
VEIN GRAFTS	↑[38, 55]	↑[35, 56]

↑= increased risk; - = no increase

Based on the comparative restenosis rates from Table 1.1, primary stent placement may be better than balloon angioplasty in specific situations where the restenosis rates between the techniques are the most disparate. For example, in locations where vascular recoil or remodeling is most severe, such as left main disease, ostial lesions, saphenous vein grafts, and the proximal anterior descending, stent implantation would be preferred. In situations where the local milieu of ruptured plaque or thrombus is associated with high restenosis rates after balloon angioplasty, stenting also enjoys an advantage. For chronic total occlusions, the need to minimize the effects of remodeling as well as the need to treat the high incidence of dissection after angioplasty of these lesions also favors stents.[58] On the other hand, because of the increased rates of both subacute occlusion and restenosis of stents in small vessels, stenting provides no differential benefit in this setting.

In-Stent Remodeling

In the Benestent trial, only 10% of patients receiving stents required further revascularization.[59] It is apparent that not all angiographic restenosis is clinically important since only 50% of patients with QCA criteria of restenosis develop ischemic symptoms. At follow-up, an MLD of 1.45mm correlates with the threshold for a recurrence of symptoms after angioplasty.[60] Patients with asymptomatic restenosis after angioplasty have an excellent prognosis, especially if their exercise test fails to demonstrate ischemia.[61] A similar prognosis would be expected after coronary stent implantation. The restenosis incidence after stent placement in native vessels plateaus at 6 months, similar to that after balloon angioplasty.[35] Despite angiographic evidence of lumen narrowing at six months, remodeling may develop in some of these patients such that at later angiography the restenosis has improved or vanished.[62]

The importance of late remodeling after angioplasty is highlighted by Mehta et al.[63] in which 12 of 15 patients who demonstrated restenosis at six month angiography showed a significant (58%) regression of stenosis at late follow-up study.[63] The mechanism of this improvement is unknown but it can be postulated that, in the same way that scar tissue contracts during the final phases of wound healing, the hyperplastic neointima of restenosis may retract during the chronic phase after angioplasty causing a regression of the restenotic lesion. This type of late remodeling may differ in that the remodeling of the contraction of intimal scar occurs but not that of the internal elastic lamina. Preliminary reports suggest that a similar type of late remodeling or late improvement occurs after stent placement.[64] Late phase follow-up data have revealed a progressive increase in the luminal dimension between six months and three years after stent placement consistent with remodeling or contraction of the hypertrophied intima.[65]

Treatment of In-stent Restenosis

Since the mechanism of intrastent restenosis is primarily intimal hyperplasia, the process can be easily and safely treated by angioplasty. There is a notion that angioplasty within stents is safer than routine angioplasty due to the protection offered by the stent.[66] Careful angiographic review of the stent dimensions before and after angioplasty for in-stent restenosis has confirmed that the improved lumen results from extrusion of the hypertrophied intimal tissue through the stent struts rather than any further dilation of the stent.[25] The rate of second restenosis after an initial in-stent restenosis depends on the morphology of the recurrence. Second in-stent restenosis rates range from 40-50%.[67,68] Focal restenoses may recur less frequently. Diffuse restenoses may recur 80% of the time.[69] The choice of treatment for stent restenotic lesions should be individualized based on both lesion and stent morphology and the specific clinical requirements.

Stent Design and Restenosis

It is not yet clear whether different stent designs will produce different rates of restenosis. A preliminary trial comparing Palmaz-Schatz and Wiktor stents in the right coronary artery suggested that the Wiktor stent had twice the rate of both clinical events and of angiographic restenosis (48% versus 23%).[70] Laboratory evidence suggests that stent modifications, such as reducing the number of strut-strut intersections, may reduce the severity of vascular injury, thrombosis and neointimal hyperplasia.[71,72] Tubular stent designs appear to decrease flow velocity and turbulence within the treated artery while helical and loop designs may increase one or both of these characteristics.[73] As these factors affect shear rates and platelet residence times, specific design features may be predicted to result in different rates of restenosis.

SUMMARY

The pathophysiology of restenosis and remodeling after stenting remains under study. Stents reduce the initial recoil after angioplasty but induce a greater amount of intimal hypertrophy during the restenosis period. Because of a much greater initial luminal gain, the stent restenosis rate is generally reduced by 30% compared to balloon angioplasty. Only 50% of those with angiographic restenosis develop symptoms resulting in a reintervention rate after stenting of about 10% across many trials. There may be further late remodeling or contraction of neointimal matrix within restenosed stents allowing a late resorption of the restenotic lesion between six months and three years. The prognosis of asymptomatic stent restenosis is excellent and medical management of these patients is appropriate pending further information. Repeated angioplasty of asymptomatic restenotic lesions before there has been time for late remodeling could result in unnecessary procedures to treat angiographic restenosis with little or no clinical benefit.

References

1. Serruys PWS, Foley DP, Kirkeeide RL, King SB III. *Restenosis revisited: Insights provided by quantitative coronary angiography.* Am Heart J 126:1243-1267 (1993).
2. Serruys PW, Luijten HE, Beatt KJ, et al. *Incidence of restenosis after successful angioplasty: a time related phenomenon. A quantitative angiographic study in 342 consecutive patients at 1, 2, 3, and 4 months.* Circulation 77:361-371 (1988).
3. Harrison DG, White CW, Hiratzka LF, et al. *Can the significance of a coronary stenosis be predicted by quantitative coronary angiography.* Circulation 64:160-168 (1981).
4. Beatt KJ, Luijten HE, de Feyter PJ, van den Brand M, Reiber JHC, Serruys PW. *Change in diameter of coronary artery segments adjacent to stenosis after percutaneous transluminal coronary angioplasty: failure of percent diameter stenosis measurement to reflect morphologic changes induced by balloon dilation.* J Am Coll Cardiol 12:314-323 (1988).
5. Foley JB. *Alterations in reference vessel diameter following intracoronary stent implantation: important consequences for restenosis based on percent diameter stenosis.* Cathet Cardiovasc Diagn 35:103-109 (1995).
6. Beatt KJ, Serruys PW, Hugenholtz PG, et al. *Restenosis after coronary angioplasty: new standards for clinical studies.* J Am Coll Cardiol 15:491-498 (1990).
7. Forrester JS, Fishbein M, Helfant R, Fagin J. *A paradigm for restenosis based on cell biology: clues for the development of new preventive therapies.* J Am Coll Cardiol 17: 758-769 (1991).
8. Carter AJ, Laird JR, Farb A, et al. *Morphologic characteristics of lesion formation and time course of smooth muscle cell proliferation in a porcine proliferative model.* J Am Coll Cardiol 24:1398-1405 (1994).
9. Currier JW, Faxon DP. *Restenosis after percutaneous transluminal coronary angioplasty: have we been aiming at the wrong target?* J Am Coll Cardiol 25:516-520 (1995).
10. Glagov S, Weisenberg BA, Zarins CK, et al. *Compensatory enlargement of human atherosclerotic coronary arteries.* N Engl J Med 316:1371-1375 (1987).
11. Heermiller JB, Tenaglia AN, Kisslo KB, et al. *In vivo validation of compensatory enlargement of atherosclerotic coronary arteries.* Am J Cardiol 71:665-668 (1993).
12. Kakuta T, Currier JW, Haudenschild CC, et al. *Differences in compensatory vessel enlargement, not neointimal formation, account for restenosis following angioplasty in the hypercholesterolemic rabbit model.* Circulation 89:2809-2815 (1994).
13. Mintz GS, Kovach JA, Javier SP, et al. *Geometric remodeling is the predominant mechanism of late lumen loss after coronary angioplasty [abstr].* Circulation 88 (suppl I):I-654 (1993).
14. Rodriguez A, Santaera O, Larribeau M, et al. *Early decrease in minimal luminal diameter after successful percutaneous transluminal coronary angioplasty predicts late restenosis.* Am J Cardiol 71:1391-1395 (1993).

15. Waller BF, Pinkerton CA, Orr CM, et al. *Restenosis 1 to 24 months after clinically successful coronary balloon angioplasty: a necropsy study of 20 patients.* J Am Coll Cardiol 17:58B-70B (1991).

16. Mintz GS, Pichard AD, Kent KM, et al. *Intravascular ultrasound comparison of restenotic and de novo coronary artery narrowings.* Am J Cardiol 74:1278-1280 (1994).

17. Rozenman Y, Gilon D, Welber S, et al. *Clinical and angiographic predictors of immediate recoil after successful coronary angioplasty and relation to late restenosis.* Am J Cardiol 72:1020-1025 (1993).

18. Kuntz RE, Safian RD, Levine MJ, et al. *Novel approach to the analysis of restenosis after the use of three new coronary devices.* J Am Coll Cardiol 19:1493-1499 (1992).

19. Karas SP, Gravanis MB, Santoian EC, et al. *Coronary intimal proliferation after balloon injury and stenting in swine: an animal model of restenosis.* J Am Coll Cardiol 20:467-474 (1992).

20. Keane D, de Jaegere P, Serruys PW, et al. *Structural design, clinical experience and current indications of the coronary Wallstent.* Cardiol Clin 12:689-697 (1994).

21. Beatt KJ, Bertrand M, Puel J, et al. *Additional improvement in vessel lumen in the first 24 hours after stent implantation due to radial dilation force [abstract].* J Am Coll Cardiol 13:224A (1989).

22. Leon MB, Popma JF, Fischman DL, et al. *Vascular recoil immediately after implantation of tubular slotted metallic coronary stents [abstr].* J Am Coll Cardiol 19:109A (1992).

23. Popma JJ, White CH, Pinkerton CA, et al. *Effect of balloon expandable stent design on vascular recoil and lesion-site morphology after intracoronary placement [abstr].* Circulation 86:1321A (1992).

24. deJaegere P, Serruys PW, van Es GA, et al. *Recoil following Wiktor stent implantation for restenotic lesions of coronary arteries.* Cathet Cardiovasc Diagn 32:147-156 (1994).

25. Gordon P, Gibson M, Cohen DJ, Carrozza JP, Kuntz RE, Baim DS. *Mechanisms of restenosis and redilation within coronary stents—quantitative angiographic assessment.* J Am Coll Cardiol 21:1166-1174 (1993).

26. Haude M, Erbel R, Issa H, Meyer J. *Quantitative analysis of elastic recoil after balloon angioplasty and after intracoronary implantation of balloon-expandable Palmaz-Schatz stents.* J Am Coll Cardiol 21:26-34 (1993).

27. vanBeusekom H, van der Giessen WJ, Suylen RJ, et al. *Histology after stenting of human saphenous vein bypass grafts: observations from surgically excised grafts 3 to 320 days after stent implantation.* J Am Coll Cardiol 21:45-54 (1993).

28. Schwartz RS, Huber KC, Murphy JG, Edwards WD, Camrud AR, Vlietstra RE, Holmes DR. *Restenosis and the proportional neointimal response to coronary artery injury: results in a porcine model.* J Am Coll Cardiol 19:267-274 (1992).

29. Erbel R, Haude M, Hopp HW, et al. *REstenosis STent (REST)-study: Randomized trial comparing stenting and balloon angioplasty for treatment of restenosis after balloon angioplasty [abstr].* J Am Coll Cardiol 27:139A (1996).

30. Serra A, Masotti M, Fernandez-Aviles F, et al. *Stent vs angioplasty restenosis trial (START). Influence of vessel size on angiographic restenosis [abstr].* Circulation 94 (suppl 1):I-92 (1996).

31. Legrand V, Serruys PW, Emanuelsson H, et al. Benestent-II Trial - final results of visit 1: a 15-day follow-up. J Am Coll Cardiol 29 (supp A): 170A (1997).

32. Stein B, Weintraub WS, Gebhart SSP, et al. *Influence of diabetes mellitus on early and late outcome after percutaneous transluminal coronary angioplasty.* Circulation 91:979-989 (1995).

33. Margolis JR, Krieger R, Glemser E. *Coronary angioplasty: increased restenosis rate in insulin dependent diabetics [abstr].* Circulation 70(suppl II):II-175 (1994).

34. Carrozza JP, Kuntz RE, Fishman RF, Baim DA. *Restenosis after arterial injury caused by coronary stenting in patients with diabetes mellitus.* Ann Intern Med 118:344-349 (1993).

35. Kimura T, Tamura T, Yokoi H, Nobuyoshi M. *Long-term clinical and angiographic follow-up after placement of Palmaz-Schatz coronary stent: a single center experience.* J Interven Cardiol 7:129-139 (1994).

36. Plokker HWT, Ernst SMPG, Bal ET, et al. *Percutaneous transluminal coronary angioplasty in patients with unstable angina pectoris refractory to medical therapy: long-term clinical and angiographic results.* Cathet Cardiovasc Diagn 14:15-18 (1988).

37. Marco JP, Caillard JB, Doucet S, et al. *Is recent myocardial infarction a worse setting for coronary stent implantation?* Circulation 21:178A (1994).

38. Holmes DR, Vliestra RE, Smith GC. *Restenosis after percutaneous transluminal coronary angioplasty (PTCA): A report from the PTCA registry of the National Heart , Lung and Blood institute.* Am J Cardiol 53:77c-81c (1984).

39. Hirshfeld JW Jr, Schwartz FS, Jugo R, et al. *Restenosis after coronary angioplasty: A multivariate statistical model to relate lesion and procedure variables to restenosis. The M-HEART Investigators.* J Am Coll Cardiol 18:647-656 (1991).

40. Reimers B, DiMario C, Nierop P, et al. *Long-term restenosis after multiple stent implantation. A quantitative angiographic study [abstr].* Circulation 92(suppl I):I-327 (1995).

41. Ellis SG, Roubin GS, King SB III, et al. *Importance of stenosis morphology in the estimation of restenosis risk after elective percutaneous transluminal coronary angioplasty.* Am J Cardiol 63:30-34 (1989).

42. de Jaegere P, Bertrand M, Wiegand V, et al. *Angiographic predictors of recurrence of restenosis after Wiktor Stent implantation in native coronary arteries.* Am J Cardiol 72: 165-170 (1993).

43. Meier B. *Total coronary occlusion: a different animal?* J Am Coll Cardiol 17:50B-57B (1991).

44. Medina A, Melian F, Suarez de Lezo J, Pan M, et al. *Effectiveness of coronary stenting for the treatment of chronic total occlusion in angina pectoris.* Am J Cardiol 73:1222-1224 (1994).

45. Ooka M, Suzuki T, Yokoya K, Huyase M, Kojima A, Kato H, Tani T, Inada T. *Stenting after revascularization of chronic total occlusion [abstr].* Circulation 92(suppl I):I-94 (1995).

46. Frierson JH, Dimas AP, Whitlow PL, et al. *Angioplasty of the proximal left anterior descending coronary artery: initial success and long-term follow-up.* J Am Coll Cardiol 19:745-751 (1992).

47. Topol EJ, Leya F, Pinkerton CA, et al. *A comparison of directional atherectomy with coronary angioplasty in patients with coronary artery disease.* N Engl J Med 329:221-227 (1993).

48. Adelman AG, Cohen EA, Kimball BP, et al. *A comparison of directional atherectomy with balloon angioplasty for lesions of the left anterior descending coronary artery.* N Engl J Med 329:228-233 (1993).

49. Boehrer JD, Ellis SG, Pieper K, et al. *Directional atherectomy versus balloon angioplasty for coronary ostial and nonostial left anterior descending coronary artery lesions: results from a randomized multicenter trial.* J Am Coll Cardiol 25:1380-1386 (1995).

50. Phillips PS, Segovia J, Alfonso F, et al. *The efficacy of stents in the proximal left anterior descending coronary artery.* Am Heart J (In Press, 1997).

51. Dimas AP, Grigera F, Arora RR, et al. *Repeat coronary angioplasty as treatment for restenosis.* J Am Coll Cardiol 19:1310-1314 (1992).

52. Ellis SG, Savage M, Fishman D, et al. *Restenosis after placement of Palmaz-Schatz stents in native coronary arteries.* Circulation 86:1836-1844 (1992).

53. Savage MP, Fischman DL, Schatz RA, et al. *Long-term angiographic and clinical outcome after implantation of a balloon-expandable stent in the native coronary circulation.* J Am Coll Cardiol 24:1207-1212 (1994).

54. Topol E, Ellis S Fishman J, et al. *Multicenter study of percutaneous transluminal angioplasty for right coronary artery ostial stenoses.* J Am Coll Cardiol 9:1214-1218 (1987).

55. Webb JG, Myler RK, Shaw RE, et al. *Coronary angioplasty after coronary bypass surgery: Initial results and late outcome in 422 patients.* J Am Coll Cardiol 16:812-820 (1990).

56. Straus BH, Serruys PW, de Scheerder IK, et al. *Relative risk analysis of angiographic predictors of restenosis within the coronary Wallstent.* Circulation 84:1636-1643 (1991).

57. Phillips PS, Alfonso F, Segovia J, et al. *The effect of rigid stents on angled coronary arteries.* Am J Cardiol 79:191-193 (1996).

58. Kereiakes DJ, Selmon MR, McAuley BJ, et al. *Angioplasty in total coronary artery occlusion: Experience in 76 consecutive patients.* J Am Coll Cardiol 6:526-533 (1985).

59. Macaya C, Serruys PW, Ruygrok P, et al. *Continued benefit of coronary stenting versus balloon angioplasty: one-year clinical follow-up of Benestent trial.* J Am Coll Cardiol 27;255-261 (1996).

60. Rensing BJ, Hermans WRM, Deckers JP, et al. *Which angiographic parameter best describes functional status 6 months after successful single vessel coronary balloon angioplasty.* J Am Coll Cardiol 21:317-324 (1993).

61. Hernandez RA, Macaya C, Iniguez A, et al. *Midterm outcome of patients with asymptomatic restenosis after coronary balloon angioplasty.* J Am Coll Cardiol 19:1402-1409 (1992).

62. Rosing DR, Cannon RO, Watson RM, et al. *Three year anatomic, functional and clinical follow-up after successful percutaneous transluminal coronary angioplasty.* J Am Coll Cardiol 9:1-7 (1987).

63. Mehta VY, Jorgensen MB, Raizner AE, et al. *Spontaneous regression of restenosis: an angiographic study.* J Am Coll Cardiol 26:696-702 (1995).

64. Hermiller J, Fry ET, Peters TF, et al. *Late coronary artery stenosis regression within the Gianturco-Roubin intracoronary stent.* Am J Cardiol 77:247-251(1996).

65. Kimura T, Hiroyoshi Y, Nakagawa Y, et al. *Three year follow-up after implantation of metallic coronary-artery stents.* N Engl J Med 334:561-566 (1996).

66. Macande PJ, Roubin GS, Agarwal SK, Cannon AD, Dean LS, Baxley WA. *Balloon angioplasty for treatment of in-stent restenosis: feasibility, safety and efficacy.* Cathet Cardiovasc Diagn 32:125-131 (1994).

67. Schomig A, Kastrati A, Rainer D, Rauch B, Neumann FJ, Katus HH, Busch U. *Emergency coronary stenting for dissection during percutaneous transluminal coronary angioplasty: angiographic follow-up after stenting and after repeat angioplasty of the stented segment.* J Am Coll Cardiol 1994; 23:1053-1060.

68. Baim DS, Levine MJ, Leon MB, et al. *Management of restenosis within the Palmaz- Schatz coronary stent (the U.S. multicenter experience).* Am J Cardiol 71:364-366 (1993).

69. Yokoi H, Kimura T, Nakagawa Y, et al. *Long-term clinical and quantitative angiographic follow-up after the Palmaz-Schatz stent restenosis [abstr].* J Am Coll Cardiol 27(suppl A): 224A (1996).

70. Goy JJ, Eeckhout E, Stauffer JC, et al. *Stenting of the right coronary artery for de novo stenoses: a comparison of the Wiktor and the Palmaz-Schatz stents [abstr].* Circulation 92 (suppl I):I-536 (1995).

71. Rogers C, Edelman ER. *Endovascular stent design dictates experimental restenosis and thrombosis.* Circulation 91:2995-3001 (1995).

72. Squire JC, Rogers C, Edelman E. *Stent geometry during inflation influences later restenosis [abstr].* Circulation 94(suppl I):I-259 (1996).

73. Woscoboinik JR, Gordov EP, Boussignac G, et al. *Difference in flow characteristics for different stent models: implications for stent design from results of an in vitro study [abstr].* Circulation 94(suppl I):I-260 (1996).

74. Versaci F, Gaspardone A, Tomai, et al. *A comparison of coronary artery stenting with angioplasty for isolated stenosis of the proximal left anterior descending coronary artery.* N Engl J Med 336: 817-882 (1997).

CHAPTER 2

ACUTE MYOCARDIAL INFARCTION

CASE 2.1: Stenting in Acute Myocardial Infarction

This 62 year old male presented with an acute anterior wall myocardial infarction, successfully treated with t-PA. Follow-up stress testing revealed no evidence of ischemia. He remained pain free for seven months when he presented with an inferior infarction, again successfully treated with t-PA. Angina recurred on the second post-infarction day. At catheterization, there was an occluded right coronary artery in association with a severely stenosed anterior descending (**Figure 2.1a, Figure 2.2a**). There was anteroapical hypokinesis with an ejection fraction of 48%.

PROCEDURE 2.1

Because of continued chest pain and electrocardiographic changes, urgent coronary angioplasty was performed. The occluded right coronary artery was presumed the most recent culprit lesion. There had been no evidence of inferior ischemia at the time of anterior wall infarction seven months earlier. This occlusion was dilated with a 3.5mm balloon. Distal thrombus was noted and further dilations were

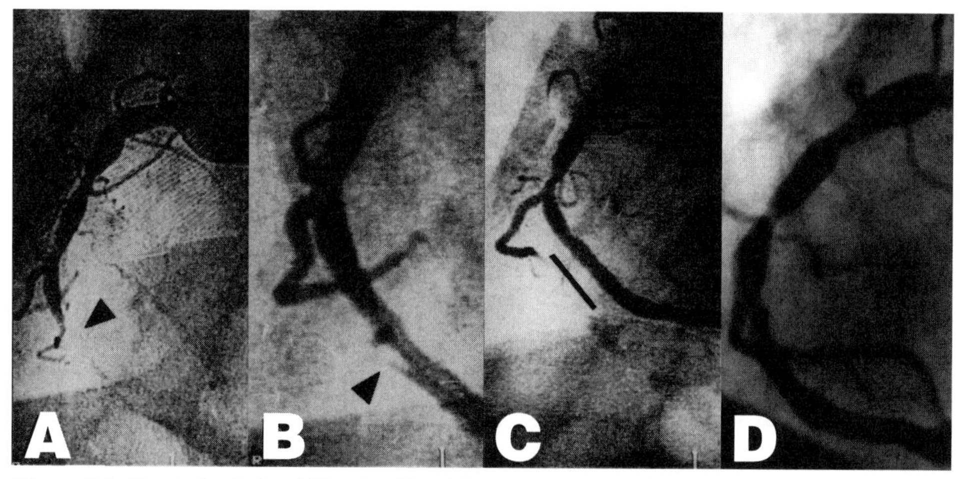

Figure 2.1 Stents for Infarct Vessels The right coronary artery, known to be the culprit, was occluded (**a;** arrow). After balloon dilation, there was a dissection at the lesion site (**b;** arrow). The dissection was treated with stent implantation (**c;** bar represents stent location). Angiography 6 months later revealed no restenosis (**d**).

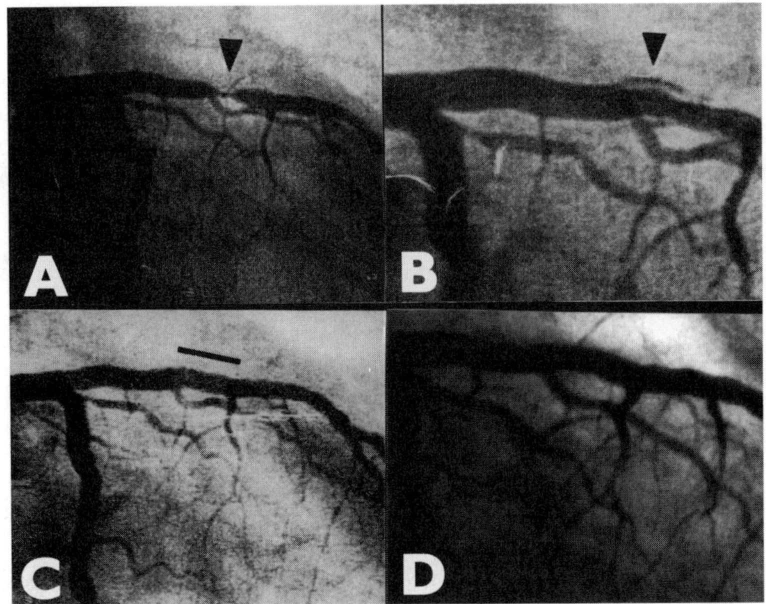

Figure 2.2 • Stents for Infarct Vessels Severe stenosis in the proximal left anterior descending artery (**a**). Angioplasty produced a dissection (**b;** arrow) treated with implantation of a stent (**c;** bar represents stent location). Angiography 6 months later reveals no stent restenosis (**d**).

performed in the occluded segment. A dissection developed proximally and was treated with a 4mm diameter Palmaz-Schatz stent (**Figure 2.1a-c**).

Despite the successful restoration of flow to the right coronary artery, the patient's chest pain persisted now with electrocardiographic changes across the anterior wall. The systolic blood pressure was 90mm Hg limiting further nitroglycerin therapy. Therefore, the left anterior descending vessel angioplasty was undertaken at the same setting.

The left anterior descending coronary stenosis, presumably present eight months earlier, was easily crossed but the lesion did not yield to a 3.5mm balloon at 12 atmospheres pressure. It responded to a 4mm balloon at the same pressure leaving a moderate linear dissection, treated with a second Palmaz-Schatz stent **(Figure 2.2a-c**).

Six months later, the patient remained asymptomatic and angiography revealed no evidence of restenosis at either stent site (**Figures 2.1d & 2.2d)**

Materials 2.1

Guiding Catheter:	Cook Lumax JR-4 & JL-4 8 French
Guidewires:	ACS Extra Support 0.14"x 175cm
Balloons:	USCI Pronto Rely 3.5 x 20 mm; Schneider Chubby 4.0 x 9mm
Stents:	Johnson & Johnson P-S 153 (15mm) (2)

DISCUSSION

Stent placement has traditionally been avoided in thrombus-related settings, such as acute myocardial infarction. Acute occlusion is more common after stent implantation for unstable angina with the attendant high incidence of thrombus.[1,2] It was thought that subacute stent closure would be even more common in acute infarction than in the setting of unstable angina. However, better stent implantation techniques[3] and antiplatelet strategies[4] have allowed a dramatic reduction in the rates of subacute stent occlusion, permitting consideration of stenting in the setting of thrombus,[5-7] thus, the original taboo of stent implantation during acute myocardial infarction has been reconsidered. This section will review primary angioplasty as an important part of the management of acute myocardial infarction and situations in which stenting may improve upon the results of direct angioplasty in this setting.

Angioplasty for Acute Myocardial Infarction

In the current era of thrombolysis, survival after myocardial infarction is less closely related to ejection fraction than it was in the pre thrombolytic era.[8-10] The patency of the infarct vessel seems to be important and beneficial, independent of both myocardial salvage and post infarction ventricular function.[10] Even the best thrombolytic therapies produce 90 minute patency of only 75-85%.[11] Angioplasty in the setting of acute infarction is successful in 94-97% of patients.[13,14] Furthermore, despite the advent of new techniques to assess reperfusion, there is no uniformly reliable means to determine which patient has been successfully reperfused by thrombolysis. The information provided by early angiography appears to predict mortality three times better than clinical risk factors.[12] Even when thrombolysis is successful, over 75% of patients have a significant residual stenosis[15] and over 50% have less than TIMI grade 3 flow[11] in the early phase post-infarction. Late reocclusion may occur 10-30% of the time after thrombolysis.[16] The long- term infarct-artery patency may persist in only 50% of patients after thrombolysis[17], compared with 95% long-term patency after direct angioplasty for myocardial infarction.[18] An improvement in long-term patency has been suggested to reduce late adverse ventricular remodeling and may improve survival. Up to 20% of patients treated with thrombolysis will suffer another ischemic event during their hospitalization, requiring revascularization.[13,19] Recent studies indicate that direct angioplasty can improve upon the results of thrombolysis for acute myocardial infarction.[14,20,21]

The PAMI (Primary Angioplasty for Myocardial Infarction) trial demonstrated that primary angioplasty without prior thrombolysis was safe and superior to thrombolytic therapy in patients with anterior infarction, especially women or those of advanced age with symptoms of cardiac insufficiency. Mortality and non-fatal infarctions were decreased. Although there was an increase in vascular repair and an increase in ventricular fibrillation at reperfusion, there were no hemorrhagic cerebrovascular accidents in the angioplasty group.[14,20,21] In one study, left ventricular function at discharge was better in the group receiving direct angioplasty.[21] These trials have demonstrated that direct angioplasty is not only safe and feasible but in certain high risk subgroups, the results are significantly better than thrombolysis. The 63% relative reduction in mortality by angioplasty was far greater than the 12% benefit provided by accelerated t-PA over streptokinase in earlier thrombolytic trials.[23]

More recent trials have allowed us to refine the benefit of direct angioplasty over thrombolysis. A meta-analysis of the pooled data of 7 randomized trials confirmed a nearly 50% reduction in death and recurrent infarction in the angioplasty group.[24] The GUSTO IIb angiographic substudy in which a broader group of centers performed angioplasty on average 80 minutes after arrival in the hospital (compared to 60-70 minutes in the earlier studies) reiterated the survival benefit of primary angioplasty over the best thrombolytic therapies when the 30-day results became available.[25] The community-based MITI registry where patients were recruited for direct angioplasty or thrombolysis in a non-randomized fashion revealed no survival difference between the therapies.[26] However, the time from hospital arrival to angioplasty in this study averaged over 100 minutes. Procedural heparin was not monitored and non-ionic contrast agents were used, which may have increased thrombotic complications in the angioplasty group. Furthermore, some centers favored angioplasty for the majority of their patients while others had no catheterization laboratory available making it difficult to compare the results of this retrospective review with previous randomized studies.

Clinical Exclusions from Acute Infarction Trials

A significant number of patients were excluded from acute myocardial infarction trials because of thrombolytic ineligibility, prior bypass surgery or cardiogenic shock. These are the very patients who might be expected to derive the greatest benefit from immediate reperfusion. Depending upon the criteria used, between 20% and 70% of patients presenting with infarction are not candidates for thrombolysis.[27] The mortality rate in this thrombolytic non-eligible group is four times that in the group eligible for thrombolysis.[27,28]

In the subgroup of patients who have had previous bypass surgery, a new infarction is caused by occlusion of a bypass graft 76% of the time.[29] Patency of that occluded vein graft is restored only 25-50% of the time by thrombolytic therapy[29,30] and may be improved by direct angioplasty. Patients presenting in cardiogenic shock represent the highest risk group. The traditional mortality exceeds 80% in this group and is not significantly reduced by thrombolytic therapy, but may be reduced to 50% by direct angioplasty.[31,77]

Thus, the case for primary or direct angioplasty in acute myocardial infarction can be made when a catheterization laboratory with an experienced team is readily available. In the setting of an active atherosclerotic coronary stenosis, fibrinolysis and the trauma of balloon angioplasty may produce less optimal results because of hemorrhage into plaques and dissected arterial segments. Both of these pathological findings (plaque hemorrhage and dissection) have been reported in angioplasty following thrombolysis but not in primary angioplasty. The prothrombotic effects of thrombolytic therapy[34] may be accentuated by the mechanical irritation of balloons upon ruptured plaques and freshly lysed thrombi. Thus, while "salvage angioplasty" may have a clear role in patients with continued pain and hemodynamic compromise associated with a closed artery after thrombolytic therapy,[35] most operators avoid angioplasty of vessels which are open and providing TIMI grade 3 flow during the first 48 hours after thrombolysis. The platelet glycoprotein IIb/IIIa inhibitors (GP IIb/IIIa antibodies) reduce thrombus propagation and may markedly improve the appearance of lesions remaining after thrombolysis.[79]

Stenting for Acute Infarction

Despite the advantages of angioplasty for acute myocardial infarction, there are procedural problems which have led to the application of stent implantation in this adverse setting. Dissection may occur more frequently during angioplasty of occluded vessels because of the inability to assess vessel size distal to the site of occlusion.[36,37] Intimal dissection, as well as residual thrombus, are the predictors of reocclusion in this setting.[38,39] Even though initial success for primary angioplasty is high, there is an in-hospital reocclusion rate of 10-15%.[13]

Restoration of flow, in addition to vessel patency, is strongly correlated with myocardial salvage.[40,4] Vessels showing TIMI grade 3 flow demonstrate two times more myocardial salvage than vessels with TIMI grade ≤ 2 flow.[42] Although direct angioplasty may leave a less than perfect result, TIMI grade 3 flow could be established in 100% of 74 patients in whom stenting was performed after coronary angioplasty with TIMI grade ≤ 2 flow in the infarct artery.[43] Stent placement after suboptimal angioplasty results was not associated with an increase in subacute stent thrombosis.[42,44-50] While suboptimal angiographic results and the increased incidence of acute closure after angioplasty for acute myocardial infarction patients are important reasons to consider stent implantation. An equal or more important reason would be improving long-term outcome. Angioplasty of infarct vessels is associated with a restenosis rate approaching 50%.[51] Stent placement in these same vessels seems to be associated with the same low restenosis rates as elective stenting.[43,52,78]

Stenting in No-reflow Conditions

The case for stent placement after suboptimal primary angioplasty of an infarct-artery must be carefully considered. Stents should not be placed in this thrombotic milieu when balloon angioplasty can provide an adequate lumen. More importantly, if angioplasty has provided a good lumen and distal flow remains TIMI grade ≤ 2, the "no-reflow" phenomenon is probably in progress. Stenting will have no effect to reduce no-reflow after infarction.[53,54] Slow angiographic flow is a chief determinant for stent placement in acute myocardial infarction. Whether the post-angioplasty flow is inadequate because of an inadequately dilated lumen or because of extensive microvascular damage and no-reflow is the key question in this setting. Intravascular ultrasound and contrast echocardiographic techniques to assess microvascular function may help determine the cause of slow flow in a patent infarct-artery.[5] If there is no evidence of lumen compromise, intracoronary verapamil to treat possible microvascular spasm rather than stenting has been used.[55] Unless the poor flow in an infarct-related artery can be clearly attributed to an inadequate lumen, a stent placed in this setting will be of little benefit.

Addressing the Non-Infarct Vessel

While stent placement provides a level of security not afforded by angioplasty for infarct-related artery patency, the non-infarct arteries should rarely, if ever, be approached in the setting of an acute myocardial infarction. Continued refractory shock may be an exception to this rule. In Case 2.1 above, the right coronary artery was presumed to be the culprit vessel. The left anterior descending artery stenosis was only approached when persistent anterior ischemia, hypotension, and chest pain appeared. When the culprit vessel is not obvious in acute infarction patients with multivessel disease, surgical revascularization may be the best option. Patients with multivessel coronary artery disease have a higher post-procedural mortality rate despite successful angioplasty of the culprit lesion.[13]

Use of Adjunctive Techniques

There are other technical issues which may be important during interventions for acute myocardial infarction. While intra-aortic balloon counterpulsation has been shown to reduce early reocclusion in direct and salvage angioplasty of myocardial infarction,[56] its role in a stented infarct artery has not yet been defined.

With regard to radiographic contrast agents, the low osmolality, ionic contrast agents are less thrombogenic than nonionic contrast agents. Ionic contrast media inhibit both platelet aggregation and coagulation to a greater extent than nonionic media.[57-59] Animal models of angioplasty-like arterial injury indicate more anticoagulant activity with ionic than with nonionic contrast media.[60,61] Most importantly, clinical evaluations of different contrast media during high risk angioplasty have confirmed that these theoretic advantages of ionic contrast media translate into clinical benefit.[62, 63] Patients receiving low osmolar ionic contrast (Hexabrix) were less likely to experience reduced blood flow during the procedure and had fewer post procedure ischemic events.[64,65]

Anticoagulation and Stenting

Traditionally interventionalists insisted on 2 to 7 days of heparinization after stenting for acute infarctions. However, preliminary findings from the ISAR (Intracoronary Stenting and Antithrombotic Regimen) study suggest that the differential benefit of antiplatelet therapy over heparin and warfarin is even more pronounced in patients stented for myocardial infarction than for elective cases.[67] This randomized trial of 123 patients stented during acute myocardial infarction showed that the subacute thrombosis rate for patients treated with only 12 hours of intravenous heparin followed by aspirin and ticlopidine was 0% compared with a rate of 10% in the group given intravenous heparin until the INR was raised by warfarin derivatives to 3-5 times normal. Thus, the traditional period of anticoagulation with warfarin may be deleterious for these stented vessels.[68]

Role of Urokinase

In angioplasty for unstable angina, the use of prophylactic urokinase resulted in more adverse clinical and angiographic outcomes than when it was avoided.[69] Urokinase given during angioplasty for acute infarction has been reported to result in angiographic deterioration which required stent implantation.[70] This result may have been due to intraplaque hemorrhage or incomplete sealing of dissections after thrombolytic administration. Currently, there is no established role for adjunctive thrombolysis in the setting of direct angioplasty.[71] Most operators would reserve this therapy for cases with persistent or worsening thrombus.

Role of IIb/IIIa Receptor Antagonists

Findings in the EPIC trial emphasized the value of platelet glycoprotein IIb/IIIa inhibitors for angioplasty of high-risk lesions. The clinical event rate was significantly reduced with 26% fewer of the treated lesions requiring revascularization at 6 months (**Figure 2.3**)[72] Preliminary data from the IMPACT II trial suggest that GP IIb/IIIa inhibitors may reduce the rate of non-Q-wave infarction after bailout stenting by 50%.[73] Others have shown that GP IIb/IIIa receptor expression on the platelet surface before stent placement is a significant predictor of subacute thrombosis[74] The EPILOG trial confirmed a marked reduction in ischemic complications for routine angioplasty.[81] These agents have been shown to dissolve thrombus prior to angioplasty in acute myocardial infarction.[79] While awaiting confirmation of larger trials, many investigators are sufficiently compelled by the data to apply these agents in all interventions involving acute myocardial infarction.[80]

The mortality rate of patients who cannot be successfully treated by angioplasty for acute myocardial infarction is especially high[13,75] In some of these patients the problem is dissection or recoil which will be responsive to stenting. In others the problem will be slow flow due to thrombosis, the "no-reflow phenomenon"[53,54] and persistent shock.

SUMMARY

Stenting for acute myocardial infarction addresses the issues of residual lumen material and guarantee of satisfactory epicardial transitive flow. Primary stenting for acute infarction has the potential to improve outcomes and sustain reperfusion. Studies using primary stenting compared to traditional methods are in progress.

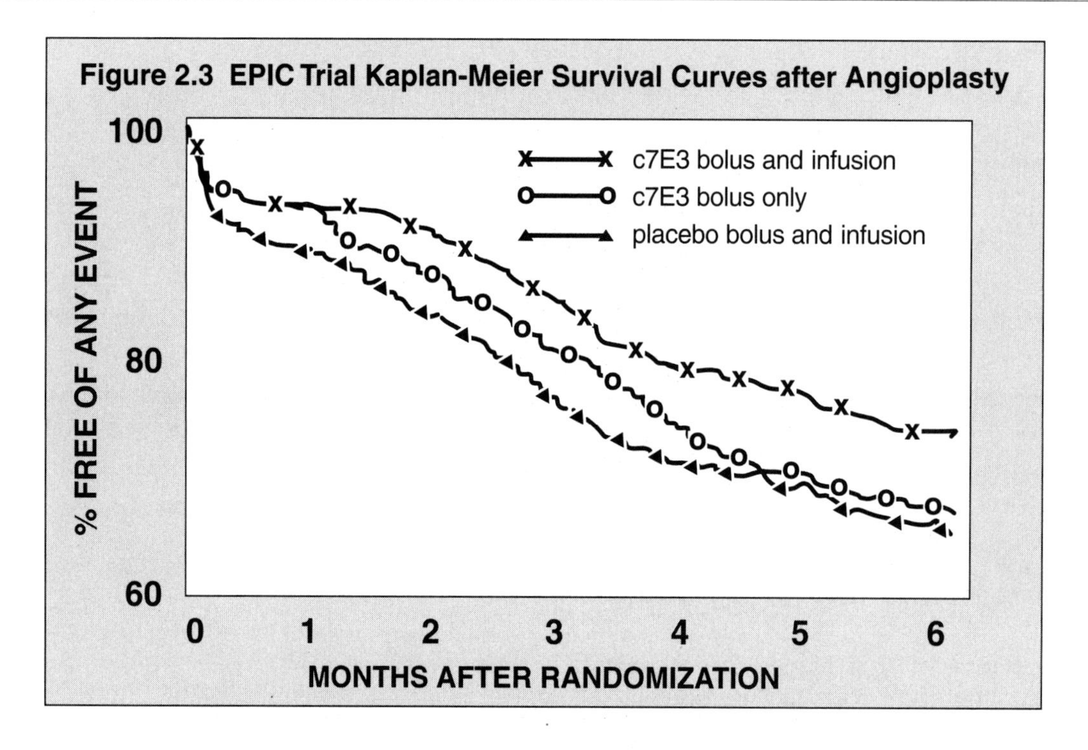

Figure 2.3 EPIC Trial The use of GP IIb/IIIa platelet inhibitors in angioplasty of high risk lesions in the EPIC trial resulted in a 26% reduction in revascularization in the treated group at 6 months. Note that while bolus administration alone provided early benefit, bolus and infusion of the platelet inhibitor was required to maintain and perhaps increase the benefit by 6 months.Adapted with permission from Dr EJ Topol and The Lancet (*Lancet* 1994;343:883).

References

1. Haude M, Erbel R, Issa H et al. *Subacute thrombotic complications after intracoronary implantations of Palmaz-Schatz stent.* Am Heart J 126:15-22 (1993).
2. Nath FC, Muller DWM, Elllis SG, et al. *Thrombosis of a flexible coil coronary stent: predictors, frequency, and clinical outcome.* J Am Coll Cardiol 21:622-627 (1993).
3. Colombo A, Hall P, Nakamura S, et al. *Intracoronary stenting without anticoagulation accomplished with intravascular ultrasound guidance.* Circulation 91:1676-1688 (1995).
4. Mehan VK, Salzman C, Kauffman U, Meier B. *Coronary stenting without anticoagulation.* Cathet Cardiovasc Diagn 34:137-141 (1995).
5. Kaul U, Agarwal R, Jain P, Wasir H. *Safety and efficacy of intracoronary stenting for thrombus containing lesions.* Am J Cardiol 77:425-427 (1996).
6. Romero M, Medina A, Suarez de Lezo J, et al. *Elective stent placement in acute coronary syndromes induced by thrombus containing lesions [abstr].* J Am Coll Cardiol 27:69A (1996).
7. Alfonso F, Rodrieguez P, Phillps P, et al. *Clinical and angiographic implications of coronary stenting in thrombus-containing lesions.* J Am Coll Cardiol 29: 725-733 (1997).
8. van de Werf F. *Discrepancies between the effects of coronary reperfusion on survival and left ventricular function.* Lancet 1:1367-1369 (1989).
9. Braunwald E. *Myocardial reperfusion, limitation of infarct size, reduction of left ventricular dysfunction and improved survival: should the paradigm be expanded?* Circulation 79:441-444 (1989).

10. Kim CB, Braunwald E. *Potential benefits of late reperfusion of infarcted myocardium—the open artery hypothesis.* Circulation 88:2426-2436 (1993).

11. The GUSTO Angiographic Investigators. *The effects of tissue plasminogen activator, streptokinase or both on coronary artery patency, ventricular function and survival after acute myocardial infarction.* N Engl J Med 329:1615-1622 (1993).

12. Grines CL. *Aggressive intervention for myocardial infarction: angioplasty, stents, and intra-aortic balloon pumping.* Am J Cardiol 78(suppl 3a):29-34 (1996).

13. O'Keefe J, Bailey WJ, Rutherford BD, Hartzler GO. *Primary angioplasty for acute myocardial infarction in 1,000 consecutive patients.* Results in an unselected population and high-risk subgroups. Am J Cardiol 72:107G-115G (1993).

14. Grines CL, Browne KF, Marco JP, and the Primary Angioplasty in Myocardial Infarction Study Group. *A comparison of immediate angioplasty with thrombolytic therapy for acute myocardial infarction.* N Engl J Med 328:673-679 (1993).

15. Topol EJ, Califf RM, George BS, and the Thrombolysis and Angioplasty in Myocardial Infarction (TAMI) Study Group. *A randomized trial of immediate versus delayed elective angioplasty after intravenous tissue plasminogen activator in acute myocardial infarction.* N Eng J Med 312:932-936 (1985).

16. Meijer A, Verheught FWA, Werter CJPS, et al. *Aspirin versus coumadin in the prevention of reocclusion and recurrent ischemia after successful thrombolysis: a prospective placebo-controlled angiographic study.* Circulation 87:1524-1530 (1993).

17. Grines C. *Primary angioplasty—the strategy of choice.* N Engl J Med 335:1313-1316 (1996).

18. Zijlstra F, Jan de Boer M, Hoortntje JCA, et al. *A comparison of immediate coronary angioplasty with intravenous streptokinase in acute myocardial infarction.* N Eng J Med 328:680-684 (1993).

19. Barbagelata A, Granger CB, Topol EJ, et al. *Frequency, significance, and cost of recurrent ischemia after thrombolytic therapy for acute myocardial infarction.* Am J Cardiol 76:1007-10013 (1995).

20. Gibbons RJ, Holmes DR, Reeder GS, et al. *Immediate angioplasty compared with the administration of a thrombolytic agent followed by conservative treatment for myocardial infarction.* N Eng J Med 328:685-691 (1993).

21. Zijlstra F, Jan de Boer M, Hoortntje JCA, et al. *A comparison of immediate coronary angioplasty with intravenous streptokinase in acute myocardial infarction.* N Eng J Med 328:680-684 (1993).

22. Stone GW, Grines CL, Browne KF, et al. *Predictors of in-hospital and 6-month outcome after acute myocardial infarction in the reperfusion era: the primary angioplasty in myocardial infarction (PAMI) trial.* J Am Coll Cardiol 25:370-377 (1995).

23. Goldman L. *Cost and quality of life: thrombolysis and primary angioplasty.* J Am Coll Cardiol 25(suppl S):38S-41S (1995).

24. Michels KB, Yusuf S. *Does PTCA in acute myocardial infarction affect mortality and reinfarction rates? A quantitative overview (meta-analysis) of the randomized clinical trials.* Circulation 91:476-485 (1995).

25. *The Global Use Of Strategies To Open Occluded Coronary Arteries in Acute Coronary Syndromes (Gusto IIb). The GUSTO Investigators. A clinical trial comparing primary coronary angioplasty with tissue plasminogen activator for acute myocardial infarction.* N Engl J Med 336: 1621-1628 (1997)

26. Every NR, Parsons LS, Hlatky M, et al. *A comparison of thrombolytic therapy with primary coronary angioplasty for acute myocardial infarction.* N Engl J Med 335:1253-1260 (1996).

27. Cragg DR, Freidman HZ, Bonema JD, et al. *Outcome of Patients with Acute Myocardial Infarction Who Are Ineligible for Thrombolytic Therapy.* Ann Int Med 115:173-177 (1991).

28. Himbert D, Juliard JM, Steg PG, et al. *Primary coronary angioplasty for acute myocardial infarction with contraindications to thrombolysis.* Am J Cardiol 71:377-381 (1993).

29. Grines CL, Booth DC, Nissen, et al. *Mechanism of acute myocardial infarction in patients with prior coronary artery bypass grafting and therapeutic implications.* Am J Cardiol 65:1292-1296 (1990).

30. Reiner JS, Lundergan CF, Kopecky SL, et al. *Ineffectiveness of thrombolysis for acute MI following vein graft occlusion. Circulation* 94(suppl I):I-570 (1996).

31. O'Neil WW. *Angioplasty therapy of cardiogenic shock: are randomized trials necessary?* (Editorial Comment). J Am Coll Cardiol 19:915 (1992).

32. Meier B. *Balloon angioplasty for acute myocardial infarction. Was it buried alive?* Circulation 82:2243-2245 (1990).

33. Waller BF, Rothbaum DA, Pinkerton CA, et al. *Status of the myocardium and infarct- related coronary artery in 19 necropsy patients with acute recanalization using pharmacologic (streptokinase, r-tissue plasminogen activator), mechanical (percutaneous transluminal coronary angioplasty) or combined types of reperfusion therapy.* J Am Coll Cardiol 9:785-801 (1987).

34. Eisenberg PR, Sobel BE, Jaffe AS. *Activation of prothrombin accompanying thrombolysis with recombinant tissue-type plasminogen activator.* J Am Coll Cardiol 19: 1065-1069 (1992).

35. Califf RM, Topol EJ, Stack RS et al. *An evaluation of combination thrombolytic therapy and timing of cardiac catheterization in acute myocardial infarction: the TAMI-5 randomized trial.* Circulation 83:1543-1556 (1991).

36. Kereiakes DJ, Selmon MR, McAuley BJ, et al. *Angioplasty in total coronary artery occlusion: Experience in 76 consecutive patients.* J Am Coll Cardiol 6:526-533 (1985).

37. Hamm CW, Kupper W, Kuck KH, et al. *Recanalization of chronic, totally occluded coronary arteries by new angioplasty systems.* Am J Cardiol 66:1459-1463 (1990).

38. Kahn JK, Rutherford BD, McCohahay DR, et al. *Results of primary angioplasty for acute myocardial infarction in patients with multivessel coronary artery disease.* J Am Coll Cardiol 16:1089-1096 (1990).

39. Kahn JK, Rutherford BD, McCohahay DR, et al. *Catheterization laboratory events and hospital outcome with direct angioplasty for acute myocardial infarction.* Circulation 82:1910-1915 (1990)

40. Karagounis L, Sjorensen SG, Menlove RL, et al. *Does thrombolysis in myocardial infarction (TIMI) perfusion grade 2 represent a mostly patent artery or a mostly occluded artery? Enzymatic and electrocardiographic evidence from the TEAM-2 study.* J Am Coll Cardiol 19:1-10 (1992).

41. Anderson JL, Karagounis LA, Califf RM. *Metaanalysis of five reported studies on the relation of early coronary patency grades with mortality and outcomes after acute myocardial infarction.* Am J Cardiol 78:1-8 (1996).

42. Laster SB, O'Keefe JH, Gibbons RJ. *The Incidence and importance of TIMI-3 flow following primary infarct angioplasty.* Circulation 90(suppl I):I-221 (1994).

43. Neumann FJ, Walter H, Schmitt C, et al. *Coronary stenting as an adjunct to direct balloon angioplasty in acute myocardial infarction [abstr].* Circulation 92(suppl I):I-609 (1995).

44. Marco JP, Caillard JB, Doucet S, et al. *Is recent myocardial infarction a worse setting for coronary stent implantation?* J Am Coll Cardiol 747:178A (1993).

45. Levy G, de Boisgelin X, Volpiliere R et al. *Intracoronary Stenting in Direct Infarct Angioplasty: Is it Dangerous?* [abstr] Circulation 92(suppl I):I-139 (1995).

46. Monassier JP, Elias J, Raynaud P, Joly P. *Results of early (<24h) and late (>24h) implantation of coronary stents in acute myocardial infarction* [abstr]. Circulation 92 (suppl I):I-609 (1995).

47. Lefevre T, Morice MC, Karrillon G, et al. *Coronary stenting during acute myocardial infarction. Results from the stent without coumadin French registry* [abstr]. J Am Coll Cardiol 27:69A (1996).

48. LeMay M, Labinaz M, Beanlands RSB, et al. *Intracoronary stenting in the setting of myocardial infarction* [abstr]. J Am Coll Cardiol 27:69A (1996).

49. Garcia-Cantu E, Spaulding C, Corcos T, et al. *Stent implantation in acute myocardial infarction.* Am J Cardiol 77:451-454 (1996).

50. Rodriguez AE, Fernandez M, Santaera O, et al. *Coronary stenting in patients undergoing percutaneous transluminal coronary angioplasty during acute myocardial infarction.* Am J Cardiol 77:685-689 (1996).

51. Brodie BR, Grines CL, Ivanhoe R, et al. *Six-month clinical and angiographic follow-up after direct angioplasty for acute myocardial infarction.* Circulation 90:156-162 (1994).

52. Ong LY, Katz S, Green J, et al. *Routine stenting for acute myocardial infarction results in 6 month outcomes comparable to patients with elective stenting.* Circulation 94(suppl I):I-577 (1996).

53. Kloner RA, Ganote CE, Jennings RB, et al. *The 'no-reflow' phenomenon following temporary coronary occlusion in the dog.* J Clin Invest 54:1496-1508 (1974).

54. Baim DS, Carroza JP. *Understanding the "no-reflow" problem.* Cathet Cardiovasc Diag 39:7-8 (1996).

55. Piana RN, Paik GY, Moscucci M, et al. *Incidence and treatment of "no-reflow" after percutaneous coronary intervention.* Circulation 89:2514-2518 (1994).

56. Ishiara M, Sato H, Tateishi H, et al. *Intraaortic balloon pumping as the postangioplasty strategy in acute myocardial infarction.* Am Heart J 122:385-389 (1991).

57. Dawson P, Hewitt P, Mackie JJ, et al. *Contrast, coagulation, and fibrinolysis.* Invest Radiol 21:248-252 (1986).

58. Grabowski EF. *Effects of contrast media on endothelial cell monolayers under controlled flow conditions.* Am J Cardiol 64:10E-15E (1989).

59. Stormorken H Skalpe IO, Testart MC, et al. *Effect of various contrast media on coagulation, fibrinolysis, and platelet function an in vitro and in vivo study.* Invest Radiol 21:348-354 (1986).

60. Grines CL, Diaz C, Mickelson J. *Acute thrombosis in a canine model of arterial injury: effect of ionic versus nonionic contrast media* [abstr]. Circulation 80 (suppl II):II-411(1989).

61. Hwang MH, Piao ZE, Murdock DK, et al. *Risk of thromboembolism during diagnostic and interventional cardiac procedures with nonionic contrast media.* Radiology 174:459-461 (1990).

62. Gasperetti CM, Feldman MD, Burwell LR, et al. *Influence of contrast media on thrombus formation during coronary angioplasty.* J Am Coll Cardiol 18:443-450 (1991).

63. Grines CL, Schreiber TL, Savas V, et al. *A randomized trial of low osmolar ionic versus nonionic contrast media in patients with myocardial infarction or unstable angina undergoing percutaneous transluminal coronary angioplasty.* J Am Coll Cardiol 27:1381-1386 (1996).

64. Esplugas E, Cequier A, Jana A, et al. *Risk of thrombosis during coronary angioplasty with low osmolality contrast media.* Am J Cardiol 68:1020-1024 (1991).

65. Jost S, Rafflenbeul W, Gerhardt U, et al. *Influence of ionic and non-ionic radiographic contrast media on the vasomotor tone of epicardial coronary arteries.* Eur Heart J 10(suppl F):60-65 (1989).

66. Schomig A, Neumann FJ, Kastrati A, et al. *A randomized comparison of antiplatelet and anticoagulant therapy after the placement of coronary-artery stents.* N Engl J Med 334:1084-1089 (1996).

67. Schomig A, Neumann FJ, Walter H, et al. *Coronary stent placement in patients with acute myocardial infarction: Comparison of clinical and angiographic outcome after randomization to anti-platelet or anti-coagulant therapy.* J Am Coll Cardiol 29: 28-34 (1997)

68. Gawaz M, Neumann FJ, Ott I, et al. *Platelet activation and coronary stent implantation— Effect of antithrombotic therapy.* Circulation 94:279-285 (1996).

69. Ambrose JA, Almeida OA, Sharma SK, et al. *Adjunctive thrombolytic therapy during angioplasty for ischemic rest angina (results of the TAUSA trial).* Circulation 90:69-77 (1994).

70. Salton AS, Oesterle SN, Yeung AC. *Coronary artery stenting for acute closure complicating primary angioplasty for acute myocardial infarction.* Cathet Cardiovasc Diag 34:142-146 (1995)

71. Vaitkus PT, Laskey WK. *Efficacy of adjunctive thrombolytic therapy in percutaneous transluminal coronary angioplasty.* J Am Coll Cardiol 24:1415-1423 (1994).

72. Topol EJ, Califf RM, Weisman HF, et al. *Randomized trial of coronary intervention with antibody against platelet IIb/IIIa integrin for reduction of clinical restenosis: results at six months.* Lancet 343:881-886 (1994).

73. Ellis S. GP *IIb/IIIa antagonists: a new actor in stenting.* Rotterdam Stent Course 1995.

74. Neumann, FJ, Gawaz M, Ott I et al. *Prospective evaluation of hemostatic predictors of subacute stent thrombosis after coronary Palmaz-Schatz stenting.* J Am Coll Card 27:15-21 (1996).

75. Ellis SG, van de Werf F, Ribeiro-daSilva E, Topol EJ. *Present status of rescue coronary angioplasty: current polarization of opinion and randomized trials.* J Am Coll Cardiol 19: 681-686 (1992).

76. Quigley RL, Milano CA, Smith R, et al. *Prognosis and management of anterolateral myocardial infarction in patients with severe left main disease and cardiogenic shock: the left main shock syndrome.* Circulation 88[part 2]:65-70 (1993).

77 Berger PB, Holmes DR, Stebbins AL, et al. *Restoration of coronary flow in myocardial infarction by intravenous chimeri 7E3 antibody without exogenous plasminogen activators.* Circulation 95: 1755-1759 (1997).

78 Spaulding C, Codor R, Benhamda K, et al. *One week and six-month angiographic controls of stent implantation after occlusive and non-occlusive dissection during primary balloon angioplasty for acute myocardial infarction.* Am J Cardiol 79: 1592-1595 (1997)

79 Gold HK, Garabedian HD, Dinemore RE, et al. *Impact of an aggressive invasive catheterization and revascularization strategy on mortality in patients with cardiogenic shock in the GUSTO-I trial.* Circulation 96:122-124 (1997)

80 van de Werf F. *More evidence for a beneficial effect of platelet glycoprotein IIb/IIIa-blockade during coronary interventions. Latest results from the EPILOG and CAPTURE trials.* Eur Heart J. 1996; 17:325-326

81 The EPILOG Investigators. *Platelet glycoprotein IIb/IIa receptor blockade and low-dose heparin during percutaneous coronary revascularation.* N Engl J Med 336: 1689-1695 (1997)

CHAPTER 3

OSTIAL STENOSES

CASE 3.1: Stenting of Ostial Stenoses

This 76 year old former smoker with severe chronic lung disease and a prior anterior myocardial infarction presented with angina at rest. He underwent cardiac catheterization which identified a severe ostial stenosis of the right coronary artery and an occluded left anterior descending coronary artery. The left ventricular ejection fraction was 30%. The ostial lesion was discrete (6mm), eccentric, and heavily calcified (**Figure 3.1a**). The patient had been denied surgery because of his resting hypercapnia and severe pulmonary dysfunction.

PROCEDURE 3.1

A percutaneous procedure was considered high risk because of diminished ventricular function, severe chronic lung disease, and unstable angina. Because of the significant eccentricity and associated calcium, rotablation followed by stent implantation was weighed against primary stent implantation. It was elected

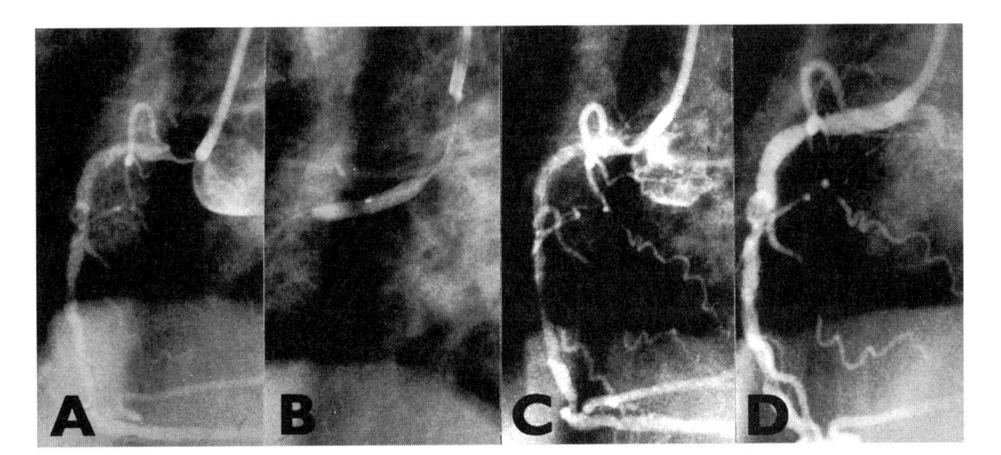

Figure 3.1 Stenting the Ostium The ostial right coronary artery lesion was severe, discrete and associated with heavy calcification (**a**). Predilation resulted in complete balloon expansion at 8 atmospheres (**b**). Note that the guiding catheter is positioned in the ascending aorta during ostial manipulations. After balloon dilation there was lesion recoil resulting in a 60% residual stenosis (**c**). There was no residual stenosis after implantation of a Rigid-Flex (NIR) stent (**d**).

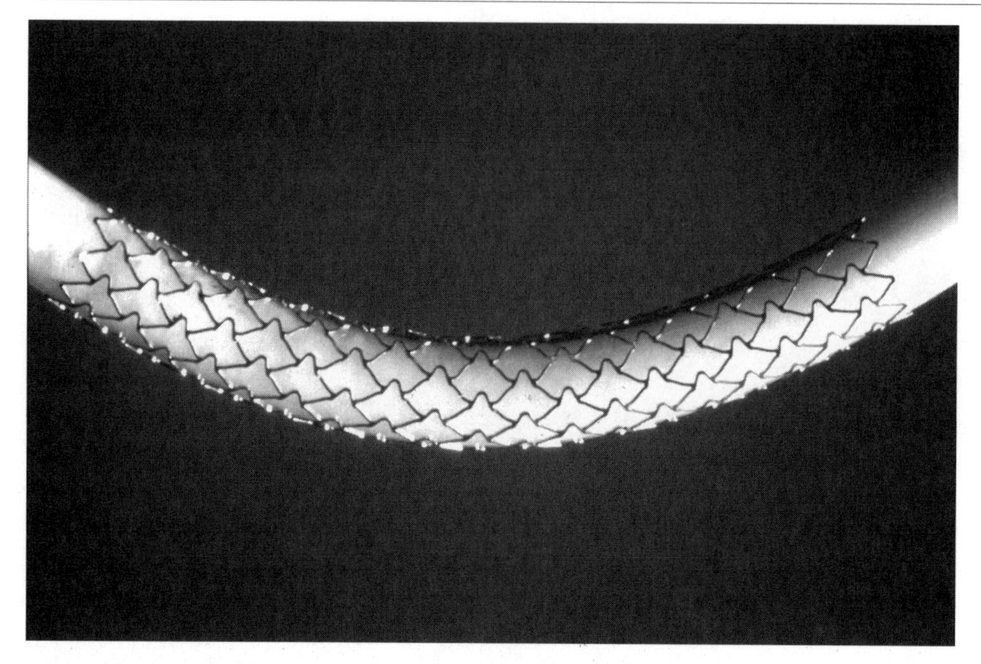

Figure 3.2 The Rigid-Flex (NIR) Stent A continuous multicellular uniform design.

to proceed with balloon dilation first and assess the amount of lesion recoil. If there was severe recoil, rotablation would be considered prior to stent implantation.

The lesion was easily crossed with an extra support guidewire. Pre-stent dilatation was performed with the guiding catheter withdrawn and the balloon straddling the ostium (**Figure 3.1b**). Although the 4.0mm balloon expanded completely at 8 atmospheres, there was considerable haziness with a residual stenosis of 60% (**Figure 3.1c**). A Rigid-Flex (NIR) 9mm stent (**Figure 3.2**) was mounted on the predilation balloon and passed across the ostial lesion. With the guiding catheter again withdrawn from the coronary ostium, the stent was positioned so that its proximal end was just extending into the aortic root. The stent was then deployed at 16 atm with the proximal end of the deployment balloon flaring the stent into the aortic root. The final angiographic images were obtained by advancing the guiding catheter back toward the ostium over the post dilatation balloon as it was deflating, thus, minimizing the likelihood of stent trauma. There was no residual stenosis (**Figure 3.1d**). The patient was discharged and remained asymptomatic at follow-up 3 months later.

MATERIALS 3.1

Guiding Catheter:	Cook Lumax JR-4 8 French
Guidewires:	ACS Extra Support 0.014"x 300cm
Balloons:	SciMed Viva 4.0 x 20mm
Stents:	Boston Scientific/SciMed Rigid-Flex NIR 9mm

CASE 3.2: Stents for Recoil

The patient is a 52 year old smoker with, hyperlipidemia, and hypertension who presented with crescendo angina, despite intravenous nitrates and heparin. Coronary angiography demonstrated a critical ostial narrowing of the right coronary artery (**Figure 3.3a**). There was no associated calcification.

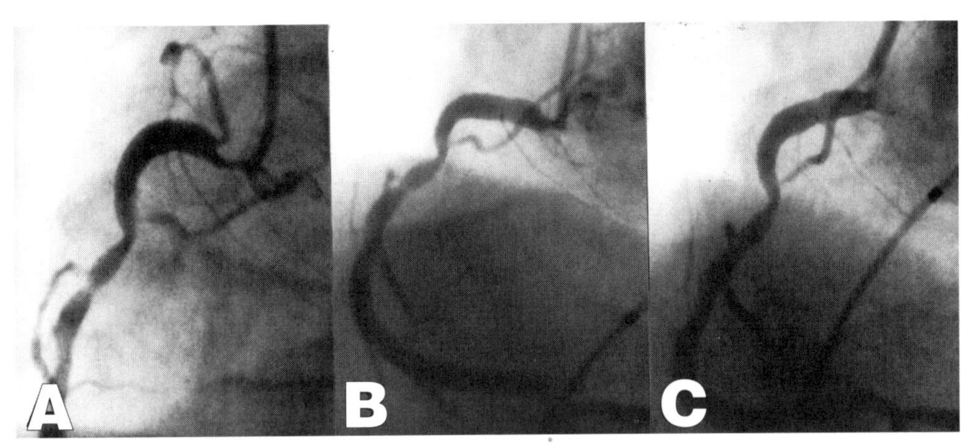

Figure 3.3 Stents for Recoil Severe ostial right coronary artery stenosis was not associated with calcification (**a**). After predilation and implantation of a Palmaz-Schatz I stent there was significant recoil (**b**). A Palmaz biliary stent, placed within the original stent, abolished the recoil. No residual stenosis remained (**c**).

PROCEDURE 3.2

Using a standard Judkins Right guiding catheter with side holes, an extra-support guidewire was easily passed into the posterior descending artery. Pre-stent balloon dilations were performed with a non-compliant 4mm balloon which reached full expansion at 5 atm. With the guiding catheter withdrawn, a Palmaz-Schatz stent was deployed leaving 1mm of the stent within the aortic root. Despite post-dilations to 18 atm, significant recoil resulted in a significant residual stenosis within the stent (**Figure 3.3b**). A 10mm Palmaz biliary stent was mounted on the post-dilation balloon and passed within the ostial portion of the original stent and deployed at 18 atm leaving less than 10% residual narrowing (**Figure 3.3c**). The patient was discharged and has remained pain free with a negative exercise test for 24 months.

MATERIALS

Guiding Catheter:	Medtronic Ascent JR 4 8 French with side holes
Guidewires:	SciMed Platinum Plus 0.014"x 300cm
Balloons:	SciMed NC Cobra 4.0 x 20mm
Stents:	Johnson & Johnson PS-153, P-100 (biliary)

DISCUSSION

Aorto-ostial lesions occur within 3mm of the aortic root and often involve the origin of saphenous vein grafts, as well as the right and left coronary arteries. Coronary branch-ostial lesions are those within 3mm of the origin of the major coronary branch vessels. Since both types of ostial lesions behave differently than standard coronary lesions within the body of the coronary arteries, they will be discussed together.

Aorto-ostial Stenoses

Aorto-ostial lesions are encountered less frequently than lesions in the body of the coronary arteries.[1] As an isolated finding apart from multivessel disease, these lesions are rare and more commonly found in women.[2,3] Ostial lesions are caused by different processes than stenoses within the body of the coronary system. Aortitis, homozygous familial hypercholesterolemia, trauma from aortic valve surgery or prior percutaneous angioplasty procedures, and mediastinal or thoracic irradiation have been associated with aorto-ostial lesions. These lesions are commonly composed of large amounts of fibrocellular material and less often contain the compliant lipid-rich material which typifies intracoronary lesions.[4,5] The ostial region is often calcified. High pressure balloon inflations are frequently required to obtain even marginally acceptable angioplasty results.[6] The extra rigidity and elasticity at these sites, as well as the difficulty in maintaining coaxial guiding catheter support without deep intubation, has often been responsible for the suboptimal balloon approach.

Results of Ostial Coronary Angioplasty

Because of the special patho-anatomic features of ostial lesions, angioplasty in the aorto-ostial location has been associated with reduced success, increased restenosis, and most importantly, a significantly increased incidence of acute complications.[6] Trauma resulting from poorly seated guiding catheters results in increased rates of severe dissection. Technological advances have improved the success rate for ostial angioplasty (success as high as 94% when both aorto and branch ostial lesions are included)[7] and, in selected cases, the restenosis rates have been reported as low as 34%.[8] Nonetheless, the residual stenosis and restenosis rates remain significant after conventional ostial angioplasty.[9-11] Consequently, a variety of percutaneous devices have been tested at this location (**Table 3.1**).

Rotational Ablation for Ostial Stenoses

Rotational atherectomy has several advantages for aorto-ostial lesions. The passage of the device is less dependent on firm guiding catheter support. Atherosclerotic plaque, especially calcific material, is selectively ablated. Smaller guiding catheters are needed than for other ablative procedures. The incidence of major complications appears to be lower than for other debulking procedures.[21] Adjunctive angioplasty is required in 85% of rotablator procedures and the exact restenosis rate remains unknown because of incomplete angiographic follow-up.[21] Nonetheless, in comparisons to balloon dilation, rotational atherectomy

Table 3.1 Comparison of Success and Restenosis Rates After Percutaneous Therapies for Ostial Lesions

TECHNIQUE	AORTO-OSTIAL LESIONS (including vein grafts)		BRANCH OSTIAL LESIONS	
	SUCCESS	RESTENOSIS	SUCCESS	RESTENOSIS
Angioplasty	79%,[6] 94%[7]	73% angiographic 48% clinical[6,46] 79% in SVG[12]	90%[41]	61%,[41] 63%[13] 46%,[11] 34%[8]*
Directional Atherectomy	78%,[15] 93%[16] 89%[28]*,100%[17]*	44%[15]*, 55%,[17] 73% in SVG[18]	90%,[9] 92%[15] 86%[11]	33%,[33] 60%[41] 48%[11]
Rotablator	99%[21], 97[19]%	>32%,[21] 44%,[16] 51%[9], 55%[19]*	96%[21]	>32%[21]
Laser Angioplasty	90%[23]	39%[23]	88%[41]	59%[41]
Stents	100%[31,40,43]*, 96%[46] 93%[39]	23%[40], 28%[39] 16%[43,9]*, 24%[46]	100%[9,42]	33%,[9] 22%[42]

* Series included less than 20 patients.

appears to be more efficacious.[22] Comparing the balloon diameter to the final artery diameter before and after ablative techniques provides an index of the utility of these ablations. Using such a "balloon efficiency index" (**see Glossary**) to correct for differences in balloon and reference artery diameters and for device size, Safian et al.[22] showed that pre-angioplasty rotablator debulking resulted in larger lumens for ostial lesions than balloon angioplasty alone.[22] While rotablator followed by adjunctive balloon angioplasty also provides improved luminal gain in lesions which were eccentric, ulcerated, calcified and long (20mm), the greatest benefit was achieved for ostial stenoses. The relative merits of different ablative methods can be compared by the degree to which angioplasty was facilitated (**Figures 3.4, 3.5**).

Laser Angioplasty

Laser angioplasty also improves the efficiency of balloon dilation in aorto-ostial locations.[22] The restenosis rate is lower than after conventional balloon angioplasty at this site.[23] Laser use at the ostium is contraindicated in angulated and moderately heavily calcified lesions. Adjunctive angioplasty is almost always needed. However, laser ablation may be particularly useful in long lesions. The use of directional and eccentric lasers may alleviate technical problems, such as vessel perforation which occur on curvatures or contralateral to calcified segments, locations at which perforations have been encountered with concentric laser catheters.

Directional Coronary Atherectomy

The early indications for directional atherectomy of eccentric, proximal, large vessel lesions with minimal calcification were well suited to ostial stenoses. Current data suggest that atherectomy for ostial stenoses facilitates balloon angioplasty (**Figure 3.5.**)[22] However, interest in this technique has waned. The amount of tissue removed by atherectomy is considerably less than necessary to account for lumenal gains.[24] Since device size is the major predictor of the final lumen, the dottering effect and not tissue removal appears to be a principle mechanism of atherectomy in increasing the lumen diameter.[25,26] Importantly, data from the CAVEAT trial showed that atherectomy was not only associated with higher restenosis rates but also with a worse long-term clinical outcome than balloon angioplasty. While branch-ostial lesions were originally considered well suited to atherectomy, such patients treated with atherectomy may not do as well than those treated with conventional angioplasty.[11]

Intravascular ultrasound information argues against the traditional morphological guidelines matching different devices to specific lesion subsets. Angioplasty may actually outperform directional atherectomy in more complex lesion subtypes.[27] The argument that atherectomy is less effective in lesions with fluoroscopically apparent calcium[28] has not been borne out by subsequent studies. Results for lesions with moderate calcification favored atherectomy over balloon angioplasty.[27] Fluoroscopically apparent calcium is, in itself, a poor predictor of the need for ablative therapies although it is often cited as a reason to consider rotational atherectomy. Although fluoroscopic calcification may predict the need for a slightly higher (0.5 atm) balloon inflation pressure, 89% of calcified lesions may be treated with inflations of less than 10 atmospheres arguing against the routine use of rotational ablation for such lesions.[24] These insights raise important questions about the traditional guidelines for lesion-specific device selection and the utility of these devices for lesion debulking before stent implantation.

Device Synergy

The concept of multiple device synergy was originally proposed by the coronary interventionalists at the Washington Heart Center.[30] In their experience, the sequential use of multiple devices resulted in an improved immediate angiographic result. For rigid or nondilatable lesions that resist effective stent expansion, debulking the atheroma first may well be a reasonable strategy.[31,37] It is especially important to decide whether to ablate atheroma before stent deployment since this technique is contraindicated once the stent is in place. Because lumen size is an important determinant of both late clinical outcome and restenosis, a synergistic approach has particular appeal for ostial stenoses. Non-randomized evaluations have suggested that the application of debulking devices (directional atherectomy, rotablator and excimer laser) improves the success rate of ostial lesion angioplasty.[32] The question of whether the small luminal gains achieved by pre-angioplasty plaque ablation will translate into clinical benefit remains unanswered. So far, long-term results comparing the debulking approach to stand alone angioplasty have found no clinical or angiographic benefit at 6 months.[33]

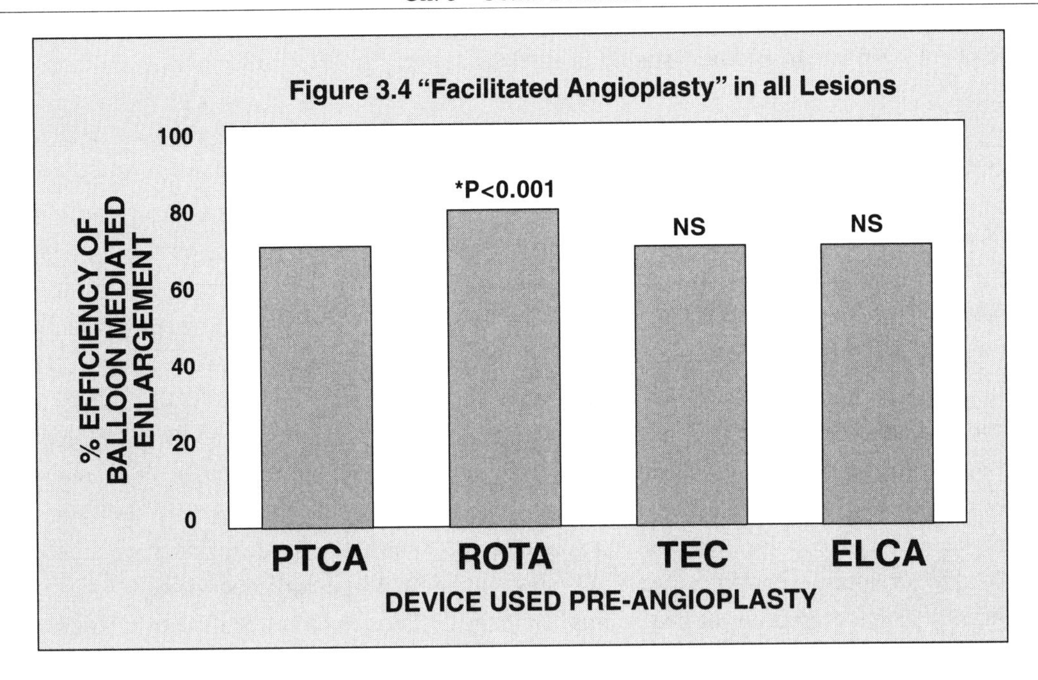

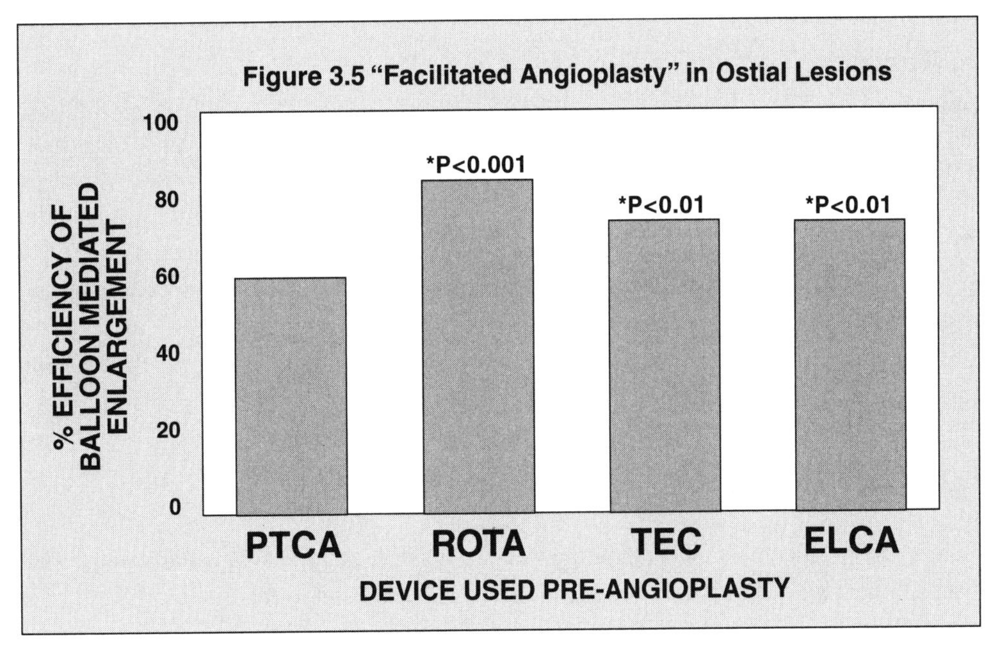

Figures 3.4, 3.5 Facilitated Angioplasty Any absolute incremental gain in arterial lumen diameter for adjunctive angioplasty after an ablative procedure compared with angioplasty alone is considered "facilitated angioplasty". When all lesions were analyzed **(Figure 3.4)** there was a 13% increment after rotational atherectomy (ROTA), but none after extraction atherectomy (TEC), or excimer laser angioplasty (ELCA). However when only ostial lesions are analyzed **(Figure 3.5)**, all three ablative techniques provide incremental gain which was as much as 41% greater after rotational atherectomy. Adapted with permission from Dr. RD Safian and The American College of Cardiology (*J Am Coll Cardiol* 1996;27:555).

The rate of non-Q-wave infarction in studies using debulking techniques for the most complex lesions is as high as 21-26%.[34-36] Non-Q-wave infarctions are important and associated with an increase in late mortality.[35] Currently, few operators are content to apply angioplasty alone to ostial lesions. It is unknown whether the excellent lumen obtained after primary stenting of ostial lesions will be improved by pre-stent debulking. Prospective data comparing standard stent implantation with stent implantation after lesion debulking is not yet available. Despite the conceptual appeal and belief that device synergy is important for improving success rates and reducing restenosis, there are no data as yet to support this concept. Observational comparisons of the multi-device debulking approach followed by selective stent implantation versus a strategy of aggressive standard stent implantation alone suggest that with optimal stent implantation, procedural success is increased and major complications are significantly reduced.[37] Another observational report of rotational atherectomy before stenting suggested that while Rotablator therapy may favorably modify vessel compliance prior to stenting and improve the procedural result, this occurred in exchange for a rather high incidence of acute stent thrombosis (1.9%).[48] Whether restenosis rates and late clinical outcomes will be favorably affected by primary stent implantation alone will be determined by prospective controlled trials. A review of alternative percutaneous therapies suggests that while the initial angiographic result may be improved, the high restenosis rates at the ostial location have not been significantly affected by these devices (**Table 3.1**).

Lesion Recoil

Even when calcium is not apparent fluoroscopically, significant recoil after angioplasty leaves a 35-45% residual stenosis.[38] The scaffolding and radial support offered by stents treats recoil of ostial lesions with little or no residual stenosis after stent implantation.[39,40] Newer stent design features have magnified this benefit. The radial force exerted by the NIR stent implanted in Case 3.1 is significantly greater than that offered even by the Palmaz-Schatz stent.[47] Confidence in this resistance to radial compression allowed the more casual approach to athero-ablation which was demonstrated in this case. With current Palmaz-Schatz designs, the 7% loss from immediate recoil after ostial stenting is superior to the 35% immediate lumen loss after ablative techniques such as laser angioplasty.[22]

Stent Designs and Recoil

While there are no prospective trials comparing stents to ablative therapies for ostial lesions, a number of small observational reports have indicated excellent stent success and restenosis rates[9,31,40,42,46] obtained with Palmaz, Palmaz-Schatz and Wallstent designs.[43] These data may not apply for other stent models. Because most coil designs provide less radial support, these stents probably should be avoided at the aorto-ostial location. The ability of coiled stent designs to prevent restenosis at this site is also unknown. The Wiktor tantalum coil stent has a tendency to unravel in aorto-ostial lesions causing major deployment complications.[44] Whether this disadvantage applies to coil devices in branch-ostial lesions is unknown. The issue of branch ostial stenting is important since increased radiopacity of the Wiktor and Cordis coil devices is a particular advantage for the precise positioning required at these sites.

Coil and woven stents may be difficult to use in some lesion subgroups. The Wallstent has been shown effective in ostial lesions, but tends to move considerably along the arterial axis during deployment making precise ostial placement a challenge. The ability to recapture the second generation (Magic) Wallstent device during deployment may alleviate this problem somewhat. Furthermore, the resistance to the extra compressive radial forces at the arterial ostium varies somewhat with the final expanded stent diameter.[45] In contrast, the AVE Micro II and GFX stents have properties of radiopacity, excellent resistance to radial compression, low profile, and short lengths and have made these the preferred ostial stent devices in many centers.

Technical Pearl: Guiding Catheters for Ostial Lesion Angioplasty

No matter which technique or combination of techniques ultimately proves superior for ostial lesions, technical challenges for this location will remain. The low success and high complication rates in ostial angioplasty were originally attributed to excessive trauma caused by the guiding catheters.[6] Contrary to most angioplasty procedures, it is essential to choose a guide which will not deep-seat. Such a tendency is counterproductive at the ostium, especially if a stent is to be deployed. Standard 8F Judkins catheters, which will not deeply intubate the ostium, are best. Side holes may be of advantage to allow perfusion during guiding catheter maneuvers and to avoid injection trauma to the diseased ostial endothelium.

For ostial coronary angioplasty, the guiding catheter will often be backed into the aorta providing even less support and backup than usual. Coaxial alignment is essential. Apposition of the guide against the opposite aortic wall or deep in the sinus of Valsalva may be necessary. These technique modifications will mean that a stent will be positioned with infrequent contrast injections. Radiopaque landmarks and a fluoroscopically visible stent become very important for correct positioning.

Technical Pearl: Pre-stent Balloon Dilations

The extra rigidity and tissue elasticity in the ostium may prevent complete balloon expansion even at high inflation pressure. On average 9 atm or higher pressures will be required to dilate ostial lesions. Therefore, only high pressure, non-compliant balloons should be selected when working in the ostium.[6] If the predilation balloon appears incompletely expanded at over 15 atm, ablative rotablator or laser techniques will be necessary before the stent can be implanted. Due to the need to maximize post-stent diameter to >3.0 mm, ablative therapies should be considered when the ostial lesion reference diameter is small (<3.0 mm). While the average length of ostial lesions is short, "watermelon seeding" or slippage of a balloon either proximal or distal to the lesion during inflation is not infrequent due to the increased lesion rigidity. The temptation to use a short balloon in ostial lesions should be resisted. The balloon should be long enough to leave a proximal portion outside the stent in the aorta, permitting stent end flaring into the aorta.

Intravascular Ultrasound (IVUS) and Ostial Stenting

Intraluminal haziness is common after ostial procedures, although less frequent with stenting, making the application of QCA problematic. IVUS may be necessary to determine if such haziness is due to residual atheroma or to an asymmetrically apposed stent. Finally, future catheterization operators must consider the possibility of stent struts protruding into the aorta or from branch-ostia into trunk arteries. When a balloon or stent does not pass easily near a previously stented segment, stop and consider whether struts of the previously deployed stent may be impeding the passage.

Key Points for Ostial Angioplasty and Stenting

1. Coaxial alignment, not deep intubation, is the objective of guiding catheter support for lesions at the coronary ostium. The guiding catheter must be withdrawn 1-2cm into the aorta during stent positioning and deployment to avoid inflating the proximal balloon within the guide.

2. Balloon predilation at the coronary ostium should always be performed with a full-sized balloon capable of high pressures. This method not only provides the greatest assurance that the stent will also pass, but also is a good index of lesion rigidity and elastic recoil. In lesions which do not fully expand despite high pressure dilation with a full-sized balloon, debulking will be required.

3. In contrast to the technique for multiple stents in the body of a coronary vessel wherein the distal stent should be placed first, the contrary approach applies to lesions of the coronary ostium. If multiple stents are needed at the coronary ostium, the most important task is to first position the proximal ostial stent precisely and then place subsequent stents distal through widely opened ostial stent.

4. The proximal 1-2mm of the stent should be flared against the wall of the aorta to ensure complete lesion coverage and prevent subsequent catheter-related strut damage.

SUMMARY

A number of technical advances have improved upon the historically poor results of angioplasty in ostial locations. While such advances as cutting and perfusion balloons have allowed increased success, the residual stenoses and increased restenosis rates warrant adjunctive therapies. Among these therapies, rotablator and laser angioplasty have proved useful in lesion debulking, but have had little impact upon the high restenosis rates. Ostial stent implantation shows promise in both increasing immediate success and in decreasing subsequent restenosis. The role of lesion debulking prior to stent implantation remains to be determined. New information suggests that the risk profile of synergistic device approaches may be of marginal benefit. It is likely, however, that a minority of highly rigid and calcified lesions will be approachable only with a stent after preliminary tissue ablation. While intracoronary ultrasound has a particularly important role in fine tuning stent deployment at the ostium of arteries, pre-deployment tests of lesion rigidity by balloon inflation are also of use.

References

1. Pritchard CL, Mudd JG, Barner HB. *Coronary ostial stenosis.* Circulation 52:46-48 (1975).
2. Thompson R. *Isolated coronary ostial stenosis in women.* J Am Coll Cardiol 7:997-1003 (1986).
3. Miller AH, Honey M, El Sayad H. *Isolated coronary ostial stenosis.* Cathet Cardiovasc Diagn 12:30-34 (1986).
4. Stewart JT, Ward DE, Davies MJ, Pepper JR. *Isolated coronary ostial stenosis: observations of the pathology.* Eur Heart J 8:917-920 (1987).
5. Popma JJ, Dick RJL, Haudenschild CC, et al. *Atherectomy of right coronary ostial stenosis: Initial and long-term results, technical features and histological findings.* Am J Cardiol 67:431-433 (1991).
6. Topol EJ, Ellis SG, Fishman J, et al. *Multicenter study of percutaneous transluminal angioplasty for right coronary artery ostial stenosis.* J Am Coll Cardiol 9:1214-1218 (1987).
7. Tan K, Sulke N, Taub N, Sowton E. *Clinical and lesion morphologic determinants of coronary angioplasty success and complications: Current experience.* J Am Coll Cardiol 25:855-865 (1995).
8. Vallbracht C, Althen D, Kneissl GD, et al. *Conventional PTCA in ostial lesions is better than its reputation.* Eur Heart J 14:247-(1993).
9. Sawada Y, Kimura T, Shinoda E, et al. *Poor outcome of balloon angioplasty for ostial left anterior descending and circumflex: Impact of new angioplasty devices* [abstr]. Circulation 90(part 2):I-436 (1994).
10. Whitworth HB, Pilcher GS, Roubin GS, et al. *Do proximal lesions involving the origin of the left anterior descending artery (LAD) have a higher rate of restenosis after coronary angioplasty (PTCA)?* [abstr]. Circulation 72 (suppl III):III-398 (1985).
11. Boehreer JD, Ellis SG, Pieper K, et al. *Directional atherectomy versus balloon angioplasty for coronary ostial and nonostial left anterior descending coronary artery lesions: results from a randomized multicenter trial.* J Am Coll Cardiol 25:1380-1386 (1995).
12. Douglas J, King S, Roubin G, Schlumpf M. *Percutaneous angioplasty of venous aortocoronary graft stenoses: late angiographic and clinical outcome* [abstr]. Circulation 74 (suppl II): II-281 (1986).
13. Whitworth HB, Pilcher GS, Roubin GS, et al. *Do proximal lesions involving the origin of the left anterior descending artery (LAD) have a higher rate of restenosis after coronary angioplasty (PTCA)?* [abstr]. Circulation 72 (suppl III):III-398 (1985).
14. Vallbracht C, Althen D, Kneissl GD, et al. *Conventional PTCA in ostial lesions is better than its reputation* [abstr]. Eur Heart J 14:247 (1993).
15. Robertson GC, Simpson JB, Velter JW, et al. *Directional coronary atherectomy for ostial lesions* [abstr]. Circulation 84 (Suppl II): II-251 (1991).

16. Bernardi MM, Cleman MW, Whitlow PL, et al. *Treatment of right coronary artery ostial stenosis with rotational atherectomy: results of a multicenter registry.* Circulation 88(suppl 1):I-546 (1993).

17. Garratt KN, Bell MR, Berger PB, et al. *Directional coronary atherectomy of saphenous vein graft ostial lesions* [abstr]. Circulation 84(suppl II):II-26 (1991).

18. Hinohara T, Robertson GC, Selmon MR, et al. *Restenosis after directional coronary atherectomy.* J Am Coll Cardiol 20:623-632 (1992).

19. Commeau R, Zimarino M, Lancelin B, et al. *Rotational coronary atherectomy for the treatment of aorto-ostial and branch-ostial lesions* [abstr]. Circulation 90(suppl 1):I-213 (1994).

20. Zampieri P, Colombo A, Almagor Y, et al. *Results of coronary stenting of ostial lesions.* Am J Cardiol 73:901-903 (1994).

21. Popma JJ, Brogan WC, Pichard AD, et al. *Rotational coronary atherectomy of ostial stenoses.* Am J Cardiol 71:436-438 (1993).

22. Safian RD, Freed M, Reddy V, et al. *Do excimer laser angioplasty and rotational atherectomy facilitate balloon angioplasty? Implications for lesion-specific coronary intervention.* J Am Coll Cardiol 27:552-559 (1996).

23. Eigler NL, Weinstock B, Douglas JS, et al. *Excimer laser coronary angioplasty of aorto- ostial stenoses-results of the excimer laser coronary angioplasty (ELCA) registry in the first 200 patients.* Circulation 88[part 1]:2049-2057 (1993).

24. Safian RD, Gelbfish JS, Erny RE, et al. *Coronary atherectomy: clinical, angiographic and histological findings and observations regarding potential mechanisms.* Circulation 82:69-79 (1990).

25. Sharaf BL, Williams DO. *"Dotter effect" contributes to angiographic improvement following directional coronary atherectomy* [abstr]. Circulation 82(supp III):III-310 (1990).

26. Popma JJ, DeCesare NB, Ellis SG, et al. *Clinical, angiographic and procedural correlates of quantitative coronary dimensions after directional atherectomy.* J Am Coll Cardiol 18:1183-1189 (1991).

27. Kimball BP, Cohen EA, Adelman AG. *Influence of stenotic lesion morphology on immediate and long-term (6 months) angiographic outcome: Comparative analysis of directional coronary atherectomy versus standard balloon angioplasty.* J Am Coll Cardiol 27:543-551 (1996).

28. Hinohara T, Rowe MH, Robertson GC, et al. *Effect of lesion characteristics on outcome of directional coronary atherectomy.* J Am Coll Cardiol 17:1112-1120 (1991).

29. Danchin N, Buffet P, Dibon O, Cuilliere M. *Should specific angioplasty techniques be used to treat calcified coronary artery lesions? A retrospective study* [abstr]. Circulation 90(suppl I):I-436 (1994).

30. Pichard AD, Mintz GS, Kent KM, et al. Transcatheter device synergy: *Preliminary experience with adjunct direction atherectomy following rotational atherectomy in treating calcific coronary artery disease [abstr].* J Am Coll Cardiol 21:227A (1993).

31. Rechavia E, Litvack F, Macko G, Eigler NL. *Stent implantation of saphenous vein graft aorto-ostial lesions in patients with unstable ischemic syndromes: immediate angiographic results and long-term clinical outcome.* J Am Coll Cardiol 25:866-870 (1995).

32. Sabri MN, Cowley MJ, DiSciascio G, et al. *Immediate results of interventional devices for coronary ostial narrowing with angina pectoris.* Am J Cardiol 73:122-125 (1994).

33. Vandormael M, Reifart N, Preussler W, et al. *Six months follow-up results following excimer laser angioplasty, rotational atherectomy, and balloon angioplasty for complex lesions: ERBAC study* [abstr]. Circulation 90(Suppl I):I-213 (1994).

34. Hong MK, Mintz GS, Popma JJ, et al. *Angiographic results and late clinical outcomes utilizing a stent synergy (pre-stent atheroablation) approach in complex lesion subsets.* J Invas Cardiol 8:15-22 (1996).

35. Abelmeguid AE, Topol EJ, Whitlow PL, et al. *Significance of mild transient release of creatinine kinase-MB fraction after percutaneous coronary interventions.* Circulation 94: 1528-1536 (1996).

36. Hinohara T, Vetter JW, Robertson GC, et al. *CK MB elevation following directional coronary atherectomy* [abstr]. Circulation 92(suppl I):I-544 (1995).

37. Hong MK, Wong SC, Kent KM, et al. *An aggressive stent strategy improves procedure success and reduces major in-hospital ischemic complications* [abstr]. Circulation 92 (suppl I):I-535 (1995).

38. Mathias DW, Fishman-Mooney J, Lange HW, et al. *Frequency of success and complications of coronary angioplasty of a stenosis at the ostium of a branch vessel.* Am J Cardiol 67:491 (1991).

39. Rocha-Singh K, Morris N, Wong C, et al. *Coronary stenting for treatment of ostial stenoses of native coronary arteries or aortocoronary saphenous venous grafts.* Am J Cardiol 75:26-29 (1995).

40. Colombo A, Itoh A, Maiello L, et al. *Coronary stent implantation in aorto-ostial lesions: immediate and follow-up results* [abstr]. J Am Coll Cardiol 27(suppl A):253A (1996).

41. Sawada Y, Kimura T, Shinoda E, et al. *Poor outcome of balloon angioplasty for ostial left anterior descending and circumflex: Impact of new angioplasty devices* [abstr]. Circulation 90(part 2):I-436 (1994).

42. De Cesare NB, Galli S, Loaldi A, et al. *Palmaz-Schatz stent for the treatment of left anterior descending ostial stenosis: Acute and long-term results* [abstr]. J Invas Cardiol 8:40(1996).

43. Nordrehaug JE, Priestley KA, Chronos NAF, et al. *Self expanding stents for the management of aorto-ostial stenoses in saphenous vein bypass grafts.* Br Heart J 72:285-287 (1994).

44. Chalet Y, Panes F, Chevalier B, et al. *Should we avoid ostial implantations of Wiktor stents?* Cathet Cardiovasc Diagn 32:376-379 (1994).

45. Jedwab MR, Clerc CO. *A study of the geometrical and mechanical properties of a self- expanding metallic stent-theory and experiment.* J of App Biomat 4:77-83 (1993).

46. Suresh PJ, Liu WM, Dean LS, et al. *Comparison of balloon angioplasty versus debulking devices versus stenting in right coronary ostial lesions.* Am J Cardiol 79: 1334-1338 (1997).

47 Almagor Y, Personal Communication October 1996; LaJolla, CA

48 Moussa I, DiMario C, Moses J, Et al. *Coronary stenting after rotational atherectomy in calcified and complex lesions.* Circulation 96: 128-136 (1997)

CHAPTER 4

SIDE BRANCHES AND STENT JAIL

CASE 4.1: Stent Migration

The patient is a 69 year old retired truck driver who had anterior myocardial infarction four years earlier. He presented with unstable angina progressing to rest angina which occurred three times on the day of admission. At angiography he was found to have a severe lesion of the distal right coronary artery crossing but not extending into the posterior descending artery (**Figure 4.1a**). There was also a

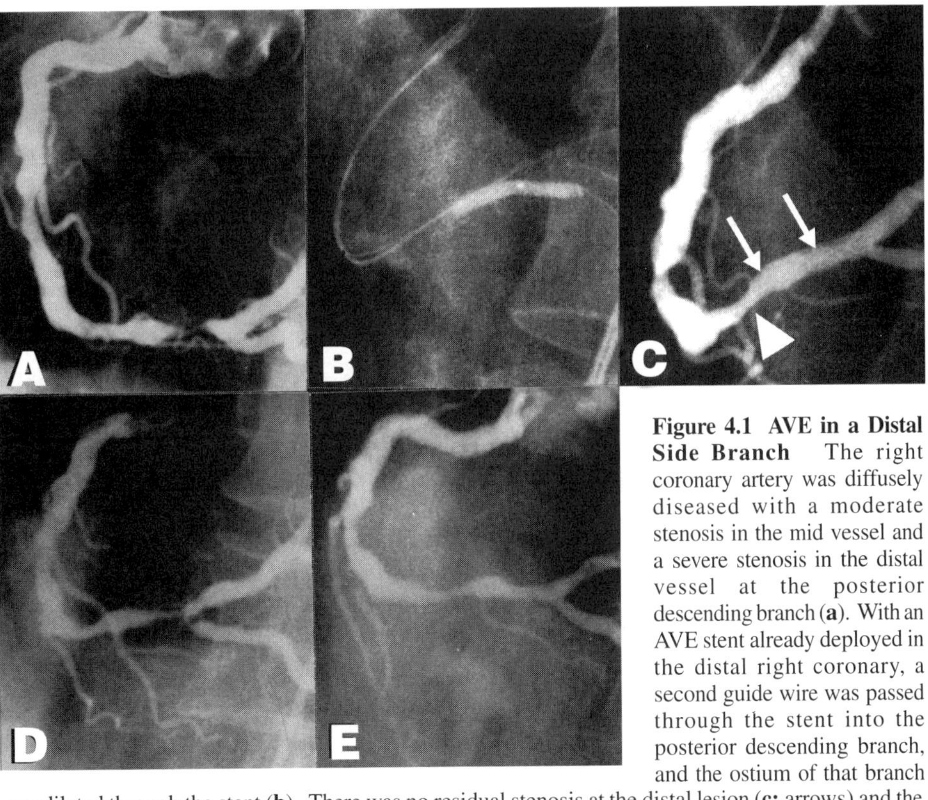

Figure 4.1 AVE in a Distal Side Branch The right coronary artery was diffusely diseased with a moderate stenosis in the mid vessel and a severe stenosis in the distal vessel at the posterior descending branch (**a**). With an AVE stent already deployed in the distal right coronary, a second guide wire was passed through the stent into the posterior descending branch, and the ostium of that branch was dilated through the stent (**b**). There was no residual stenosis at the distal lesion (**c; arrows**) and the remaining moderate stenosis (arrowhead) was treated with additional stenting. At 6 month angiography there was restenosis at both the distal right coronary and posterior branch (**d**) which was successfully treated with further dilations at both sites (**e**).

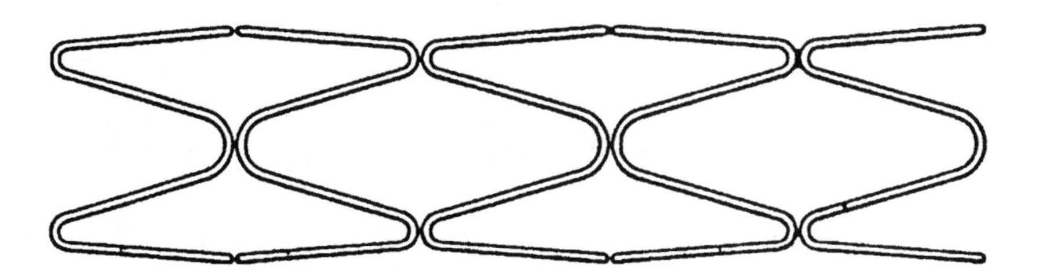

Figure 4.2 AVE Microstent A continuous zigzag wire segmented design.

moderate lesion of the mid right coronary artery and a chronic occlusion of the mid to distal left anterior descending coronary artery.

PROCEDURE 4.1

The distal right coronary artery lesion was approached first with a 2.5mm balloon. Despite balloon inflations to 12 atm, there was elastic recoil with a residual lesion of 50%. A stent was indicated for a suboptimal angioplasty result. The origin of the large posterior descending branch was in the middle of the distal right coronary artery lesion. Given the important side branch, a stent through which future procedures might be performed was selected. An Applied Vascular Engineering (AVE) Micro I stent of 3.5mm (**Figure 4.2**) was deployed with a 12 atm inflation across the origin of the posterior descending artery. The stent was over-dilated with a 3.5mm balloon to 16 atm. The distal right coronary artery was now widely patent, but disruption of the branch ostium with plaque shifting into the posterior descending artery resulted in a new 80% stenosis. An additional guidewire was easily passed through the AVE stent into the posterior descending branch. Sequential dilations were performed with a 2.5mm and then a 3.0mm balloon to 8 atm across the stent into the posterior descending artery (**Figure 4.1b**). There was no residual stenosis in either artery at the dilated sites (**Figure 4-1c**). The moderate (60%) mid right coronary lesion (**Figure 4-1c arrow, Figure 4.3a**) was predilated with the 3.5mm balloon and a 4.0mm X 16mm AVE Micro I stent was implanted. This stent was dilated with a 4.0mm balloon to 18 atm with an adequate final result (**Figure 4.3b**). The position of the portions of the AVE 4mm stent are indicated in **Figure 4.3c**. It is important to note that this stent is under-dilated angiographically (**Figure 4.3c**).

The patient was discharged after 24 hours of intravenous heparin and remained asymptomatic for six months when progressive angina and a positive stress test occurred. Repeat angiography revealed restenosis of both the distal right coronary lesion and the posterior descending ostium (**Figure 4.1d**). The proximal result remained adequate but the distal 8mm portion of the 4.0 mm X 16mm AVE Micro I stent had migrated about 1 cm down the vessel (**Figure 4.3d**). Angioplasty of the distal stent and posterior descending artery was again performed, this time using the alternating 2.5mm kissing balloon technique. Both guidewire and balloon could pass easily through the AVE stent to accomplish these dilations. The final result is portrayed in **Figure 4.1e.**

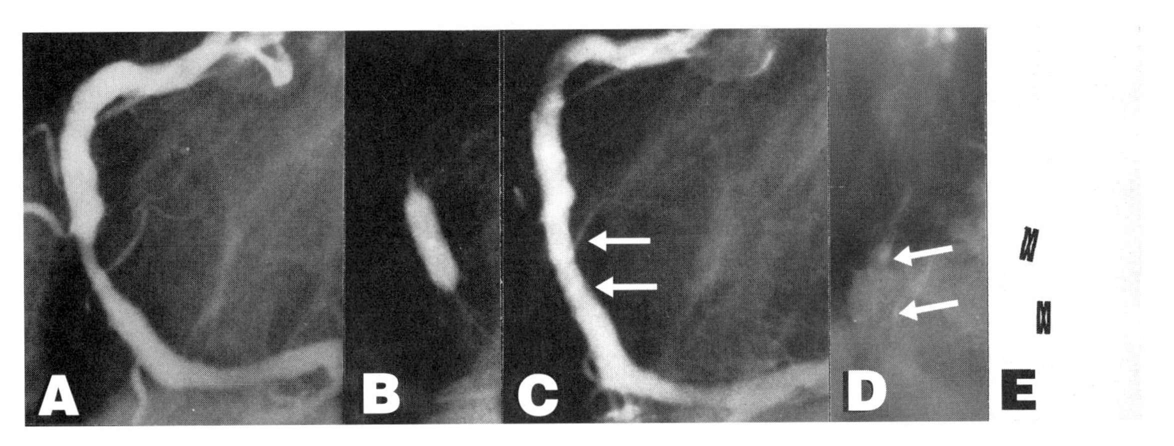

Figure 4.3 Stent Migration In the earliest AVE stents, the modular segments were not welded together. The mid vessel lesion (**a**) in the same right coronary artery depicted in **Figure 4.1** was also treated with implantation of an AVE stent. This was post dilated to 18 atm with a 4 mm balloon (**b**). The final result reveals underdilation of the diseased segment (**c**). While there was no restenosis at this location at 6 month angiography, the AVE stent segments appeared separated on fluoroscopy (**d**), with the distal segment of the underdilated stent migrating further distally (**e**).

MATERIALS 4.1

Initial Procedure

Guiding Catheter:	Right Amplatz 1
Guidewires:	ACS Extra Support 0.014" (2)
Balloons:	Schneider Goldie 2.5mm x 20mm
	Schneider Chubby 3.5mm x 9mm
	USCI Pronto Rely 3mm x 20mm
	Schneider Chubby 4.0 x 9mm
Stents:	Applied Vascular Engineering (AVE) 3.5mm x 16mm
	Applied Vascular Engineering (AVE) 4.0mm x 16mm

Follow-up Procedure (6 months later)

Guiding Catheter:	Schneider Guidezilla JR4
Guidewires:	USCI Veriflex 0.014", Hyperflex 0.014"
	ACS Extra Support 0.014"
Balloons:	Schneider Goldie 2.5 x 20mm, Cordis Passage 3.5 x 20mm
Stents:	None

CASE 4.2: Impacted Wire Side Branch Technique

The patient is a 42 year old mechanic who had an inferoposterior infarction followed by post-infarction chest pain. Cardiac catheterization two weeks after the infarction revealed preserved left ventricular function and a normal non-dominant right coronary artery. The left anterior descending artery had a 90% stenosis proximally and the large circumflex artery had a severe stenosis straddling the first obtuse marginal and the continuation of the distal circumflex (**Figure 4.4a**).

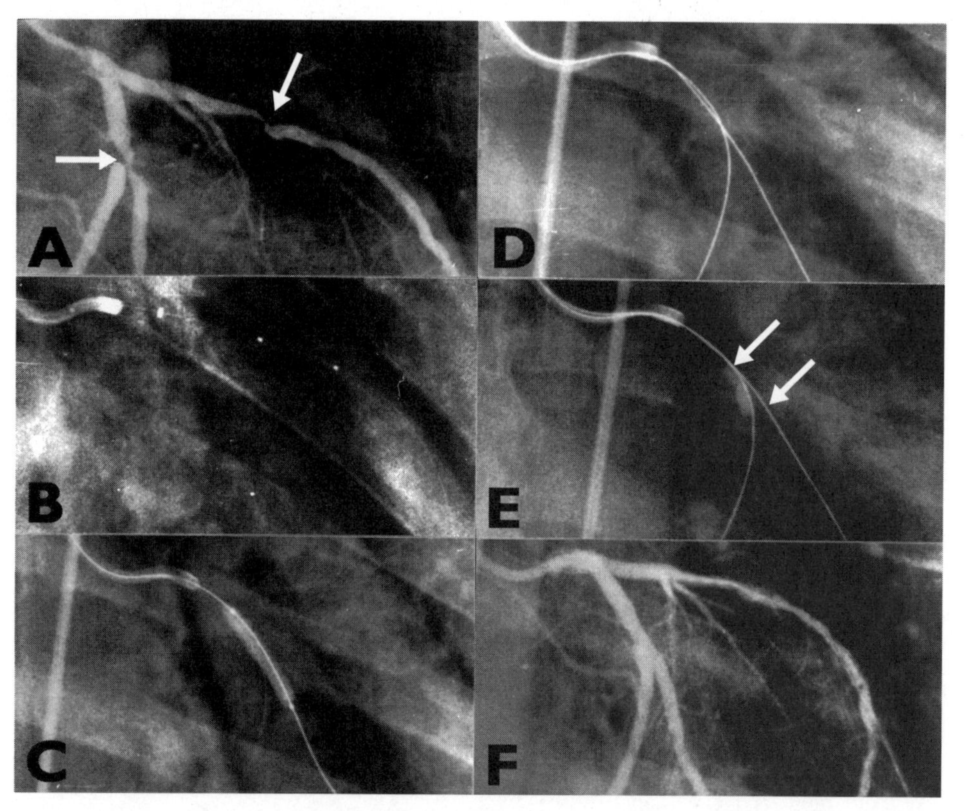

Figure 4.4 Impacted Wire Side branch Technique There is a 90% stenosis in the proximal left anterior descending and a severe stenosis of the circumflex at its bifurcation into the first obtuse marginal vessel (**a;** arrows). The markers of the ACS Multilink stent are seen during positioning prior to deployment (**b**). The Gianturco- Roubin II stent is deployed in the circumflex and first obtuse marginal simultaneously impacting a radiolucent guide wire (**c**) which remains in the distal circumflex. A third guidewire which is radiopaque has been passed through the coils of the stent into the distal circumflex and the impacted guidewire has been withdrawn (**d**). After high pressure dilations within the Gianturco- Roubin stent, a compliant balloon is passed through the coils of the stent and dilated to treat the distal circumflex (**e**). The final angiographic result revealed no residual stenosis at the ACS Multilink stent in the anterior descending artery nor at the Gianturco-Roubin stent in the circumflex and obtuse marginal arteries (**f**).

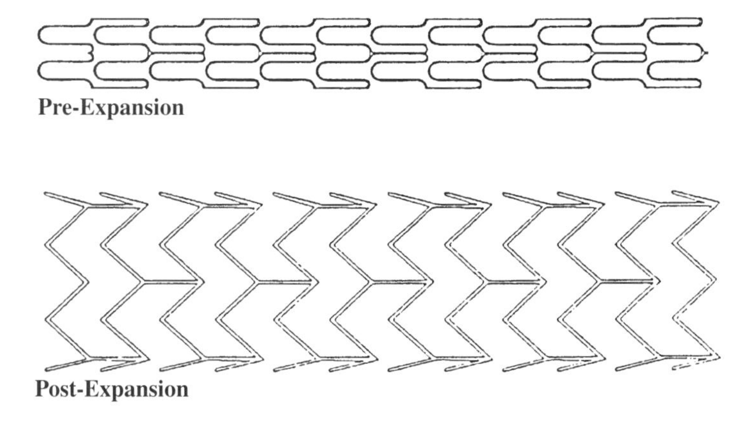

Figure 4.5 The ACS Multilink Stent – multiple zigzag rings connected with multiple links

PROCEDURE 4.2

De novo stenting of the proximal left anterior descending was performed first, so that the more demanding procedure in the circumflex artery could be undertaken with the security of an open left anterior descending coronary artery.

An extra support guidewire was easily passed across the stenosis and into the distal anterior descending artery. The lesion was predilated with a 3.0/3.5mm CAT balloon at 6 atm and an ACS multi-link stent (**Figure 4.5**) was positioned and implanted, assisted by the Multilink markers (**Figure 4.4b**). The stent was post-dilated to 15 atm leaving no residual stenosis (**Figure 4.4f**).

The complex lesion in the mid circumflex artery, the infarct artery, was addressed next. Because both the distal circumflex and the first obtuse marginal were 3mm vessels, it was important to protect both branches before approaching the high risk lesion. The extra support wire was passed into the distal circumflex vessel. Another radiopaque guidewire was passed into the distal obtuse marginal. Initial dilations in both arterial segments with the 3.0/3.5mm CAT balloon resulted in a hazy angiographic appearance (not shown). It was elected to proceed with stent implantation from the proximal circumflex extending into the obtuse marginal vessel. Because of the possible need to implant an additional stent into the distal circumflex artery, a Gianturco-Roubin II (GR II) stent (**Figure 4.6**) was chosen. An additional stent could be passed through its struts, if necessary. The GR II stent was implanted, leaving the guidewire in place in the distal circumflex, now impacted against the arterial wall by the deployed stent. A lumen was preserved through which to pass yet a third wire should the distal circumflex be compromised by the stent implantation (**Figure 4.4c**). After deployment of the stent at 6 atm and before post-implantation dilations, a third radiopaque guidewire was passed into the distal circumflex location and the impacted guidewire was withdrawn (**Figure 4.4d**). [In this case, removal of the impacted wire was quite easy.

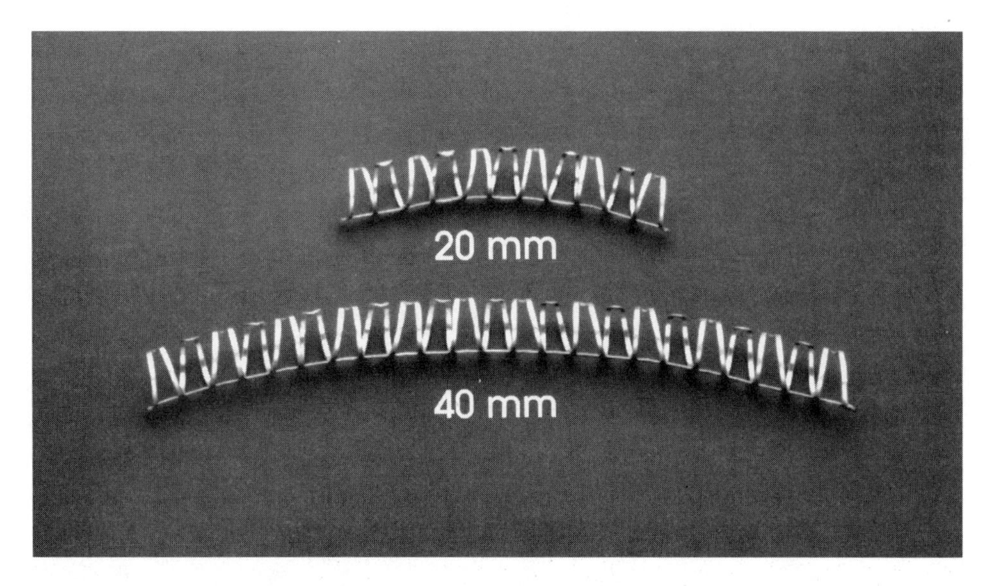

Figure 4.6 The Gianturco-Roubin II Interdigitating loops of flat wire on a longitudinal spine.

However, on previous occasions during wire removal, occasional deep intubation of the guiding catheter has been noted.] After post-stent deployment, inflations with the CAT balloon to 14 atm, an unused low profile, compliant balloon was passed through the flat coils of the stent and, while still astride the stent, was dilated to 5 atm (**Figure 4.4e**). The final result revealed neither the initial haziness nor any residual stenosis in either distal branch (**Figure 4.4f**). A third stent to be passed through the Gianturco-Roubin II was not necessary. The patient was heparinized overnight and discharged two days after the procedure.

MATERIALS 4.2

Guiding Catheter:	Cook 8F AL-3
Guidewires:	ACS Extra S'port 0.014"x300cm
	USCI Hyperflex 0.014"x300cm (2)
Balloons:	Cardiovascular Dynamics CAT 3.0/3.5mm x 20/10mm
	Schneier Goldie 3.5 x 20mm
Stents:	ACS/Guidant Multilink 3.25mm
	Cook G-R II 3.5 x 20mm

CASE 4.3: Kissing Balloons Through a Stent on a Curve

The patient is a 46 year old print shop foreman. He was a smoker with hypertension, severe hyperlipidemia, and diabetes mellitus type 1 who was referred because of two months of increasing angina and an early positive treadmill exercise test. Diagnostic angiography revealed a severe lesion on an angulated segment of the mid left anterior descending artery (**Figure 4.7a**). The 2.5mm diagonal branch was involved in the anterior descending plaque well visualized by orthogonal projections. Left ventricular function was normal. Primary stent implantation was performed because of the anticipated benefit in reducing restenosis.

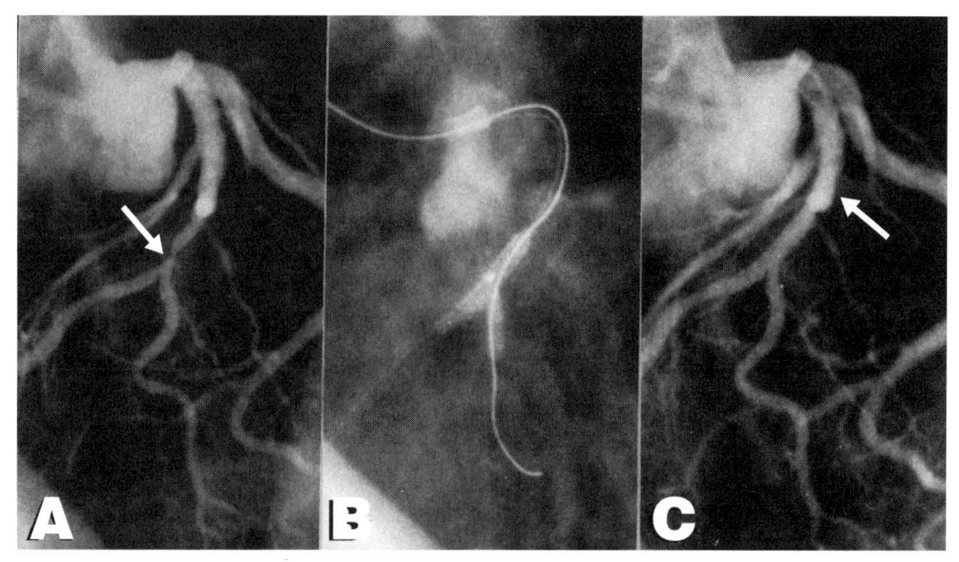

Figure 4.7 Kissing Balloons for Side branch on Curve A severe lesion is noted in an angulated segment of the left anterior descending artery at the origin of a moderate sized diagonal branch (**a;** arrow). Simultaneous or "kissing" dilations of both the XT stent within the anterior descending and the diagonal tributary were performed to treat plaque shifting (**b**). The final result reveals no stenosis within the anterior descending branch, and only a minor deformity at the ostium of the diagonal branch (**c;** arrow shows aneurysmal segment).

PROCEDURE 4.3

The large diagonal side branch was involved in the target plaque. In addition to side branch protection, the significant left anterior descending artery angulation presented an additional challenge for stent placement. Consequently, a modular coil design stent, the Bard XT (**Figure 4.8**) was chosen. Guidewires were passed into both the left anterior descending and diagonal vessels. Both vessels were alternately dilated and the diagonal wire was withdrawn prior to left anterior descending stent (16mm Bard XT stent) deployment at 10 atm. Care was taken to position the dorsal spine of the stent away from the diagonal orifice before deployment. A flexible radiopaque wire (USCI) was easily passed through the cellular units of the XT stent into the diagonal branch. Plaque shifting with contrast lucencies moving from the left anterior descending artery to diagonal branch and back during the predilation had been noted. Consequently, simultaneous "kissing" dilations of both the stented left anterior descending vessel and the diagonal branch were performed (**Figure 4.7b**). The final result revealed no residual lesion in the left anterior descending artery and a minor ostial deformity in the diagonal branch. An aneurysmal dilation just proximal to the stent was left untouched (**Figure 4.7c** arrow). The patient was discharged on the second day post-procedure on aspirin and ticlopidine. He has remained asymptomatic.

MATERIALS 4.3

Guiding Catheter:	Cook Lumax JL-4 8 French
Guidewires:	ACS Extra Support 0.014"x 175cm
	USCI Phantom 0.14"x 180cm, Hyperflex 0.014"x
Balloons:	USCI Pronto Rely 3 x 20mm
	Schneider Goldie 2.5 x 20mm
Stents:	Bard XT

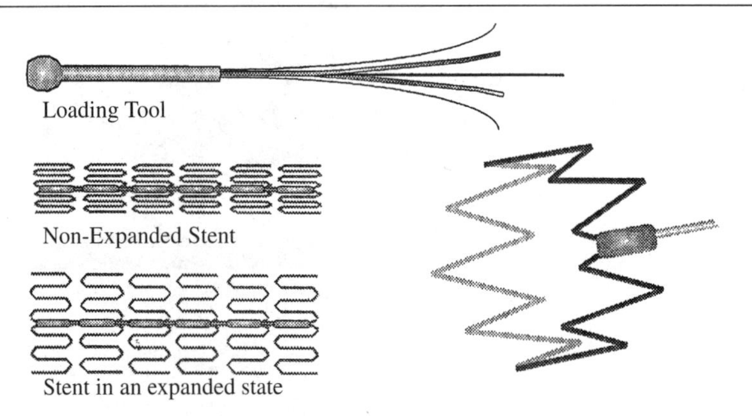

Figure 4.8 The Bard XT – Modular zigzag rings on a longitudinal spine

DISCUSSION

Stenting Side Branches and Risk of Closure

The presence of side branches has had a major influence on the strategy of angioplasty for over a decade. Over half of angioplasty procedures place a side branch in danger.[1] The presence of side branches increases procedural complications.[1,2] The occlusion rate of side branches during coronary angioplasty ranges from 3-15%, depending on the clinical and anatomic features.[3,4] Stents may improve or worsen the flow through side branches in both elective and bailout settings. The concept of "stent jail" is described as the incarceration of side branches when their ostia are covered and made inaccessible by trunk vessel stenting. A number of reports have reviewed the effects of stents on side branches both in the setting of acute closure and at elective implantation. As a result, certain guidelines and techniques have evolved for avoidance and management of stenting across side branches.

In a retrospective review of 57 elective Palmaz-Schatz stents spanning 66 side branches of greater than 1mm size, Fischman et al[5] demonstrated that acute occlusion of side branches was uncommon (≤5%). In this series, the presence of disease in the ostium of the side branch was the major determinant of subsequent branch occlusion. While only 3% of side branches having a less than 50% ostial stenosis occluded after preparatory angioplasty or stenting, 30% of the side branches having a greater than 50% ostial lesion became occluded. Interestingly, the three side branches that became occluded after stenting were all patent at six month follow-up and there were no new late occlusions. The occlusion of these side branches was of little clinical significance as there was neither electrocardiographic nor enzymatic evidence of myocardial infarction. These favorable results have been amplified for Palmaz-Schatz stents applied in bailout as well as elective situations.[6,7] While the rate of side branch occlusion may rise to 14% when vessels of less than 1mm are included, there is again little clinical significance to these occlusions.[7] As in the original study[5] a significant proportion of the vessels occluded at stenting were found patent at six month follow up.[7]

Stent Designs and Side Branches

The available studies principally reflect the effects of slotted tube stents on side branches.[5-7] After deployment, 20% of the arterial surface area is covered by the tube stent material. The coil design stents expose only 10-15% of the vessel surface area to stent material and the wire coil may be better molded to side branch contours. Side branches are more accessible through wire coils should this approach be necessary in the future. Consequently, coiled wire designs are preferred by many laboratories for stenting across important side branches. In a review of 129 major (>1mm) and 108 minor (<1mm) side branches whose trunk vessels were stented with the Gianturco-Roubin Flex-Stent (coiled wire), ≥1% of these branches were occluded after stenting.[8] The rate of occlusion remained exceptionally low with this coil design despite the fact that 38% of the procedures were performed as bailouts for acute occlusion.

Surprisingly, 27% of the major and 39% of the minor side branches occluded by angioplasty before the bailout stent regained their patency after stent placement. The mechanism of this early restoration of patency was felt to be the re-approximation of the dissected and displaced intima away from the obstructed branch ostia and toward its original position.[8] As in previous series with the slotted tube stents, stenting also facilitated late opening of occluded side branches with two-thirds of those remaining occluded after stenting having been opened at follow-up angiography. Loss of a side branch was again not associated with clinically significant events.

These series[5-8] were not designed to compare the performance of wire coil and slotted tube type stents with respect to side branch occlusion. The study protocols, side branch sizes, and patient groups are entirely different. However, it is notable that although the Gianturco-Roubin study selected a patient group with high percentages of closed and nearly closed vessels, the rate of further side branch closure was significantly lower, attributed, in part, to the bailout setting where many of the side branches were already closed by the pre-stent procedure. On the other hand, this finding may support the clinical intuition of many centers that the coil design is preferable in the setting of important side branches.

Mechanism of Side Branch Occlusion

The mechanism of side branch obstruction includes some combination of dissection of the dilated artery into the ostium of the side branch, intimal disruption, or plaque shifting into the side branch ostium ("snow-plowing"), as well as stent strut coverage of the side branch origin. Some of these effects could be remedied if a guidewire were to be left down the side branch during stent implantation as described in the "impacted wire technique" of *CASE 4.2*. The most common techniques applied to protect side branches during stent implantations are modifications of the "kissing balloon" technique of standard balloon angioplasty.[9]

Management of Stenting Across Side Branches

The first technical consideration is to determine the clinical importance of the side branch as well as the likelihood that future disease in that vessel may ultimately require access. Side branches larger than 2mm remain a major contraindication to stenting and the trunks of these vessels may be best treated by alternate therapies. If stenting remains the preferred option, the likelihood of acute closure of the side branch during stenting must be assessed. As discussed above, the risk of side branch compromise is increased if there is a stenosis >50% in the origin of the side branch or if the trunk vessel lesion is eccentric and involves the branch. Splitting stents to avoid incarcerating the side branch has been applied but requires considerable manipulation of the stent.[10] The more common approach to reduce the risk of side branch occlusion is to use a wire coil design which will facilitate side branch access after stent deployment. If the side branch has an ostial stenosis of over 50%, it and the trunk vessel are predilated. Predilation is not performed if the side branch has no baseline stenosis. A protecting wire is left in place while the trunk vessel is dilated. Dilations may be sequential, or simultaneous ("kissing") if there is significant vessel tapering or residual plaque shifting. These preliminary dilations facilitate balloon or stent passage into the branch if there is a branch occlusion after stent deployment. The side branch wire is usually withdrawn before a stent is deployed in the trunk vessel. While slotted tube stents have been successfully crossed to allow side branch angioplasty or stent placement,[9,11] most laboratories would prefer to deploy a coil stent to ensure easy branch access.

Imbedded Branch Wire Technique

The trunk vessel stent is deployed first leaving the side branch wire in place. This wire is chosen as a radiopaque soft wire and directs the operator to the lumen if the side branch origin should become disrupted. The branch imbedded wire also prevents complete occlusion of the side branch and facilitates passage of a second side branch wire through the deployed trunk stent. The imbedded side branch wire is withdrawn only after the second protecting wire is in place. The withdrawal is not usually difficult but attention to guiding catheter traction is required to prevent deep catheter seating.

Stent implantation into a side branch prior to implantation in the trunk vessel is not advised as minor protrusion of the stent from the side branch into the trunk vessel may cause difficulties in the stenting of the more important vessel.

Balloon Compliance for Jailed Branch Angioplasty

An important point should be made about the selection of balloons to cross the struts of an implanted stent and dilate a side branch. To prevent balloon entrapment in the implanted stent, the balloon should self-wrap after inflations. The stent "crossability" of various balloons has been tested in vitro and only compliant balloons rewrap upon deflation sufficiently well to reliably retract through the stent.[13] Therefore, only compliant balloons should be used to dilate side branches through the struts or coils of a deployed stent

T-Stenting for Side Branches

Implantation of kissing or T-formation stents in both side branches and trunk vessels should be avoided whenever possible. In a non-prospective review of procedures in which a side branch also received a stent compared to procedures in which only the trunk vessel was stented, the complication rate was twice as high (11%) in the group receiving stents to both trunk and side branch vessels.[12] The increased complications for complex stenting may be related to the anatomic complexity involving both major and minor branches, or to the inadequacy of current stent technologies. To address stenting for bifurcations and side branches, the NIR Rigid-flex, Bard XT, Cardiocoil, and other stent designs will be available in a bifurcated "trouser" configuration. In bifurcation stent devices, a proximal stent will fork into two "pants legs" distally, facilitating implantation in these lesions.

The recent introduction of coiled Cordis, (carved tube or corrugated ring with coil-like flexibility) ACS/ Guidant Multilink, continuous wire subunits AVE-Micro, short wave wire coil Wiktor, and cellular mesh NIR Rigid-Flex stents provides a number of stent designs with features permitting easier access to side branches than the slotted tube designs. Stents with more radiopacity are also preferred when careful positioning in the ostia of side branches is required. It remains to be determined whether the various stent designs offer any difference in the rate of side branch loss or trunk vessel restenosis.

SUMMARY

Ostial stenoses have been succesfully conquered using stent techniques. Synergistic applications of devices to improve stent placement for ostial lesions may demonstrate superiority over direct stenting. This approach will require prospective randomized trials, but appears to have promise.

References

1. Meier B, Gruentzig A, King S III, et al. *Risk of side branch occlusions during coronary angioplasty.* Am J Cardiol 53:10-14 (1984).
2. Ellis GS, Roubin GS, King SB III, Douglas JS, et al. *Angiographic and clinical predictors of acute closure after native vessel coronary angioplasty.* Circulation 77:372-379 (1988).
3. Rankin J, Wijns W, Hanek C, et al. *Angioplasty of coronary bifurcation stenosis: Immediate and long-term results of the protecting branch technique.* Cathet Cardiovasc Diagn 22:167-173 (1991).
4. Arora RR, Raymond RE, Dimass AP, Bhadwar K, Simfendorfer C. *Side branch occlusion during coronary angioplasty: incidence, angiographic characteristics and outcome.* Cathet Cardiovasc Diagn 18:210-212 (1989).
5. Fischman DL, Savage MP, Leon MB, et al. *Fate of lesion-related side branches after coronary artery stenting.* J Am Coll Cardiol 22:1641-1646 (1993).
6. Iniguez A, Macaya C, Alfonso F, et al. *Early angiographic changes of side branches arising from a Palmaz-Schatz stented coronary segment: results and clinical implications.* J Am Coll Cardiol 24: 911-915 (1994).
7. Pan M, Medina A, Suarez de Lezo J, et al. *Follow-up patency of side branches covered by intracoronary Palmaz-Schatz stent.* Am Heart J 129:436-440 (1995).
8. Wojciech M, Grinstead WC, Hakim AH, et al. *Fate of side branches after intracoronary implantation of the Gianturco-Roubin flex-stent for acute or threatened closure after percutaneous transluminal coronary angioplasty.* Am J Cardiol 74:1207-1210 (1994).
9. Colombo A, Gaglione A, Nakamura S, Finci L. *"Kissing" stents for bifurcational coronary lesions.* Cathet Cardiovasc Diagn 30:327-330 (1993).
10. Medina A, Hernandez E, Suarez de Lezo, et al. *Divided Palmaz-Schatz stent for discrete coronary stenosis.* J Invasive Cardiol 4:389-392 (1992).
11. Nakamura S, Hall P, Maiello L, Colombo A. *Techniques for Palmaz-Schatz stent deployment in lesions with a large side branch. Cathet Cardiovasc Diagn* 34:353-361 (1995).
12. Colombo A, Maiello L, Itoh A, et al. *Coronary stenting of bifurcation lesions: immediate and follow-up results* [abstr]. J Am Coll Cardiol 27:277A (1996).
13. Unpublished data presented in personal communication with Dr. Erminia Guarneri October, 1996.

CHAPTER 5

STENTS IN LONG LESIONS: TOTAL VASCULAR RECONSTRUCTION

CASE 5.1: Obtuse Marginal Branch Reconstruction

The patient is a 65 year old man who had a stent placed in the right coronary artery one year earlier for unstable angina. Angina recurred two months before this procedure. Angiography revealed an excellent result in the right coronary artery but new and severe progression of disease in the first obtuse marginal artery with a 30mm segment of moderate stenosis encompassing two severe stenoses (**Figure 5.1a**). The lesion was felt to be at high risk of both complications and restenosis using conventional angioplasty techniques. Elective stent implantation was therefore performed in the long circumflex branch segment.

PROCEDURE 5.1

Because of the 3mm diameter vessel and the need to cover the diseased segment completely, a 40mm Wallstent was selected (**Figure 5.2**). A left Judkins guide catheter was chosen because the long left main and non-acute angle of the circumflex origin. The lesion was crossed with an extra support guidewire

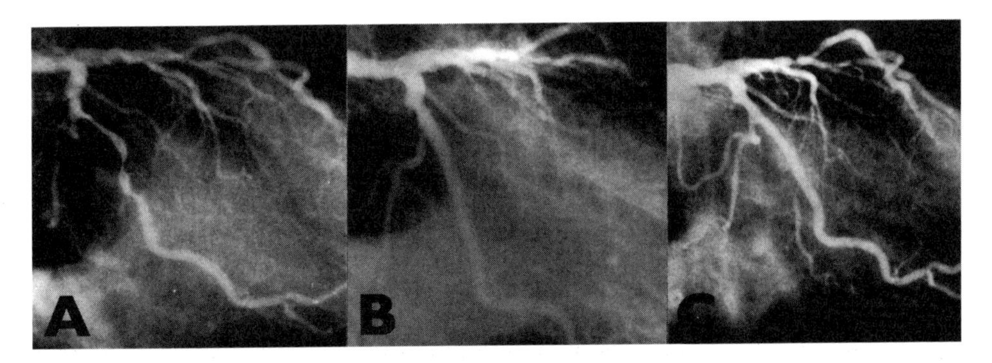

Figure 5.1 Obtuse Marginal Reconstruction A diffusely diseased segment of the first obtuse marginal artery with two severely diseased segments (**a**). The result after treatment with a long Wallstent (**b**) was maintained at 6-month angiography (**c**).

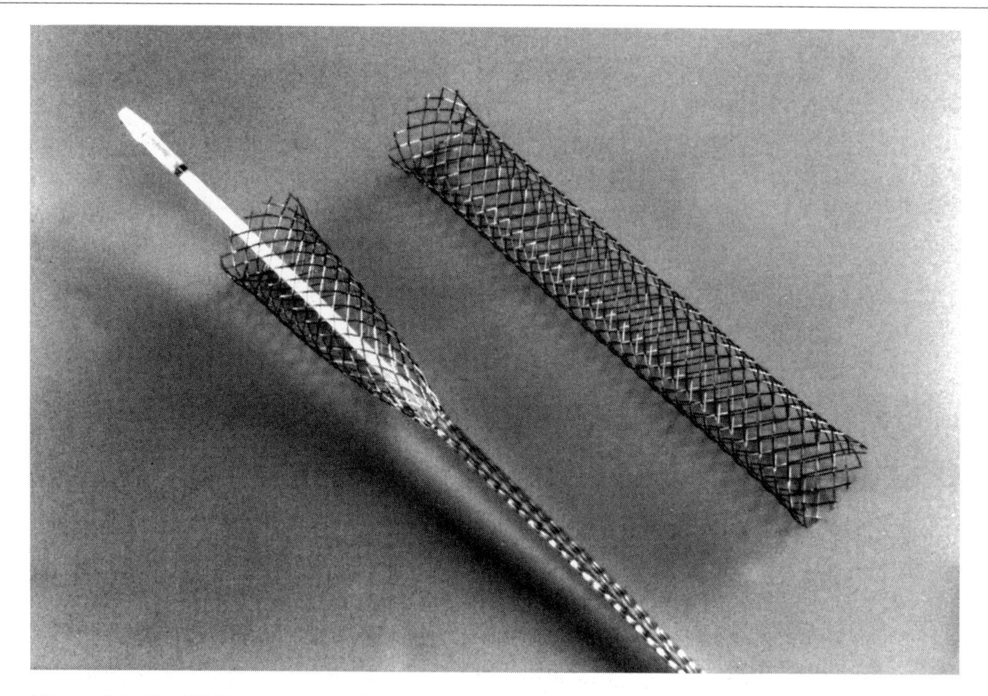

Figure 5.2 The Wallstent A self expanding wire braid.

and predilated with a long noncompliant balloon at 4 atm. A 4mm x 25mm Wallstent was positioned and deployed so that the proximal portion was several mm proximal to the lesion. The stent was dilated with a 3mm diameter balloon to 12 atm leaving no residual stenosis (**Figure 5.1b**). The patient was discharged and remained angina free at angiographic follow-up six months later. The follow-up angiogram revealed no evidence of restenosis (**Figure 5.1c**).

MATERIALS 5.1

Guiding Catheter:	Cook Lumax JL-4 8 French
Guidewires:	ACS/Guidant Extra Support 0.014" x 300 mm
Balloons:	Mansfield High Energy 3.0 x 20 mm
	Schneider Goldie 2.0 x 20 mm & 3.0 x 20 mm
Stents:	Schneider Wallstent 4.0 x 24 mm (covers 33mm length at 3.0mm diameter, 30mm length at 3.5mm diameter)

CASE 5.2: Total Vascular Reconstruction of a Right Coronary Artery

The patient is a 51 year old commercial pilot for Iberian Airlines. He suffered a myocardial infarction which was treated with thrombolysis six months earlier. During follow-up, thallium scintigraphy revealed a region of reversible ischemia in the inferior wall. Coronary angiography showed a subtotal occlusion with a recanalized appearance in the mid right coronary artery. In order to return to work, the patient was required to have no evidence of ischemia on nuclear exercise testing. He was referred for angioplasty six months after the myocardial infarction.

PROCEDURE 5.2

Initial coronary angiography showed an occluded right coronary vessel. Intracoronary nitroglycerin, however, opened the artery revealing a 50mm long lesion segment (**Figure 5.3a**). After passing the lesion with a flexible guidewire, a sequence of low profile balloons were unsuccessful in crossing the affected segment. Using a 1.5mm balloon to dilate the vessel as it was advanced, the entire lesion segment could be traversed. Predilation to 3.0mm was followed by the sequential implantation of two 32mm and one 9mm NIR Rigid-Flex stents. The radiographic appearance of the stent is demonstrated without

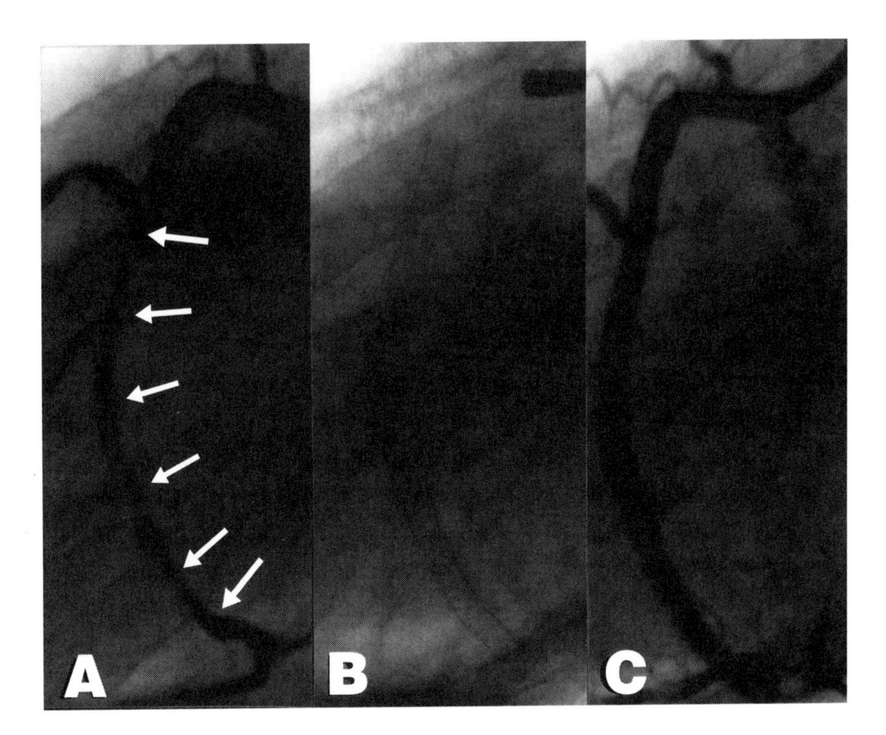

Figure 5.3 Total Reconstruction of the Right Coronary Artery After nitroglycerin, the occluded right coronary artery opened revealing a 50mm long diseased segment (**a**). The lesion was treated with serial Rigid-Flex (NIR) stents seen fluoroscopically (**b**). The final result was excellent (**c**).

contrast in **Figure 5.3b.** The stents were implanted from distal to proximal until the entire affected segment was covered leaving no residual stenosis (**Figure 5.3c**). The post-procedure thallium treadmill was normal without evidence of ischemia. The patient returned to work after a 6-month negative thallium scintigraphic study.

MATERIALS 5.2

Guiding Catheter:	Cook Lumax JR-4 8 French
	Cook Lumax AR-2 8 French
Guidewires:	ACS/Guidant High Torque Floppy 0.014"x 300cm
Balloons:	SciMed Viva Primo 3.0 x 20mm
	ACS/Guidant Rx Elipse 2.0 x 20mm
	Schneider Goldie 1.5 x 20mm
	Schneider Longie 3.5 x 35mm
Stents:	SciMed Rigid-Flex (NIR) 32mm (#20), 9mm (#1)

DISCUSSION

Long Stenoses: Issues of Morphology

The percutaneous treatment of long lesions must address a particular set of problems. How much of the artery is actually diseased? What is the true vessel diameter? Is there arterial tapering over the course of the lesion? What associated features (curves, side branches, calcification) need to be considered in selecting the appropriate therapy?

Long lesions have been defined in a variety of ways. In the Coronary Artery Surgery Study (CASS) any lesion exceeding 10mm in length was considered tubular or diffuse.[1] A more contemporary angioplasty definition describes long lesions as those between 11-20mm in length. Diffuse disease implies lesions >20mm or segments containing >3 discrete lesions. By ACC/AHA task force lesion classification criteria, all lesions over 20mm long are type C (see **Appendix II**), lesions which are associated with lower success and higher complication rates.[2] These lesions occur in distinct higher risk patient subsets, including elderly and diabetic patients, as well as patients with decreased ventricular function.

Angioplasty Results in Long Lesions

Angioplasty of long lesions is historically associated with lower rates of success and higher rates of complication.[3-5] Angioplasty success exceeding 95% in lesions <10mm falls to 78% in lesions >20 mm.[6] Lesion length is an independent predictor of acute closure requiring surgery.[4,7] Complications are more frequent in cases with disease of the entire vessel than in those with isolated long or multiple lesions.[8] Increased restenosis rates for long lesions have been repeatedly demonstrated and range from 49-58% for lesions longer than 7mm.[9-13] Of note, the restenosis lesions after angioplasty of diffusely diseased segments are often shorter than the original narrowings.[14]

Some recent studies have not confirmed a lower success rate for long and diffuse disease[8,15] possibly due to case selection, application of long angioplasty balloons, and stents for complex dissections. [14,16,17] The frequent dissections in longer lesions treated with short balloons[18] may be reduced using long balloons. It is postulated that long balloons reduce the stress at the lesion endpoint and consequently reduce dissections in diffusely diseased segments. Despite increased success with long balloons, restenosis rates of these lesions remain high (50-55%).[14]

Alternative Revascularization Techniques for Long Lesions

When considering alternative approaches, it should be noted that surgical techniques for diffusely diseased vessels are often suboptimal. The 30-day mortality of patients undergoing surgical coronary endarterectomy ranges from 6.3 to 10.4% with correspondingly increased rates of post- operative myocardial infarction.[19]

Directional atherectomy has been shown to have lower success and higher rates of acute complications in lesions longer than 10mm.[20] Lesion length, especially in smaller diameter vessels,[20] is an independent risk factor for restenosis after directional atherectomy. The procedure is not well suited to long lesions.[21]

Rotational atherectomy provides its greatest benefits in facilitating angioplasty in ostial, eccentric, ulcerated, calcified and long (>20mm) lesions.[22] Rotational atherectomy has reduced the complication rate in long lesions, but restenosis rates remain high.[23,24] Furthermore, as lesion length increases, the procedural success decreases and both complications and restenosis increase.[25-27]

Despite early increased success with excimer laser coronary angioplasty (ELCA) techniques, the restenosis rate in long lesions treated with ELCA remains high (47-59%).[28-30] In a randomized trial comparing ELCA with angioplasty in long lesions, laser offered no clinical or angiographic benefit.[31] The 6-month restenosis rate was 52% in the laser group compared to 41% in the balloon group with a trend to increased restenosis after laser treatment. The existing clinical data and the expense of ELCA make it unlikely that this technique will find broad application in this lesion subgroup.

Stents for Long Lesions

The data for stent implantation in long lesions and diffusely diseased arteries is gradually becoming available. While some investigators have shown that tandem or overlapping stents nearly double the risk for restenosis,[32-34] other studies have not shown this correlation.[35] It appears that it is the length of the lesion rather than the number of stents that predicts restenosis rates.[36]

Stents are associated with lower rates of complications than angioplasty in long lesions. In a series of 48 lesions averaging 40 ± 16mm, angiographic restenosis occurred in only 25%.[37] Stents implanted in 108 lesions of mean length of 32 ± 6mm had a 93% success and 35% angiographic restenosis rate.[38] The majority of these patients were treated with antiplatelet therapy only. While encouraging, the effect of stents on restenosis in long lesions remains under study.

There are few comparative trials of stents in long lesions. Several clinical data registries have confirmed the utility of stents in long lesions. The Rigid-Flex (NIR) stent could be deployed with 98% success in long lesions of small tortuous vessels. The restenosis rate remains unknown, but there was no subacute occlusion.[39] Although early results suggested a higher incidence of subacute thrombosis[40-42] with the long self-expanding Wallstent, recent trials using modern deployment techniques and antiplatelet therapies have not reproduced these results. Marco et al[43] showed high success and low complications in 60 patients receiving the Magic Wallstent for lesions averaging 30mm in length.[44] Restenosis rates in this group were reported between 28 and 46%.[45] In a comparison of the Palmaz-Schatz, Wiktor, and Gianturco-Roubin I stents in lesions >20mm, although the final vessel diameters were higher with the Gianturco-Roubin device, the restenosis rates among the three devices were not significantly different. The restenosis rates (24-35%) for these devices in long lesions were higher than that for stent restenosis in focal lesions.[46]

Technical Considerations

Special considerations for long lesions include conservative balloon sizing to minimize dissection. Operators should target balloon-to-artery ratios of 1:1 rather than ≥1.1:1. Longer balloon inflation times at the minimum pressure required to reduce barotrauma have been advocated by some operators.[47] Fibrosis may be distributed unevenly along the course of long lesions. To minimize over-dilation of the less calcified and fibrotic segments, noncompliant balloons are preferred.

Long lesions often involve significant vessel tapering. Specially designed decremental or tapered balloons may allow prolonged high pressure inflations without increased risk of dissection.[48] The curves and tortuosities associated with long or diffuse lesions may make assessment of the lesion length difficult. A "marker wire," which has a distal tip scaled with radiopaque bands, may avoid the situation of arriving at a distal lesion site with a device too short to cover the lesion.[49] Because calcification and side branches are frequently present along the course of diffusely diseased vessels, device selection with an optimal crossing profile and ability to access side branches will be advantageous.

SUMMARY

The limitations of standard balloon angioplasty in long and diffusely diseased segments have been partly overcome by long balloon catheters and stents [50]. Despite increased success and reduced complications, restenosis of long lesions after conventional angioplasty, DCA, and rotablator remains >50%. Currently reported stent restenosis rates in non-controlled trials in long lesions also appear to be higher than those in de novo focal disease.

References

1. Principal Investigators of CASS and their associates (Killip T, editor, Fisher LD, Mock MB, associate editors). *National Heart, Lung and Blood Institute Coronary Artery Surgery Study.* Circulation 63(suppl I):I-1(1981).
2. Ryan TJ, Faxon DP, Gunnar RM, et al. *Guidelines for percutaneous transluminal coronary angioplasty: A report of the American College of Cardiology/American Heart Association Task Force on assessment of diagnostic and therapeutic cardiovascular procedures (subcommittee on percutaneous transluminal coronary angioplasty).* J Am Coll Cardiol 12:529-545 (1988) and J Am Coll Cardiol 22:2033-2054 (1993).
3. Sharma SK, Israel DH, Kamean JL, et al. *Clinical, angiographic, and procedural determinants of major and minor coronary dissection during angioplasty.* Am Heart J 126:39-47 (1993).
4. Ellis SG, Roubin GS, King SB, et al. *Angiographic and clinical predictors of acute closure after native vessel coronary angioplasty.* Circulation 77:372-379 (1988).
5. Myler RK, Shaw RE, Stertzer SH, et al. *Lesion morphology and coronary angioplasty: current experience and analysis.* J Am Coll Cardiol 19:1641-1652 (1992).
6. Tan K, Sulke N, Taub N, et al. *Clinical and lesion morphologic determinants of coronary angioplasty success and complications: current experience.* J Am Coll Cardiol 25:855-865 (1995).
7. Detre KM, Holmes DR, Holubkov R, et al. *Incidence and consequences of periprocedural occlusion. The 1985-1986 NHLBI PTCA registry.* Circulation 82:739-750 (1990).
8. Goudreau E, DiSciascio G, Kelly K, et al. *Coronary angioplasty of diffuse coronary artery disease.* Am Heart J 121:12-19 (1991).
9. Mata LA, Bosch X, David PR, et al. *Clinical and angiographic assessment 6 months after double vessel percutaneous coronary angioplasty.* J Am Coll Cardiol 6:1339-1344 (1985).
10. Vandormael MG, Deligonul U, Kern MJ, et al. *Multilesion coronary angioplasty: clinical and angiographic follow-up.* J Am Coll Cardiol 10:246-252 (1987).
11. Ellis SG, Roubin GS, King SB, et al. *Importance of stenosis morphology in the estimation of restenosis risk after elective percutaneous transluminal coronary angioplasty.* Am J Cardiol 63:30-34 (1989).
12. Hirshfeld JW, Schwartz JS, Jugo R, et al. *Restenosis after coronary angioplasty: a multivariate statistical model to relate lesion and procedure variables to restenosis.* J Am Coll Cardiol 18:647-656 (1991).
13. Bourassa MG, Lesperance J, Eastwood C, et al. *Clinical, physiologic, anatomic and procedural factors predictive of restenosis after percutaneous transluminal coronary angioplasty.* J Am Coll Cardiol 18:368-376 (1991).
14. Tenaglia AN, Zidar JP, Jackman JD, et al. *Treatment of long coronary artery narrowings with long angioplasty balloon catheters.* Am J Cardiol 71:1274-1277 (1993).
15. Ellis SG, Vandormael MG, Cowley MJ, et al. *Coronary morphologic and clinical determinants of procedural outcome with angioplasty for multivessel coronary disease: implications for patient selection.* Circulation 82:1193-1202 (1990).
16. Kaul U, Upasani PT, Agarwal R, et al. *In-hospital outcome of percutaneous transluminal coronary angioplasty for long lesions and diffuse coronary artery disease.* Cathet Cardiovasc Diagn 35:294-300 (1995).
17. Cannon AD, Roubin GS, Hearn JA, et al. *Acute angiographic and clinical results of long balloon percutaneous transluminal coronary angioplasty and adjuvant stenting for long narrowings.* Am J Cardiol 73:635-641 (1994).

18. Hall DP, Gruentzig AR. *Influence of lesion length on initial success and recurrence rates in coronary angioplasty* [abstr]. Circulation 70:II-176 (1984).

19. Brenowitz JB, Kayser KL, Johnson D. *Results of coronary artery endarterectomy and reconstruction.* J Thorac Cardiovasc Surg 95:1-10 (1988).

20. Hinohara T, Rowe MH, Robertson GC, et al. *Effect of lesion characteristics on outcome of directional coronary atherectomy.* J Am Coll Cardiol 17:1112-1120 (1991).

21. Mooney MJ, Fishman-Mooney, Madison J, et al. *Directional atherectomy for long lesions: improved results.* Cathet Cardiovasc Diagn 29:26-30 (1993).

22. Safian RD, Freed M, Reddy V, et al. *Do excimer laser angioplasty and rotational atherectomy facilitate balloon angioplasty? Implications for lesion-specific coronary intervention.* J Am Coll Cardiol 27:552-559 (1996).

23. Warth D, Leon MB, O'Neill W, et al. *Rotational atherectomy multicenter registry: acute results, complications and 6-month angiographic follow-up in 709 patients.* J Am Coll Cardiol 24:641-648 (1994).

24. Stertzer S, Rosenblum J, Shaw R, et al. *Coronary rotational ablation: initial experience in 302 procedures.* J Am Coll Cardiol 21:287-295 (1992).

25. Tierstein PS, Warth DC, Haq N, et al. *High speed rotational coronary atherectomy for patients with diffuse coronary artery disease.* J Am Coll Cardiol 18:1694-1701 (1991).

26. Ellis S, Popma JJ, Buchbinder M, et al. *Relation of clinical presentation, stenosis morphology, and operator technique to the procedural results of rotational atherectomy-facilitated angioplasty.* Circulation 89:882-892 (1994).

27. Reisman M, Cohen B, Warth D, et al. *Outcome of long lesions treated with high-speed rotational ablation* [abstr]. J Am Coll Cardiol 21:443A (1993).

28. Karsch KR, Haase KK, Voelker W, et al. *Percutaneous coronary excimer laser angioplasty in patients with stable and unstable angina pectoris: acute results and incidence of restenosis during 6-month follow-up.* Circulation 81:1849-1859 (1990).

29. Bittl JA, Sanborn TA, Tcheng JE, et al. *Excimer laser-facilitated coronary angioplasty Relative risk analysis of acute and follow-up results in 200 patients.* Circulation 86:71-80 (1992).

30. Bittl JA, Sanborn TA, Tcheng JE, et al. *Clinical success, complications and restenosis rates with excimer laser coronary angioplasty. The percutaneous excimer laser coronary angioplasty registry.* Am J Cardiol 70:1533-1539 (1992).

31. Appleman YEA, Piek JJ, Strikwerda S, et al. *Randomised trial of excimer laser angioplasty versus balloon angioplasty for treatment of obstructive coronary artery disease.* Lancet 347:79-84 (1996).

32. Straus BH, Serruys PW, de Scheerder IK, et al: *Relative risk analysis of angiographic predictors of restenosis within the coronary* Wallstent. Circulation 84:1636-1643 (1991).

33. Ellis SG, Savage M, Fischman D, et al. *Restenosis after placement of Palmaz-Schatz stents in native coronary arteries-initial results of a multicenter experience.* Circulation 86:1836-1844 (1992).

34. Lablanche JM, Danchin N, Grollier G, et al. *Factors predictive of restenosis after stent implantation managed by ticlopidine and aspirin* [abstr]. Circulation 94(suppl I):I-256 (1996).

35. Eeckhout E, Goy JJ, Vogt P, et al. *Complications and follow-up after intracoronary stenting: critical analysis of a 6-year single-center experience.* Am Heart J 127:262-272 (1994).

36. Hall P, Nakamura S, Maiello L, et al. *Factors associated with late angiographic outcome after intravascular ultrasound guided Palmaz-Schatz coronary stent implantation: a multivariate analysis* [abstr]. J Am Coll Cardiol 25:36A (1995).

37. Reimers B, Di Mario C, Nierop P, et al. *Long-term restenosis after multiple stent implantation: a quantitative angiographic study* [abstr]. Circulation 92(suppl I):I-327 (1995).

38. Maiello L, Hall P, Nakamura S, et al. *Results of stent implantation for diffuse coronary disease assisted by intravascular ultrasound* [abstr]. J Am Coll Cardiol 25:156A (1995).

39. Almagor Y, Richter K, DiMario C, et al. *Treatment of long lesions in small tortuous coronary vessels with a new intravascular rigid-flex (NIR) stent [abstr].* J Am Coll Cardiol 27:110A (1996).

40. Serruys PW, Strauss BH, Beatt KJ, et al. *Angiographic follow-up after placement of a self-expanding coronary artery stent.* N Engl J Med 324:13-17 (1991).

41. Strauss BH, Serruys PW, Bertrand ME, et al. *Quantitative angiographic follow-up of the coronary Wallstent in native vessels and bypass grafts (European experience-March 1986-March 1990).* Am J Cardiol 69:475-481 (1992).

42. Goy JJ, Sigwart U, Vogt P, et al. *Long-term follow-up of the first 56 patients treated with intracoronary self-expanding stents (the Lausanne experience).* Am J Cardiol 67:569-572 (1991).

43. Marco J, Fajadet J, Brunel P, et al. *Anatomy reconstruction of native coronary arteries and vein grafts with the less shortening self-expandable Wallstent* [abstr]. J Am Coll Cardiol 27:179A (1996).

44. Colombo A, Itoh A, Hall P, et al. *Implantation of the Wallstent for diffuse lesions in native coronary arteries and venous bypass grafts without subsequent anticoagulation* [abstr]. J Am Coll Cardiol 27:53A (1996).

45. Marco J. *Seventh Complex Angioplasty Course*; Toulouse, France. May, 1996.

46. Akira I, Hall P, Maiello L, et al. *Coronary stenting of long lesions (greater than 20mm)— a matched comparison of different stents.* Circulation 92(suppl I):I-688 (1995).

47. Kaul U, Upasani PT, Agarwal R, et al. *In-hospital outcome of percutaneous transluminal coronary angioplasty for long lesions and diffuse coronary artery disease.* Cathet Cardiovasc Diagn 35:294-300 (1995).

48. Banka V, Baker HA III, Vemuri DN, et al. *Effectiveness of decremental diameter balloon catheters (tapered balloon).* Am J Cardiol 69:188-193(1992).

49. Oda H, Milda T, Toeda T, Higuma N. *Efficacy of marker wire for intracoronary stenting.* Cathet Cardiovasc Diagn 37:447-451 (1996).

50. Cannon AD, Roubin GS, Hearn JA, et al. A*cute angiographic and clinical results of long balloon percutaneous transluminal coronary angioplasty and adjuvant stenting for long narrowings.* Am J Cardiol 73:635-641 (1994)

CHAPTER 6

STENTS AND ARTERIAL PERFORATION

CASE HISTORY 6.1: Arterial Perforation Within a Stent

A 54 year old woman had undergone coronary artery bypass surgery 10 months previously with a left internal mammary artery to the left anterior descending artery and a saphenous vein graft to the right coronary artery. The post-operative course was complicated by mediastinitis and recurrent angina. A severe stenosis in the anastomosis of the internal mammary to the left anterior descending artery was successfully dilated one month after surgery with relief of symptoms. The patient was readmitted with recurrence of both exertional and rest angina. Coronary angiography demonstrated a new severe stenosis in the mid portion of the graft to the right coronary artery and a diffuse, moderate stenosis in the distal graft up to the anastomosis with the right coronary artery (**Figure 6.1a** arrows). Stent implantation in the vein graft to the right coronary artery was performed.

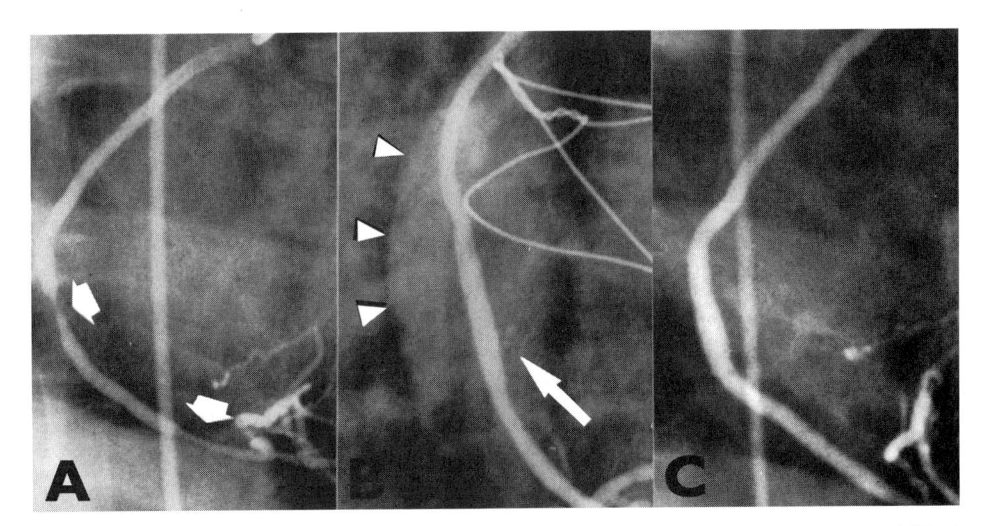

Figure 6.1 Arterial Perforation Within a Stent The vein graft to the right coronary artery exhibited a severe stenosis in its mid portion and a diffuse moderate stenosis distally (**a;** arrows). A Wallstent was deployed distally and a Palmaz- Schatz II stent was placed in the more proximal lesion. Post-dilation of the Palmaz-Schatz II stent required high pressure to resolve stent deformities. The subsequent injection revealed arterial perforation (**b**). The white arrow indicates the jet of contrast and the white arrowheads delineate the contrast stained pericardium. The perforation was adequately treated with a prolonged low pressure inflation. Angiography three days later revealed a good result (**c**).

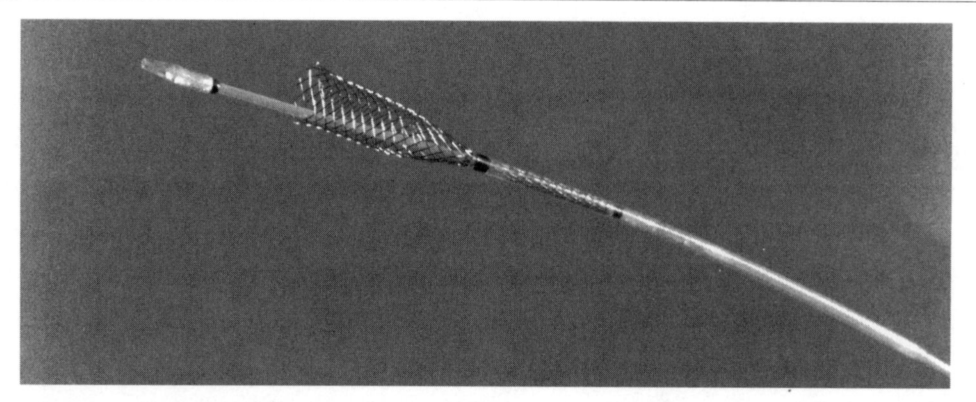

Figure 6.2a Wallstent

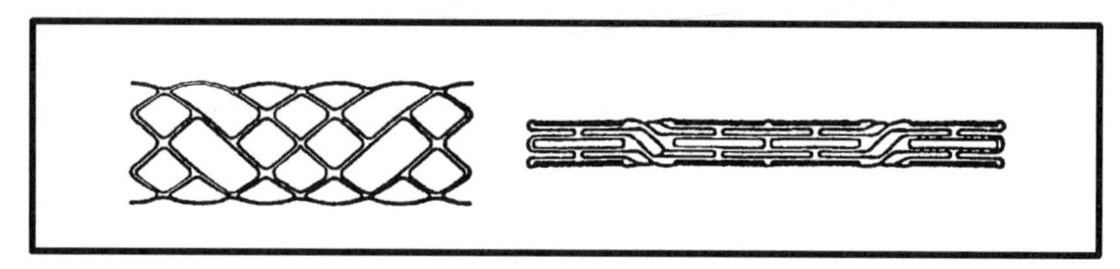

Figure 6.2b The Heparin Coated Palmaz-Schatz Stent A slotted tube with spiral articulation.

PROCEDURE 6.1

The distal moderate graft stenosis had progressed over 10 months and was felt likely to reduce the outflow of a stent placed in the mid-graft lesion. Because of lesion length, the distal lesion was treated with a Wallstent **(Figure 6.2a).** The mid-graft lesion was treated with a heparin-coated Palmaz-Schatz stent **(Figure 6.2b).** Both lesions were pre-dilated with a 2.5mm balloon. The Wallstent was easily passed to the distal site and deployed. This stent was dilated with the predilation 2.5mm balloon to 9 atm covering its entire length. Next, a Palmaz-Schatz stent was mounted on a 3.5mm non-compliant balloon, passed to the mid-graft site, and deployed at 10 atm. An indentation remained in the deployment balloon even at this pressure. Fluoroscopic inspection of this moderately radiopaque stent revealed a persistent narrowing in its mid section. Further dilatations with the non-compliant 3.5mm balloon to 14 atm a resolved the balloon and stent deformities.

The subsequent angiogram revealed a faint jet of contrast exiting the right coronary artery graft medially and entering the pericardial space **(Figure 6.1b).** The diagnosis of perforation was made and treated with a 4-minute 3.5mm balloon inflation at 2 atm over the perforation site. Heparin was immediately reversed with protamine. The patient remained asymptomatic and hemodynamically stable after the balloon deflation. The patient was observed an additional 30 minutes in the laboratory and repeat angiography revealed resolution of the extravascular contrast jet. Echocardiography identified a minimal pericardial effusion without findings of cardiac tamponade.

The patient was not heparinized after the procedure. However, aspirin and ticlopidine were continued. Coronary angiography 3 days later revealed both stents to be widely patent. No abnormality could be seen at the perforation site **(Figure 6.1c).** The patient remained angina free and at follow-up had negative exercise testing.

MATERIALS 6.1

Guiding Catheter:	Cook Lumax JR 4-8F
Guidewires:	ACS (Guidant) Extra Suppor 0.014"
Balloons:	SciMed Long Cobra 2.5 x 30mm Schneider Goldie 3.5 x 20mm
Stents:	Schneider Wallstent 4.0 Johnson & Johnson PS 204C 18mm

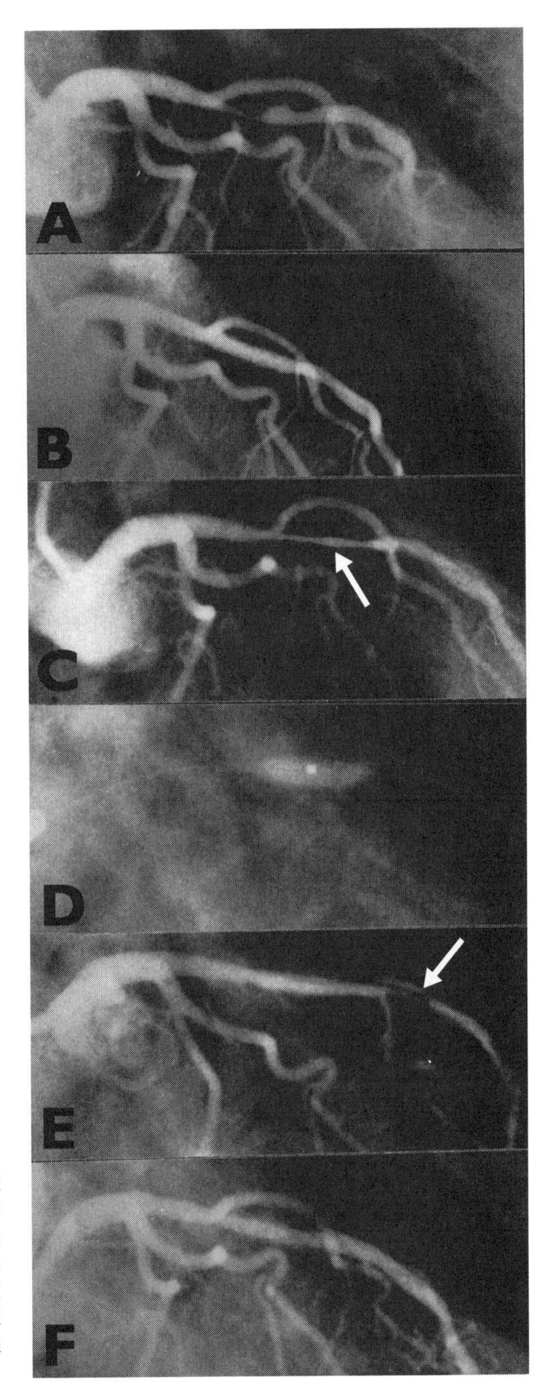

CASE 6.2: Distal Dissection During Angioplasty Within a Stent

An 82 year old widow presented with unstable angina three months earlier. A severe proximal left anterior descending artery narrowing was treated with a coated Palmaz-Schatz II stent using a 3 mm balloon with no residual stenosis **(Figures 6.3a and b).** However, rest angina recurred three months later due to restenosis in the proximal portion of the left anterior descending stent with a diffuse moderate stenosis over the rest of the stent length **(Figure 6.3c** arrow). Angioplasty redilation was performed to treat the stent restenosis.

Figure 6.3 Distal Dissection During Angioplasty Within a Stent A severe proximal anterior descending stenosis (**a**) was initially treated with implantation of a Palmaz-Schatz stent (**b**). When restenosis developed (**c;** arrow), it was treated with balloon dilation using a short balloon within the stent (**d**). A dissection (NHLBI type B) developed further distal in the artery well beyond the dilated stent segments(**e;** arrow). This was successfully treated with implantation of a Palmaz-Schatz articulated stent (**f**).

PROCEDURE 6.2

An extra support guidewire was passed across the stenosed segment of the stent and into the transapical portion of the left anterior descending. A 3.5mm short (9mm) balloon was chosen and dilations were carefully performed within the stent (Figure 6.3d). The restenosis lesion was surprisingly hard and residual asymmetry persisted in the short balloon until a pressure of 16 atm had been reached. Resolution of the restenosis was now accompanied by a new, linear type B dissection distal to the stent (Figure 6.3e arrow). The dissection did not improve after several prolonged dilations with a 20mm balloon at 3 atm. A second Palmaz-Schatz I articulated stent was passed easily through the dilated lumen of the first stent and was deployed distally with a final result of ≤10% residual stenosis (Figure 6.3f). The patient was discharged two days later with no further angina.

MATERIALS 6.2

Guiding Catheter:	Cook Lumax JL4-8 French
Guidewires:	ACS Extra Support 0.014"
Balloons:	Schneider Chubby 3.5 x 9 mm, Goldie 3.5 x 20 mm
Stents:	Johnson & Johnson PS-153

DISCUSSION

In-Stent Restenosis

Angioplasty is commonly performed within previously implanted stents for symptomatic restenosis. One of the mechanisms of in-stent restenosis involves the encroachment of intimal proliferative tissues into the arterial lumen within the stent.[1] The stent itself prevents the vascular recoil, commonly present after conventional angioplasty. In the case of bypass grafts, only rarely does a fibrotic compression of the stent account for restenosis. Lumen enlargement during angioplasty for in-stent restenosis can be achieved by extrusion of the proliferated tissue through the stent struts.[1] The considerable amount of tissue which must be extruded through an embedded stent may be one of the reasons for an increased recurrence rate of restenotic lesions treated within stents. While focal restenotic lesions within stents have a limited second restenosis rate of only 15% and focal lesions at the stent margins have a 40% restenosis rate, diffuse restenotic lesions within stents have a recurrence of over 80%[2] with a rate of second restenosis for all lesions within stents ranging from 40-50%.[3,4] When compared to the second restenosis rates (<20%) for stent treatment of angioplasty restenosis, the extruded material outside the stent appears to be an important limitation of successful treatment of in-stent restenosis.

Table 6.1 Arterial Perforation after Percutaneous Therapy

DEVICE	WM. BEAUMONT[10] (n=116)	REGISTRY[8] (n=771)
PTCA	0.1	0.1
TEC	1.3	2.1
DCA	0.3	0.7
EXCIMER LASER	2.0	1.9
ROTABLATOR	0	1.3

PTCA: percutaneous transluminal coronary angioplasty; TEC: transluminal extraction catheter; DCA: directional coronary atherectomy

Safety of Angioplasty within Stents

There is a general perception that angioplasty within stents is safer than routine angioplasty. The structural support offered by the stent seems to protect the vessel from balloon barotrauma and results in a lower complication rate. Baim et al[4] reported a 100% angioplasty success rate in these lesions within the Palmaz-Schatz stent,[4] and Macande et al[6] suggested that angioplasty within Gianturco-Roubin stents is safer than routine angioplasty. These data, and the drive to optimize stent deployment, have promoted dilations with larger and higher pressure inflations for in-stent restenosis. The aggressive use of large balloons and high pressure inflations to optimize the results in *CASES 6.1 and 6.2* emphasizes that such vessels are not immune to dissection and perforation.

Arterial Perforation

Arterial perforation during angioplasty is uncommon. In the NHLBI registry the incidence was 2 in 3079 procedures.[8] In the era of aggressive multi-device intervention, the occurrence of arterial perforation remains infrequent but is increased, especially in the elderly and in women.[9] In retrospective reviews of 8,932 percutaneous interventions at William Beaumont Hospital and of 12,900 procedures in the Perforation Registry (groups overlap), arterial or saphenous vein graft perforation occurred in 1.3 and 1.4% of patients, respectively. Table 6.1 lists the incidence of perforation by device.

The rate of perforation during high pressure stent implantation techniques is 2%.[11,12] In these series, perforation was apparent at the time of angiography 90% of the time, but importantly, it presented as delayed cardiac tamponade in about 10% of patients. However, even when perforation occurs, it is not usually associated with hemodynamic compromise. Thus, management depends largely on the extent of pericardial communication.

Table 6.2 The Classification of Coronary Artery Perforations[9]

TYPE	DESCRIPTION
Type I	Extraluminal crater without extravasation
Type II	Pericardial or myocardial blush without contrast jet extravasation
Type III	Extravasation through frank (1mm) perforation
Cavity Spilling	Perforation into an anatomic cavity chamber, coronary sinus, etc.

Perforation Classification

A perforation classification has been devised based on this concept in order to best direct therapy (Table 6.2).

In treating class I and II perforations, prolonged inflations are usually sufficient to stop the contrast extravasation. Anticoagulation with aspirin and heparin can be continued. Management of more severe perforations includes reversal of heparin anticoagulation and prolonged dilations with perfusion balloons to seal the perforation.[13] Immediate two-dimension echocardiography is important to assess the pericardial space. Occasionally, pericardiocentesis is necessary for cardiac tamponade.[14] Late tamponade remains a significant potential problem. Patients who may exhibit late tamponade with hemodynamic compromise should be sent for revascularization.

In the William Beaumont experience, conservative techniques were successful in 63% of cases. Surgery was required in 37% (with or without bypass).[10] The perforation registry data revealed that certain class III ruptures with leakage into other cardiac "cavities" carried a more benign prognosis. The "Cavity Spilling" category was devised for this group who may be monitored conservatively. From these two series, 10% of patients with perforations may not present with tamponade until late after the procedure. Patients undergoing ablative rather than compressive therapies and patients suspected of possible perforation during their procedure are at risk of late tamponade and should be observed for a minimum of 24 hours in-hospital.

Covered Stents

Stents have been implanted to scaffold and to control the disrupted artery without surgery.[15] Vein covered stents provide an impermeable barrier and structural support. They have been applied to pseudoaneurysms both after controlled and uncontrolled perforations.[16-19] Endoluminal grafts, such as covered stents, may well be an ideal transcatheter technique for arterial perforation with continued leakage.

SUMMARY

Despite the perception that angioplasty within stents is safer than routine angioplasty procedures, the cases presented demonstrate that it is not risk free. Distal dissection and arterial perforation may result from the attempts to optimize the in-stent angiographic result. Complications must be anticipated and treated promptly to avoid adverse patient outcomes.

References

1. Gordon P, Gibson M, Cohen DJ, Carrozza JP, Kuntz RE, Baim DS. *Mechanisms of restenosis and redilation within coronary stents—quantitative angiographic assessment.* J Am Coll Cardiol 21:1166-1174 (1993).
2. Kimura T, Tamura T, Yokoi H, Nobuyoshi M. *Long-term clinical and angiographic follow-up after placement of Palmaz-Schatz coronary stent: a single center experience.* J Interven Cardiol 7:129-139 (1994).
3. Schomig A, Kastrati A, Rainer D, Rauch B, Neumann FJ, Katus HH, Busch U. *Emergency coronary stenting for dissection during percutaneous transluminal coronary angioplasty: angiographic follow-up after stenting and after repeat angioplasty of the stented segment.* J Am Coll Cardiol 23:1053-1060 (1994).
4. Baim DS, Levine MJ, Leon MB, et al. *Management of restenosis within the Palmaz- Schatz coronary stent (the U.S. multicenter experience).* Am J Cardiol 71:364-366 (1993).
5. Erbel R, Haude M, Hopp HW, et al. *REstenosis STent (REST)-study: randomized trial comparing stenting and balloon angioplasty for treatment of restenosis after balloon angioplasty* [abstr]. J Am Coll Cardiol 27:139A (1996).
6. Macande PJ, Roubin GS, Agarwal SK, Cannon AD, Dean LS, Baxley WA. *Balloon angioplasty for treatment of in-stent restenosis: feasibility, safety and efficacy.* Cathet Cardiovasc Diagn 32:125-131 (1994).
7. Moris C, Alfonso A, Lambert JL, et al. *Stenting for coronary dissection after balloon dilation of in-stent restenosis: stenting a previously stented site.* Am Heart J 131:834-836 (1996).
8. Cowley MJ, Dorros G, Kelsey SF, et al. *Acute coronary events associated with percutaneous transluminal coronary angioplasty.* Am J Cardiol 53:12c-16c (1984).
9. Ellis SG, Ajluni S, Arnold AZ, et al. *Increased coronary perforation in the new device era—incidence, classification, management, and outcome.* Circulation 90:2725-2730 (1994).
10. Ajluni SC, Glazier S, Blankenship L, O'Neill WW, Safian RD. *Perforations after percutaneous coronary interventions: clinical, angiographic, and therapeutic observations.* Cathet Cardiovasc Diagn 32:206-212 (1994).
11. Benzuly KH, Glazier S, Grines CL, et al. *Coronary perforation: an unreported complication after intracoronary stent implantation* [abstr]. J Am Coll Cardiol 27:252A (1996).
12. Alfonso F, Goicolea J, Hernandez R, et al. *Arterial perforation during optimization of coronary stents using high-pressure balloon inflations.* Amer J Cardiol 78:1169-1172 (1996).
13. Parker JD, Ganz P, Selwyn AP, et al. *Successful treatment of an excimer laser-associated coronary artery perforation with the Stack perfusion catheter.* Cathet Cardiovasc Diagn 22:118-122 (1991)
14. Teirstein PS, Hartzler GO. *Nonoperative management of aortocoronary saphenous vein graft rupture during percutaneous transluminal coronary angioplasty.* Am J Cardiol 60: 377-378 (1987).
15. Thomas MR, Wainwright RJ. *Use of an intracoronary stent to control bleeding during coronary artery rupture complicating coronary angioplasty.* Cathet Cardiovasc Diagn 30: 169-172 (1993).
16. Wong SC, Kent KM, Mintz GS, et al. *Percutaneous transcatheter repair of a coronary aneurysm using a composite autologous cephalic vein-coated Palmaz-Schatz biliary stent.* Am J Cardiol 76:990-991 (1995).
17. Colon PJ, Ramee SR, Mulingtapang R, et al. *Percutaneous bailout therapy of a perforated vein graft using a stent-autologous vein patch.* Cathet Cardiovasc Diagn 38:175-178 (1996).
18. Dorros G, Jain A, Kumar K. *Management of coronary artery rupture: covered stent or microcoil embolization.* Cathet Cardiovasc Diagn 36:148-154 (1995).
19. Colombo A, Itoh A, Di Mario C, et al. *Successful closure of a coronary vessel rupture with a vein graft stent: case report.* Cathet Cardiovasc Diagn 38:172-174 (1996).

CHAPTER 7

STENTING TOTAL OCCLUSIONS

CASE 7.1: Arterial Reconstruction for Total Coronary Occlusion

The patient is a 64 year old man who had angioplasty of a long right coronary artery stenosis one year earlier. He returns with progressive exertional angina and an abnormal exercise test. At angiography, the right coronary artery was occluded in its mid portion with a faint bridging pattern of branching collaterals (Figure 7.1a). There was good left-to-right collateral flow. The occluded segment appeared to be <20mm in length.

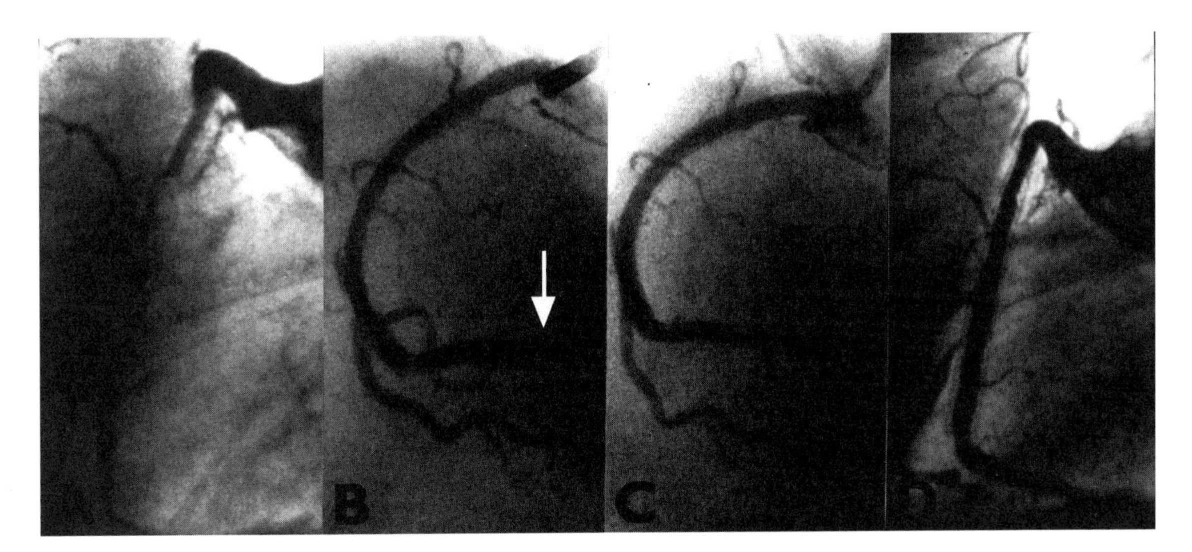

Figure 7.1 • Arterial Reconstruction The occluded right coronary artery exhibited bridging collaterals (**a**) associated with chronic obstruction. After crossing the obstruction with a stiff wire and implanting a Wallstent, a short but severe distal stenosis was apparent for the first time (**b; arrow**). This lesion was treated by passing a short AVE Micro I stent through the long Wallstent to the distal lesion and deploying (**c**). Eight months later there was no restenosis (**d**).

PROCEDURE 7.1

Despite the chronicity of the occlusion suggested by the plexus of collaterals, the occluded segment appeared relatively short. The procedure was started with a 0.014" standard guidewire. Using orthogonal projections to position the distal wire tip, the occluded segment was crossed and dilated with a 2.0mm balloon. As flow improved, the length of the diseased segment was found to be about 30mm. The distal vessel was 3.0mm in diameter. After dilating with a 3.0 x 35mm balloon, a Wallstent was implanted covering the entire length of the diseased segment. After post-stent dilation (12 atm), a 70% stenosis of the distal right coronary artery within the Wallstent became apparent (**Figure 7.1b arrow**). The stenosis did not respond until an inflation pressure of 14 atm was reached. A 6mm long Micro I stent was passed through the Wallstent to the site of the distal lesion and deployed with a single 10 atm inflation. The final angiogram revealed <10% residual stenosis at both stented sites (**Figure 7.1c**). The patient has remained symptom free. Angiography 8 months after the procedure revealed no evidence of lesions at either stent site (**Figure 7.1d**).

MATERIALS 7.1

Guiding Catheter:	Cook Lumax JR-4 8 French
Guidewires:	ACS/Guidant Standard 0.014"x 300cm
Balloons:	SciMed Cobra 2.0 x 20mm
	Schneider Speedy Longy 3.0 x 35 mm
	Mansfield High Energy 3.0 x 20 mm
Stents:	Schneider Wallstent 5.5 x 35 mm (> 45 mm length when deployed to 3.0mm)
	AVE Micro I 3.0 x 6mm

CASE 7.2: Stent Recanalization for Thrombotic Occlusion

An 80 year old man had an acute anteroseptal myocardial infarction. His peak CPK was 800 IU/L and he did not develop Q-waves. He developed recurrent angina six weeks later. At angiography, an occluded left anterior descending artery with thrombus propagating proximally toward the ostium was seen. There was collateral flow from both the right and left coronary circulations. The occluded segment was estimated to be 10 to 20mm in length. Left ventricular function was normal (65%). The patient was placed on heparin. Angioplasty and stenting was performed 10 days later.

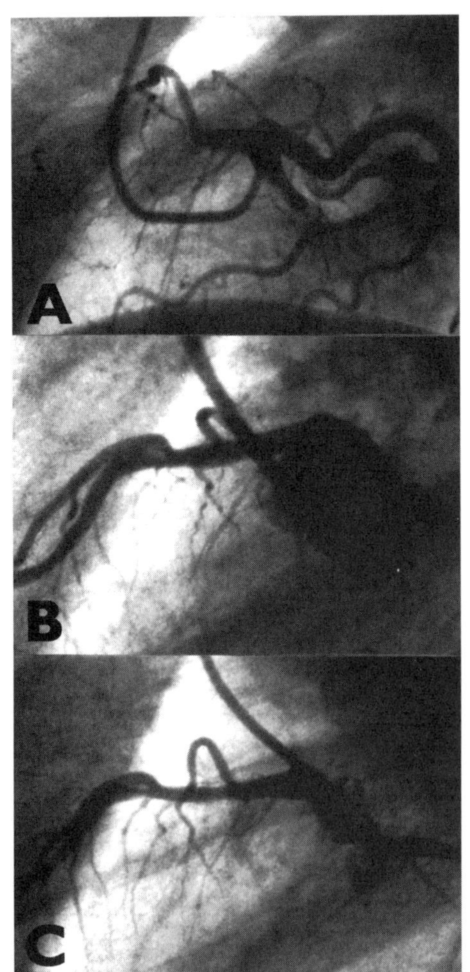

Figure 7.2 Stent Recanalization with Thrombus In the lateral projection, a flush occlusion of the left anterior descending artery is noted (**a**). After recanalization and implantation of a Palmaz-Schatz II stent there was no residual stenosis (**b**). The result was maintained at angiography six months later (**c**).

PROCEDURE 7.2

Repeat angiography showed the left anterior descending artery to be occluded prior to septal perforators. The proximal thrombus was no longer apparent (Figure 7.2a). The segment between the occlusion and resumption of the left anterior descending artery by visible collaterals was >20mm. There was no evidence of bridging collaterals.

The occlusion was easily crossed with a standard angioplasty guidewire. A 3.5mm x 20mm High Energy balloon (Mansfield/Boston Scientific, Watertown, MA) was passed across the occlusion and inflated to 6 atm. Antegrade TIMI grade 3 flow was restored with a 10% residual stenosis. It was elected to proceed with left anterior descending stenting. After exchanging the standard guidewire for an extra support guide wire, a Palmaz-Schatz II stent was crimped on a 3.5mm balloon. The assembly was passed easily across the previously occluded segment and deployed with 10 atm inflation. The final result showed no evidence of residual narrowing. The patient was transferred to the recovery area (Figure 7.2b).

After 12 hours of intravenous heparin, the patient was given only aspirin and ticlopidine and discharged two days later. He remained asymptomatic six months later and angiography revealed no evidence of restenosis (Figure 7.2c).

MATERIALS 7.2

Guiding catheter:	Cook Lumax JL4 8F
Guidewires:	0.014" Standard (USCI), 0.014" Extrasupport (ACS)
Balloons:	3.5 x 20mm High Energy (Mansfield/Boston Scientific)
Stent:	Palmaz-Schatz II 154A 14mm (Johnson and Johnson)

DISCUSSION

Coronary Angioplasty of Total Occlusions

Approximately 20% of patients referred for coronary angiography are found to have a chronic total occlusion of at least one vessel.[1] An occluded vessel with good collateral supply has the functional significance of a 90% stenosis.[2] Despite the frequency and physiological significance of total occlusions, the success rate for percutaneous recanalization is only 65-70%, significantly below the ≥90% success rates for non-occlusive stenoses.[3,4]

The restenosis rates after opening chronic occlusions are 50-68%, considerably higher than those for angioplasty of subtotal stenoses.[3] Total occlusions, thus, represent a lesion subset which has a poor long-term outcome with balloon angioplasty and become, at times, the defining feature in favor of coronary bypass surgery.

Although patients rarely suffer recurrent myocardial infarction in the territory of chronic occlusions, angina attributed to these vessels is common. Successful recanalization resolves angina in 70-75% of patients.[4] After angioplasty for occlusions, the resolution of symptoms and low rate of bypass surgery persist over the medium-term follow-up.[3,6] Successful recanalization also results in improved global and regional left ventricular function.[7] which becomes apparent at follow-up (averaging 9 months) when associated with persistent vessel patency.[5] Diastolic indices of ventricular function are also improved immediately as reflected by decreased left ventricular end diastolic pressures, increased synchrony of relaxation and improved regional wall motion response to tachy-pacing.[5]

Benefits of an Open Artery

In consideration of total occlusion angioplasty, an open artery confers several theoretical benefits compared to a persistently occluded vessel. A patent vessel may prevent ventricular dilation, aneurysm formation, and myocardial rupture. A patent vessel may also provide a protective effect through future collaterals should progression of atherosclerosis result in the occlusion of another coronary artery. Evidence from acute myocardial infarction trials shows that vessel patency with TIMI grade 2 flow or better is a major predictor of survival and left ventricular function both early and late post-infarction.[8] Much of the evidence of the "open artery hypothesis" pertains to acute occlusions and acute myocardial infarction. However, the successful opening of chronic occlusions has also resulted in improved survival.[3,9,10]

Angiographic Predictors of Angioplasty Success

Several large series have demonstrated the angiographic predictors of successful recanalization for total occlusions (Table 7.1).

Table 7.1 Angioplasty of Total Occlusions: Predictors of Success

PARAMETER	SUCCESS RATE (%)		SUCCESS RATE (%)	
Chronicity of occlusion	<3 months	75%	>3 months	37%
Antegrade Flow	Present (TIMI 1)	76%	Absent (TIMI 0)	58%
Vessel Cut-o ff	Tapering	77%	Abrupt	50%
Bridging Collaterals*	Absent	71%	Present	23%
Lesion Length	<15mm	increased	>15mm	decreased
Right Coronary**	Present	decreased	Absent	—
Retrograde Collaterals**	Present	increased	Absent	decreased
Coronary Calcium**	Present	decreased	Absent	increased

* A "medusa head" of bridging collaterals is a particularly poor harbinger of procedural success. This plethora of enlarged vasa vasorum predicts a success rate of only 20% by conventional techniques even in the most experienced centers.[12]

** These categories reflect a different prediction profile when using newer recanalization devices.[11] Data compiled in the review of Puma et al.[4]

Devices for Chronic Total Occlusions

The most common cause of failure of angioplasty for a chronic occlusion is the inability to cross the occlusion with a guidewire. The increased technical demands have led to the development of devices specifically for chronic occlusions.[13,14] The Magnum/Magnarail system (Schneider, Switzerland), the Rotacs device (Oscor Medical Corp, Palm Harbor, FL), and the Prima Total Occlusion Device (Spectranetics, Colorado Springs, CO) are three such devices.

The Magnum/Magnarail system consists of a 0.021"or 0.014" steel shaft affixed to a guidewire with a 1mm diameter olive shaped tip. A monorail or Magnarail balloon provides increased pushing power for the blunt tip. The system purportedly finds the path of least resistance through the lumen while minimizing intimal trauma and lowering the risk of perforation.

The Rotacs device consists of a motorized catheter rotating a 1.3mm blunt tip at 100-200 rpm. It is intended to gently negotiate passage through occlusions.

The Prima device consists of excimer laser energy transmitted through a 0.018" hypotube. The device is directed fluoroscopically in the direction of the intended target occlusion and advanced as tissue is ablated. It has allowed passage of a guidewire in occlusions which could not be crossed by conventional wires. However, there is an increased risk of perforation.[15]

One randomized trial has suggested conventional guidewires offer the highest primary success rate (66%) when compared to the Magnum system (39%) and Rotacs device (30%).[16] Another study compared the Magnum system to conventional guidewires and demonstrated a significantly higher success rate (67% vs 45% primary success).[17] Although both trials[16,17] were prospective and randomized, it appears that the relative success rate of these devices may be operator-dependent. No trial has compared the excimer laser system to other devices. Preliminary investigations have confirmed the success of laser in crossing lesions which could not be crossed by conventional wires.[11,18] Current practice in many laboratories initiates the procedure with a conventional wire, progressing to stiffer guidewires or the Magnum system. Alternate devices are reserved for vessels which cannot be crossed with these wire systems.[19]

Complications of Total Occlusion Angioplasty

While these specialized devices have allowed success rates for total occlusions to rise to 75%, complications have increased.[20] Although excellent pre-procedural collaterals provide protection against infarction, the subacute closure of vessels may still result in acute myocardial infarction with loss of collateral supply.[21,22] The increased complication may be due to the increased rate of intimal dissection associated with angioplasty of chronic occlusions.[13,19,23] Furthermore, while newer approaches have increased procedural success rates, the high restenosis rates for total occlusions remain unchanged. The increased restenosis rate is attributed predominantly to reocclusion at follow-up rather than to increased late luminal loss,[24] the increased likelihood of dissection, late occlusion, and restenosis rates have provided the impetus for stenting of chronically occluded arteries.

Stenting Total Coronary Occlusions

Stenting reduces restenosis of de novo, non-occluded vessels by 20-30%.[25,26] In 1994, the first report of stenting for chronic total occlusion in 30 patients indicated there was a 22% restenosis rate at 6-month follow-up, significantly lower than the >60% rate expected with balloon angioplasty in this setting.[27] Subsequently, stenting has been proven safe and effective in the setting of chronic coronary occlusion.[28-30] In one study, there was a 36% crossover rate to stenting from the angioplasty control group because of inadequate angiographic results.[28] A retrospective analysis reported that the stent restenosis rate may be reduced to as low as 20%,[30] while other studies report rates closer to 40%.[29] Although the rate of post-procedure acute and subacute closure is also improved by stenting,[29,30] the presence of a severe dissection before stent implantation may predict a higher percent residual stenosis and clinical event rate at follow-up.[30]

Several randomized trials, such as TOSCA (Total Occlusion Stenting vs Coronary Angioplasty) and SICCO (Stenting In Chronic Coronary Occlusion using heparin-coated Palmaz-Schatz stents),[31,32] have evaluated the efficacy of stenting for total occlusions. Recurrence of angina and restenosis are 50% less common in the stented groups.[31]

SUMMARY

The available data for stenting of chronic occlusions shows improved long-term outcomes compared to traditional balloon angioplasty and is especially important in the sealing of dissections or suboptimal angiographic results. Stents for total occlusions will likely be a routine part of clinical practice after presentation of appropriately sized prospective studies.

References

1. Baim DS, Ignatius EJ. *Use of coronary angioplasty: results of the current survey.* Am J Cardiol 3G-8G (1988).
2. Flamerg HW, Schwartz F, Hehrelein FW. *Intraoperative evaluation of the functional significance of coronary collateral vessels in patients with coronary artery disease.* Am J Cardiol 42:187-192 (1978).
3. Bell MR, Berger PB, Bresnahan JF, Reeder GS, Barly KR, Holmes DR. *Initial and long-term outcome of 354 patients after balloon angioplasty of total coronary artery occlusions.* Circulation 85:1003-1011 (1992).
4. Puma JA, Sketch MH, Tchang JE, Harrington RA, Phillips HA, Stack RS, Califf RM. *Percutaneous revascularization of chronic coronary occlusions: an overview.* J Am Coll Cardiol 26:1-11(1995).
5. Meier B. *Total coronary occlusion: a different animal?* J Am Coll Cardiol 17:50B-57B (1991).
6. Finci L, Meier B, Righetti A, Rutishauser W. *Long-term results of successful and failed angioplasty for chronic total occlusion.* Am J Cardiol 66:660-662 (1990).
7. Sabia PJ, Powers ER, Ragosta M, et al. *An association between collateral blood flow and myocardial viability in patients with recent myocardial infarction.* N Engl J Med 327: 1825-1831 (1992).
8. *Kim CB, Braunwald E. Potential benefits of late reperfusion of infarcted myocardium—the open artery hypothesis.* Circulation 88:2426-2436 (1993).
9. Ivanhoe RJ, Weintraub WS, Douglas JS et al. *Percutaneous transluminal coronary angioplasty of chronic total occlusions: primary success, restenosis, and long-term follow-up.* Circulation 85:106-115 (1992).
10. Moliterno DJ, Lange RA, Willard JE, Boehrer JD, Hillis LD. *Does restoration of antegrade flow in the infarct-related coronary artery days to weeks after myocardial infarction improve long-term survival?* Coronary Art Dis 3:299-304 (1990).
11. Holmes DR, Forrester JS, Litvak F, et al. *Chronic total obstruction and short-term outcome: The excimer laser coronary angioplasty registry experience.* Mayo Clin Proc 68:5-10 (1993).
12. Stone GW, Rutherford BD, McConahay DR, et al. *Procedural outcome of angioplasty for total coronary artery occlusion: An analysis of 971 lesions in 905 patients.* J Am Coll Cardiol 15:849-856 (1990).
13. Meier B, Conlier M, Finci L, Nukta E, Urban P, Niedenhauser W, Favre J. *Magnum wire for balloon recanalization of chronic total coronary occlusions.* Am J Cardiol 64: 148-154 (1989).
14. Danchin N, Julliere Y, Cassagnes J et al. *Randomized multicenter study of low speed rotational angioplasty versus standard angioplasty for chronic total coronary occlusion* [abstr]. Circulation 88 (suppl I):I-504 (1993).
15. Sievert H, Rohde S, Ensslen R, et al. *Recanalization of chronic coronary occlusions using a laser wire.* Cathet Cardiovasc Diagn 37:220-222 (1996).
16. Jacksch R, Papadakis E, Rosanowski C, Toker Y. *Comparison of three different techniques in reopening chronic coronary artery occlusion* [abstr]. Circulation 86(Suppl I):I-781 (1992).
17. Pande AK, Meier B, Urban P, de la Serna F, Villavicencio R, Dorsaz PA, Favre J. *Magnum/Magnarail versus conventional systems for recanalization of total chronic coronary occlusions: a randomized comparison.* Am Heart J 123:1182-1186 (1992).
18. Sanborn TA, Spokojny AM, Bergman GW, Cohen B, Power J. *A 0.018" excimer laser guidewire to recanalize chronic total occlusions and guide conventional angioplasty catheters* [abstr]. Circulation 88(Suppl I):I-504 (1993).
19. Hamm CW, Kupper W, Kuck KH, et al. *Recanalization of chronic, totally occluded coronary arteries by new angioplasty systems.* Am J Cardiol 66:1459-1463 (1990).

20. Kaltenbach M, Vallbracht C, Hartmann A. *Recanalization of chronic coronary occlusions by low speed rotational angioplasty* (ROTACS). J Interven Cardiol 4:155-165 (1991).

21. Andreae GE, Myler RK, Clark DA, et al. *Acute complications following coronary angioplasty of totally occluded vessels.* Circulation 76(suppl IV):IV-400 (1987).

22. Smyth DW, Thomas S, Jewitt DE. *Recanalization of chronic coronary angioplasty of totally occluded vessels* J Invas Cardiol 7:98-106 (1995).

23. Kereiakes DJ, Selmon MR, McAuley BJ, et al. *Angioplasty in total coronary artery occlusion: experience in 76 consecutive patients.* J Am Coll Cardiol 6:526-533 (1985).

24. Laris AG, Melkert R, Serruys PW. *Long-term luminal renarrowing after successful elective coronary angioplasty of total occlusions—a quantitative angiographic analysis.* Circulation 91:2140-2150 (1995).

25. *Fischman DL, Leon MB, Baim DS, et al. A randomized comparison of coronary-stent placement and balloon angioplasty in the treatment of coronary artery disease.* N Engl J Med 331:496-501 (1994).

26. *Serruys PW, De Jaegere P, Kiemeneij F, et al. A comparison of balloon-expandable-stent implantation with balloon angioplasty in patients with coronary artery disease.* N Engl J Med 331:489-495 (1994).

27. Medina A, Melian F, Suarez de Lezo J, Pan M, et al. *Effectiveness of coronary stenting for the treatment of chronic total occlusion in angina pectoris.* Am J Cardiol 73:1222-1224 (1994).

28. Sato Y, Kimwa T, Nosaka H, Nobuyoshi M. *Randomized comparison of balloon angioplasty (BA) versus coronary stent implantation (CS) for total occlusion (TO): preliminary results* [abstr]. Circulation 92 (Suppl I):I-475 (1995).

29. Ooka M, Suzuki T, Yokoya K, Huyase M, Kojima A, Kato H, Tani T, Inada T. *Stenting After Revascularization of Chronic Total Occlusion* [abstr]. Circulation 92(Suppl I):I-94 (1995).

30. Goldberg SL, Colombo A, Maiello L, Borrione M, Finci L, Almagor Y. *Intracoronary stent insertion after balloon angioplasty of chronic total occlusions.* J Am Coll Cardiol 26:713-719 (1995).

31. Simes PA, Golf S, Myreng Y, et al. *Stenting in chronic coronary occlusion (SICCO): a randomized, controlled trial of adding stent implantation after successful angioplasty.* J Am Coll Cardiol 28:1444-1451 (1996).

32. Thomas M, Hancock J, Holmberg S, et al. *Coronary artery stenting following successful angioplasty for total occlusions: preliminary results of a randomized trial* [abstr]. J Am Coll Cardiol 27:153A (1996).

CHAPTER 8

HIGH PRESSURE, LARGE BALLOONS AND ARTERIAL INJURY

CASE 8.1: Atherectomy Through a Stent for Recurrent Stenosis

A 58 year old woman presented with unstable angina due to a solitary severe stenosis in the right coronary artery (**Figure 8.1a**).

PROCEDURE 8.1

The lesion was dilated with a 3.0mm x 20mm balloon (Cobra, Scimed, USA) with a 4 atm inflation for 120 seconds, resulting in a class B dissection [1]. The dissection did not resolve after a 240 second 4 atm

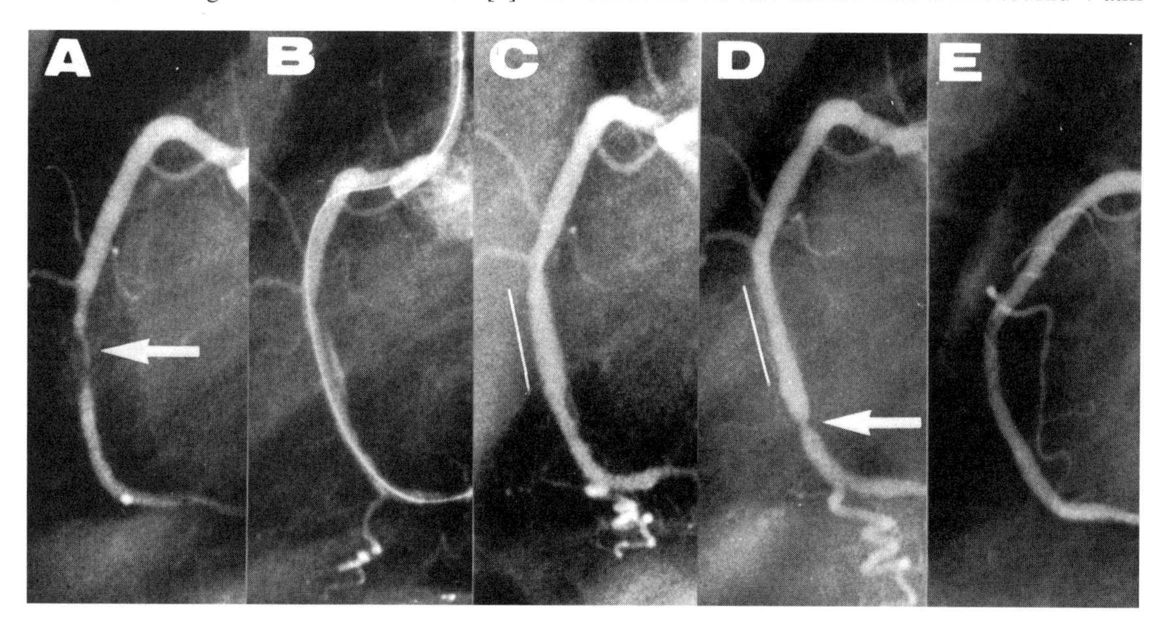

Figure 8.1 Atherectomy through a Stent. A severe mid right coronary artery lesion is seen (**a;** arrow). A type B dissection resulted after angioplasty (**b**) and was treated with stent implantation (**c;** bar represents stent location). A small residual dissection was left untreated distally. Six months later the new lesion (**d;** arrow) was distal to both the original lesion and to the stent (**d;** bar). There is no residual lesion after successful atherectomy through the stent (**e**). Reprinted with permission from Futura Publishing Co. (J. Interven Cardiol 1996; 9: 303).

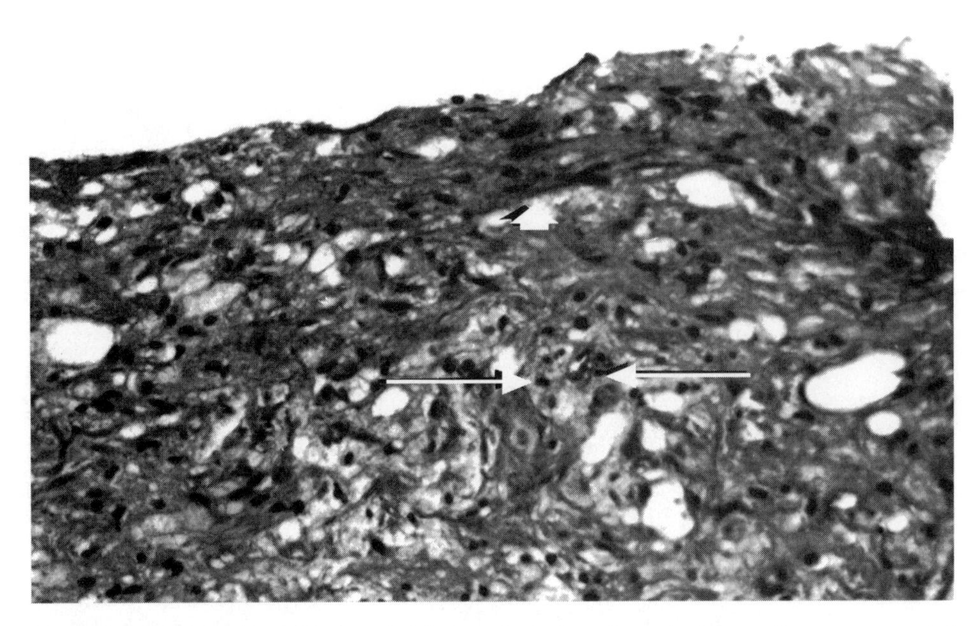

Figure 8.2 The Pathology of Restenosis The pathological specimen obtained at atherectomy revealed an aggressive proliferative response with numerous smooth muscle cells (short arrow) and foam cells (long arrows) consistent with restenosis. Sparse fibrotic tissue and no cholesterol clefts are seen. Reprinted with permission from Futura Publishing Company (*J Interven Cardiol* 1996;9:303).

balloon inflation (**Figure 8.1b**). A 14mm Palmaz-Schatz stent (PS 154A) was deployed without difficulty with a 3.5 x 20mm balloon (Goldie, Schneider, Switzerland) inflated at 9 atm. The post-deployment balloon extended 5mm beyond the stented segment where a minimal residual dissection was apparent (**Figure 8.1c**). The patient was discharged on ticlopidine 250mg daily for one month and aspirin 200mg daily.

Six months later the patient returned again with unstable angina. A new, severe lesion was now present 10mm distal to the stented segment (**Figure 8.1d**). There was no stenosis within the stent. The new lesion was treated with directional coronary atherectomy (DCA, 7 French Simpson Atherocath, Devices for Vascular Interventions, USA) passing the DCA catheter through the stented segment. Multiple longitudinal cuts resulted in <10% residual stenosis (**Figure 8.1e**). The tissue specimens were sent for routine pathological review.

Histopathological examination revealed a moderate to severe proliferative response of smooth muscle cells (**Figure 8.2**) with no evidence of cholesterol clefts, atheromatous plaque nor thrombus. There was a moderate lymphocytic infiltrate and occasional foam cells were noted (**Figure 8.2**). The patient was discharged and remains asymptomatic.

MATERIALS 8.1

Guiding Catheter:	DVI JR-4ST 9.5 French
Guidewires:	ACS/Guidant Extra Support 0.014"x 300cm
Balloons:	Scimed
Stents:	Johnson & Johnson
Device:	DVI 7 French GTO atherotome

DISCUSSION

The current case demonstrates the pathologic characterization of a new lesion appearing distal to a stent for angioplasty-induced dissection.[2] Coronary dissection is the most frequent cause of acute coronary occlusion after angioplasty,[3] a complication which has been dramatically reduced by stenting.[4,5] The prognosis of distal dissection left uncovered by a stent is usually benign and has little effect on the restenosis rate.[6] The new severe stenosis at a site distal to the region of stent contact is an unusual site for restenosis and raises the possibility that the new lesion was due to plaque activation and rupture rather than the more common proliferative mechanism of most restenotic lesions. The new lesion was treated with atherectomy through the stent to allow a pathological assessment. Examination of the tissue revealed a proliferative response suggesting that the new lesion was the result of arterial injury rather than a plaque rupture with or without thrombus, a finding which has important implications for stenting and the treatment of distal dissection after stent placement.

Restenosis After Stenting

Restenosis after coronary stenting occurs within the stent in the vast majority of cases.[5,7] It remains controversial whether stent restenosis occurs more at the articulation site[5] or within the proximal or distal stent segments.[7] Typically, the restenosis process occurs within and not distal to the stent, thus, the lesion which developed in this patient distal to the stent was unusual. Angiographically, this lesion was classified as a distinct, focal and de novo lesion. The possible etiologies included not only a new plaque with rupture and thrombus but also restenosis due to angioplasty trauma to a distal angiographically normal segment.

Pathology of New Lesions After Stenting

The pathology of atherosclerotic lesions differs from that of restenosis. The histology of de novo atherosclerotic lesions nearly always contains lipid-rich or fibrotic plaque material with or without cholesterol clefts and lymphocytes.[8,9] Restenotic lesions histologically nearly always demonstrate intimal proliferation with proliferation of stellate or spindle-shaped smooth muscle cells within a fibrotic myxoid stroma [8,9]. Although found in 30-40% of primary or de novo lesions,[10,11] intimal proliferation is not usually the predominant feature. In one of the few studies in which de novo lesions had evidence of intimal proliferation, nearly half of the lesions were proximal or distal to a site of previous angioplasty or atherectomy.[10] Thus, the new lesion distal to the stent site in the current patient was pathologically more like a restenotic than a de novo lesion. The lesion location suggests that the rapid intimal proliferation was a response to balloon injury rather than directly to stent implantation. Platelet-rich thrombus associated with initial stent deployment could be an additional catalyst to active vascular proliferation. However, there was no angiographic evidence of thrombus.

Angioplasty Trauma and Restenosis

The arterial damage of balloon angioplasty is a result of both balloon pressure and size, and the specific histologic characteristics of the target lesion. This arterial injury acts as a stimulus for intimal hypertrophy and initiates the restenosis process.[12] The degree of arterial injury has been related to restenosis through several parameters, including balloon-to-artery ratio, severity of initial stenosis, size of arterial lumen after angioplasty, and acute complications.[13-16] The relation of balloon pressure to arterial injury indicates that the most arterial damage occurs within the first several atmospheres of applied pressure. Controversy exists regarding the importance of maximal balloon pressure, number of inflations, and maximal balloon inflation time to restenosis.[17-19] In general, increasing balloon diameter is more likely to lead to complications of dissection or vessel rupture than increasing pressure.[20-22] The use of oversized balloons (balloon/artery ratio > 1.3) is a clear predictor of increased dissection,[14] myocardial infarction and the need for urgent surgery.[15]

At follow-up angiography, the reference vessel segment adjacent to angioplasty sites responds to balloon angioplasty trauma with the same proliferative response which occurs in the lesion itself.[23] In animal models, the severity of neointimal thickening of restenosis is directly proportional to the degree of arterial injury incurred during the procedure.(**Figure 8.3**).[12]

The Paradox of High Pressure Stent Deployment and Restenosis

Despite the desire to minimize arterial trauma, contemporary stent implantation and optimization technique requires high pressure dilations with optimally sized balloons to insure complete and symmetric stent apposition. Intracoronary ultrasound imaging evaluations have confirmed suboptimal stent implantation after low pressure dilations in over two thirds of patients.[24,25] Colombo et al report that patients having stents implanted with high pressure normal-sized balloons have fewer complications than when stents are implanted with high pressure oversized balloons, but higher restenosis rates. The fourth phase of the Benestent II Pilot study, the phase using the most generous balloon sizing method, had significantly reduced restenosis.[26] The routine use of high pressure maximally sized balloon inflations appears to optimize stent deployment. To improve distal blood flow through the stent, regions of mild atherosclerosis

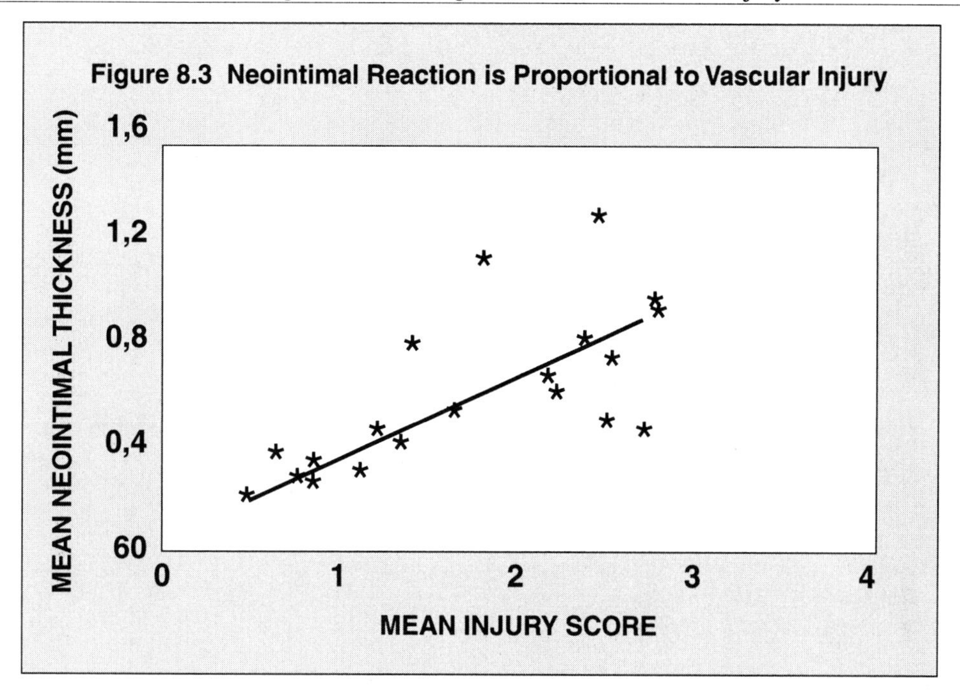

Figure 8.3 Neointimal Reaction is Proportional to Vascular Injury. Schwartz has demonstrated that the amount of neointimal proliferation is proportional to the degree of arterial injury in a stent over-expansion model. The thickness of the neointima which develops after stent implantation is compared to the degree of arterial injury induced by the procedure. Reprinted with permission from Dr. RS Schwartz and The American College of Cardiology (*J Am Coll Cardiol* 1992; 19:270).

and minimal narrowing outside the end of the stent are often dilated increasing the degree of arterial injury compared to conventional balloon angioplasty. Aggressive angioplasty techniques may result in arterial rupture and patient death.[27-29] The paradox of minimizing trauma while optimally expanding the stent must be managed on an individual patient basis. The interventionalist must weigh the increased risks of subacute thrombosis and restenosis for untreated suboptimal results against the risks of increased restenosis in distal segments treated by high pressure inflations or large balloons.

Management of Stent Edge Dissections

Small dissections or "edge tears" occur in 17% of arterial segments after stent implantation using modern techniques.[32] These dissections are usually invisible angiographically, but may be apparent by intracoronary ultrasound imaging. Edge dissections are not associated with adverse early clinical consequences. When intracoronary ultrasound is used to assess restenosis after angioplasty, dissection and plaque fracture are <u>not</u> predictors of restenosis.[33] Further, the prognosis of untreated distal dissections after balloon angioplasty is benign when clinical outcomes of small and moderate dissections were reviewed.[6] Dissections which typically resolved without restenosis[6] were associated with the following characteristics: satisfactory coronary flow, a stable dissection, and no associated stenosis of >50% diameter. The decision to treat a residual dissection distal to the stent should be individualized, depending on the relative importance of factors such as the difficulty of passing another stent distal to the first, the clinical importance and consequences of ischemia in the arterial territory, and operator experience.

SUMMARY

Modern stent optimization requires larger balloons at higher pressures to obtain more anatomically perfect results at a cost of traumatized distal arterial segments. Addressing the paradox between reducing complications and restenosis is an individualized decision based on clinical and anatomic factors, as well as operator experience in managing post-stent implantation complications.

References

1. *Coronary Artery Angiographic Changes after PTCA: Manual of Operations* NHLBI PTCA Registry, 1985; pp6-9.
2. Phillips PS, Alfonso F, Aragoncillo P, et al. *Characterization of a precocious new lesion distal to a stent site by atherectomy.* J Interventional Card 9:301-304 (1996).
3. deFeyeter PJ, van den Brand M, Jaarman G et al. *Acute coronary occlusion during and after percutaneous transluminal coronary angioplasty.* Circulation 83:927-936 (1991).
4. Maude M, Erbel R, Straub U, et al. *Results of intracoronary stents for management of coronary dissection after balloon angioplasty.* Am J Cardiol 67:691-696 (1991).
5. Herrman HC, Buchbinder M, Clemen MW, et al. *Emergent use of balloon-expandable coronary artery stenting for failed percutaneous transluminal coronary angioplasty.* Circulation 86:812-819 (1992).
6. Alfonso F, Hernandez R, Goicolea J, et al. *Coronary stenting for acute coronary dissection after coronary angioplasty: implications of residual dissection.* J Am Coll Cardiol 24:989-995 (1994).
7. Gordon P, Gibson M, Cohen DJ, et al. *Mechanisms of restenosis and redilation within coronary stents—quantitative angiographic assessment.* J Am Coll Cardiol 21:1166-1174 (1993).
8. Miller MJ, Kuntz RE, Friedrich SP, et al. *Frequency and consequences of intimal hyperplasia in specimens retrieved by directional atherectomy of native primary coronary artery stenoses and subsequent restenoses.* Am J Cardiol 71:652-658 (1993).
9. Waller BF, Johnson DE, Schnitt SJ, et al. *Histologic analysis of directional coronary atherectomy samples: a review of findings and their clinical relevance.* Am J Cardiol 72: 80E-87E (1993).
10. Johnson DE, Hinohara T, Robertson GC, et al. *Coronary vascular lesions resected by directional atherectomy: the histology of 328 successfully excised primary and recurrent stenoses.* Unpublished observations.
11. Schnitt SJ, Safian RD, Kuntz RE, et al. *Histologic Findings in specimens obtained by percutaneous directional coronary atherectomy.* Hum Pathol 23:415-420 (1992).
12. Schwartz R, Huber KC, Murphy JG, et al. *Restenosis and the proportional neointimal response to coronary artery injury: Results in a porcine model.* J Am Coll Cardiol 19: 267-274 (1992).
13. Ellis SG, Shaw RE, Gershony G, et al. *Risk factors, time course, and treatment effect after successful percutaneous transluminal angioplasty of chronic total occlusion.* Am J Cardiol 63:897-901(1989).
14. Nichols A, Smith R, Berke A, Schlofmitz R, Powers E. *Importance of balloon size on initial success, acute complications, and restenosis after percutaneous transluminal coronary angioplasty. A prospective, randomized study.* J Am Coll Cardiol 13:1094-1100 (1989).

15. Roubin GS, Douglas JS, King SB, et al. *Influence of balloon size on initial success, acute complications, and restenosis after percutaneous transluminal coronary angioplasty: A prospective, randomized study.* Circulation 78:557-565 (1988).

16. Beatt KJ, Serruys PW, Luijten HE, et al. *Restenosis after coronary angioplasty: the paradox of increased lumen diameter and restenosis.* J Am Coll Cardiol 19:258-266 (1992).

17. Bourassa MG, Lesperance J, Eastwood C, et al. *Clinical, physiologic, anatomic and procedural factors predictive of restenosis after PTCA.* J Am Coll Cardiol 18:368-376 (1991).

18. Sarembock IF, La Veau PJ, Sigal SL, et al. *Influence of inflation pressure and balloon size on the development of intimal hyperplasia after balloon angioplasty.* Circulation 80: 1029-1040 (1989).

19. Mathews BJ, Ewels CJ, Kent KM, et al. *Coronary dissection: A predictor of restenosis?* Am Heart J 115:547-554 (1988).

20. Sarembock IJ, SaVeau PJ, Sigal SL, et al. *The influence of inflation pressure and balloon size on the development of intimal hyperplasia following balloon angioplasty. A study in the atherosclerotic rabbit.* Circulation 80:1029-1040 (1989).

21. Nakamura S, Colombo A, Gaglione A, et al. *Intracoronary ultrasound observations during stent implantation.* Circulation 89:2026-2034 (1994).

22. Mudra H, Klauss V, Blasini R, et al. *Ultrasound guidance of Palmaz-Schatz intracoronary stenting with a combined intravascular ultrasound balloon.* Circulation 90:1252-1261 (1994).

23. Beatt KJ, Luijten HE, de Feyter PJ, et al. *Change in diameter of coronary artery segments adjacent to stenosis after percutaneous transluminal coronary angioplasty: failure of percent diameter stenosis measurement to reflect morphologic changes induced by balloon dilation.* J Am Coll Cardiol 12:314-323 (1988).

24. Colombo A, Hall P, Nakamura S, et al. *Intracoronary stenting without anticoagulation accomplished with intravascular ultrasound guidance.* Circulation 91:1676-1688 (1995).

25. Nakamura S, Colombo A, Gaglione A, et al. *Intracoronary ultrasound observations during stent implantation.* Circulation 89:2026-2034 (1994).

26. Carlos Macaya, personal communication, Madrid, August, 1996.

27. Alfonso F, Goicolea J, Hernandez R, et al. *Vessel perforation during optimization of coronary stents using high-pressure balloon inflations.* Am Heart J (In press, 1997).

28. Colombo A, Hall P, Nakamura S, et al. *Intracoronary stenting without anticoagulation accomplished with intravascular ultrasound guidance.* Circulation 91:1676-1688 (1995).

29. Nakamura S, Colombo A, Gaglione A, et al. *Intracoronary ultrasound observations during stent implantation.* Circulation 89:2026-2034 (1994).

30. Andersen HR, Maeng M, Thorwest M, Falk E. *Remodeling rather than neointimal formation explains luminal narrowing after deep vessel wall injury—insights from a porcine coronary (re)stenosis model.* Circulation 93:1716-1724 (1996).

31. Merino A, Cohen M, Badimon JI, et al. *Synergistic action of severe wall injury and shear forces on thrombus formation in arterial stenosis: definition of a thrombotic shear rate threshold.* J Am Coll Cardiol 24:1091-1094 (1994).

32. Metz JA, Mooney MR, Walter PD, et al. *Significance of edge tears in coronary stenting: Initial observations from the STRUT registry* [abstr]. Circulation 92 (suppl I):I-546 (1995).

33. Peters JK, Kok WEM, DiMario C, et al. *Prediction of restenosis after coronary balloon angioplasty. Results of PICTURE (Post-Intra Coronary Treatment Ultrasound Result Evaluation), a prospective multicenter intracoronary ultrasound imaging study.* Circulation 95: 2254-2261 (1997)

CHAPTER 9

PSEUDOSTENOSES DURING STENTING: WRINKLES AND INTUSSUSCEPTIONS

CASE 9.1: Vascular Wrinkles

A 42 year old man presented with unstable angina and a prior non-Q-wave inferior infarction. Angiography revealed occlusion of a non-dominant right coronary artery with a severe stenosis of the proximal circumflex immediately distal to a severe (>90°) curve.

PROCEDURE 9.1

After predilation with a 3.5mm balloon, a 3.5mm Palmaz-Schatz stent was positioned and dilated with a 15 x 4mm balloon to 14 atm with an excellent intrastent angiographic appearance. However, a new 50% stenosis was now apparent immediately proximal to the stent. This lesion was suspected to be an intimal wrinkle

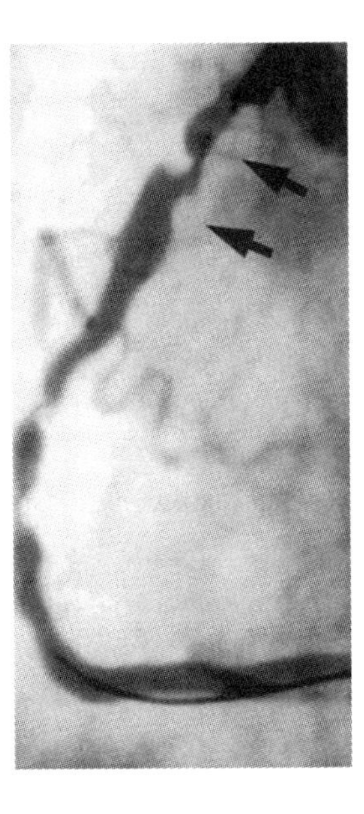

Figure 9.1 Cineangiogram of RCA demonstrates wrinkling due to stiff angioplasty guide wire used for PTCA. New lesion wire resolves on removal.

caused by unnatural straightening of the artery. Without further balloon therapy, the extra support guidewire was withdrawn leaving only the floppy portion across the new lesion and stent. At this point, the lesion was no longer apparent and the entire angioplasty system was withdrawn. Figure 9.1 demonstrates pseudostenoses due to wrinkling of a tight coronary artery by a stiff guidewire during PTCA.

MATERIALS 9.1

Guiding catheter:	Cook Lumax AL2, 8F
Guidewires:	ACS Extra support 0.014"
Balloons:	Baxter Quick 3.5mm, Schneider Chubby 4mm(9mm long)
Stent:	Palmaz-Schatz 1535AH (Benestent II, Johnson and Johnson)

CASE 9.2: Vessel Intussusception

The patient is a 59 year old man with progressive exertional angina and a positive exercise test on nitrates and beta-blockers. Coronary angiography revealed a 75% diameter narrowing in the mid portion of the second obtuse marginal artery.

PROCEDURE 9.2

An extra support guide was passed across the lesion located at the bifurcation of the second obtuse marginal and distal circumflex vessels. Angioplasty resulted in a type C dissection. A 16mm NIR stent was selected to permit access to the distal circumflex vessel. The distal circumflex vessel was not considered large enough to warrant protection with a separate guide wire. After deployment of the NIR Rigid-flex stent (16 atm), eccentric contrast lucencies appeared proximally and distally in regions which had not been dilated (similar to those in Figure 9.1). These lesions extended inward from the regions exhibiting the greatest curvature prior to wire passage and suggested vascular intussusceptions. To confirm this suspicion, the extra stiff support guide wire was withdrawn until only its flexible tip was across the distal new lesion which immediately resolved. The guidewire was then completely withdrawn and final angiographic images were obtained. The patient has remained asymptomatic with a negative exercise test.

MATERIALS 9.2

Guiding Catheter:	Cook Lumax JL-4
Guidewires:	ACS Extra Support 0.014"x
Balloons:	SciMed/Boston Scientific Viva 3.0 x 20mm
Stents:	SciMed/Boston Scientific Rigid Flex NIR 16mm

DISCUSSION

Vessel wall invaginations and wrinkles (pseudostenoses) occur when the arterial conduit is unnaturally straightened by stiff guidewires and devices. This phenomenon has been described by Tenaglia[1] and others.[2-8] It has also been described as "pseudo narrowing," "accordion effect," "crumpled coronary," "vessel wall invagination," and as "pseudo-transection".[2-8] These invaginations usually occur in tortuous vessels proximal to the target lesion. Their hallmark is typically a lucency extending inward from the outer wall of the most curved segment in a perpendicular fashion. They often occur in segments which have been untouched by balloon dilations, thus, giving a clue to their benign nature. Another important indicator of their presence is the marked straightening of the affected segment when compared to the pre procedural image of that same segment. In CASES 9.1 & 9.2 the operator immediately identified the exaggerated straightening of the target segments and confirmed the suspicion by withdrawing the stiff guidewire.

In the current era, it is important to remain alert to inducing pseudo-complications, especially when using stiffer guidewires for stent passage. The presence of other stents may have already straightened an arterial segment, predisposing to vessel wrinkling. If the operator remains unconvinced that a new lesion is indeed wrinkling, he may test for invagination before committing his patient to further dilations or stents. The easiest test for this artifact is to withdraw the guidewire until only the soft distal tip traverses the affected area as was done in *CASE 9.2*. If the lesion is truly an invagination, it will disappear when the vessel is allowed to resume its natural curve. At times it may be advisable to exchange the stiff guidewire for a softer guidewire to demonstrate that the defect is only an invagination. Intravascular ultrasound imaging has not yet been reported with this problem, but can be of assistance in excluding both plaque and dissection at these sites.

Some vascular folds resulting from long stents may be avoided if two shorter stents of the same design are placed. It is unknown if vascular pseudolesions and resulting intimal disruption or intimal stress will result in a new variant of restenosis; new lesions distal to stents placed on curves.

SUMMARY

Pseudostenoses may appear during vessel straightening using stiff guidewires for stent support. Vascular pseudolesions must be differentiated from intimal disruptions. Replacement of stiff guidewires with more flexible guidewires is often needed. Wire removal may be essential to assess the pseudolesions. Consideration of these problems should be made before stent implantation.

References

1. Tenaglia AN, Tcheng JE, Phillips HR, Stack RS. Creation of pseudo narrowing during coronary angioplasty. Am J Cardiol 67:658-659 (1991).
2. Rauh RA, Ninneman RW, Joseph D, Gupta VK, Senior DG, Millier WP. Accordian effect in tortuous right coronary arteries during percutaneous transluminal coronary angioplasty. Cathet Cardiovasc Diagn 23:107-110 (1991).
3. Shea PJ. Mechanical right coronary artery shortening and vessel wall invagination: a fourth cause of iatrogenic coronary obstruction during coronary angioplasty. A case report and review of the literature. Cathet Cardiovasc Diagn 26:136-139 (1992).
4. Mascarenhas DAN, Silver KH, Heller LI, Folland ED. Intimal invagination due to coronary artery straightening: a temporary iatrogenic cause of proximal artery narrowing during angioplasty. J Invas Cardiol 5:302-305 (1993).
5. Lau KW, Ding ZP, Gao W, Susan Q, Abdullah J. Pseudo-dissection in percutaneous coronary angioplasty. J Invas Cardiol 6:296-299 (1994).
6. Hays JT, Stein B, Raizner AE. The crumpled coronary: an enigma of arteriographic pseudopathology and its potential for misinterpretation. Cathet Cardiovasc Diagn 31:293-300 (1994).
7. Blankenship JC. Right coronary artery pseudo-transection due to mechanical straightening during coronary angioplasty. Cathet Cardiovasc Diagn 36:43-45 (1995).
8. Deligonul U, Tatineni S, Johnson R, Kern MJ. Accordian right coronary artery: An unusual complication of PTCA guidewire entrapment. Cathet Cardiovasc Diagn 23:111- 113 (1991).
9. Mata LA, Bosch X, David PR, et al. Clinical and angiographic assessment 6 months after double vessel percutaneous coronary angioplasty. J Am Coll Cardiol 6:1339-1344 (1985).
10. Vandormael MG, Deligonul U, Kern MJ, et al. Multilesion coronary angioplasty: clinical and angiographic follow-up. J Am Coll Cardiol 10:246-252 (1987).
11. Ellis SG, Roubin GS, King SB, et al. Importance of stenosis morphology in the estimation of restenosis risk after elective percutaneous transluminal coronary angioplasty. Am J Cardiol 63:30-34 (1989).

CHAPTER 10

STENTS AND CORONARY ANEURYSMS

CASE 10.1: Stenting in a 6mm Aneurysm

The patient is a 57 year old man who presented with unstable angina and new anterior T-wave inversions. Coronary arteriography demonstrated an isolated severe left anterior descending coronary artery stenosis in the middle of a fusiform aneurysmal dilatation 6 mm in diameter. Because of the aneurysm, it was elected to treat the lesion with balloon angioplasty rather than primary stenting. The stenosis was dilated with a 4.5mm balloon leaving a 30% diameter residual narrowing. His symptoms resolved and a thallium treadmill was negative ten days later.

Two weeks later, he had acute onset of chest pain and a non-Q-wave myocardial infarction. At catheterization he was found to have a severe renarrowing at the site of the initial lesion **(Figure 10.1a)**.

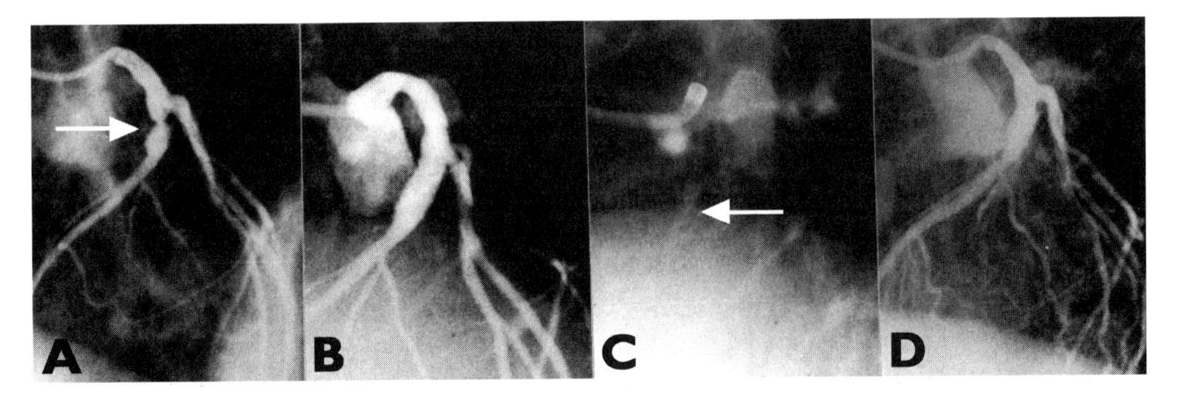

Figure 10.1 • Stenting in an Aneurysm A lesion in an aneurysm of the anterior descending artery (**a**) was found 10 days after an angioplasty at that site. The result after stent implantation within the aneurysm was good (**b**). The Palmaz-Schatz II stent can be seen fluoroscopically (**c**). Six month angiography revealed no restenosis (**d**).

PROCEDURE 10.1

The presence of an aneurysm was a cause of concern for stent placement but the rapid restenosis suggested stenting might now be a better revascularization option. The lesion was easily crossed with an extra support guidewire. Pre-stent dilation was performed with a 6mm balloon at 2 atm. The precise positioning of a stent between a proximal diagonal branch and the distal segment of the aneurysm (which demonstrated significant tapering) was most important. The precise localization was dependent on an understanding of the degree of stent shortening when expanded to a large diameter. A 20mm Palmaz-Schatz stent will shorten to approximately 17.8mm length at 6mm diameter. The stent was hand-wrapped on the original 6mm balloon and passed to the site of stenosis. The stent was deployed with an 8 atm inflation for 30 seconds.

Final angiograms revealed no residual stenosis **(Figure 10.1b & c).** The patient remained symptom free and at 6-month follow-up angiography, there was no evidence of restenosis (Figure 10.1d).

MATERIALS 10.1

Guiding Catheter:	Cook Lumax JL-4 8F
Guide wires:	ACS Extra Support 0.014"x 175cm
Balloons:	Schneider Speedy Bypass 6mm x 20mm
Stents:	Johnson & Johnson Palmaz-Schatz II 204 (20 mm)

CASE 10.2: Aneurysm after Angioplasty Despite Stenting

A 54 year old man presented with prolonged angina and anterior wall electrocardiographic changes three years earlier due to a 50% diameter left anterior descending stenosis. The patient was treated medically. He returned with progressive angina and an early positive treadmill stress test. Angiography now revealed a new severe left anterior descending lesion proximal to the older moderate mid vessel stenosis **(Figure 10.2a).**

PROCEDURE 10.2

Balloon dilation of the left anterior descending stenosis resolved the narrowing but produced a type C coronary dissection which persisted after prolonged balloon inflations **(Figure 10.2b;** arrow**).** Because of the very proximal location of the dissection, a non-articulated Palmaz-Schatz II stent was implanted. This stent was easily positioned because of its increased radiopacity and post-dilated to 10 atm **(Figure 10.2c).** The patient became asymptomatic.

As part of a protocol 6 months later, follow-up angiography revealed a saccular dilation at the site of the original dissection consistent with a pseudoaneurysm (Figure 10.2d). The aneurysm could not be well imaged by transesophageal echocardiography. An additional angiogram in one year after the original procedure is planned to evaluate the long-term result.

MATERIALS 10.2

Guiding Catheter:
- Schneider Guide Zilla
- JL-4 8 French

Guidewires:
- ACS Extra Support
- 0.014"x 175cm

Balloons:
- Schneider Goldie 3.5 x 20mm

Stents:
- Johnson & Johnson
- P-S 204 (18mm)

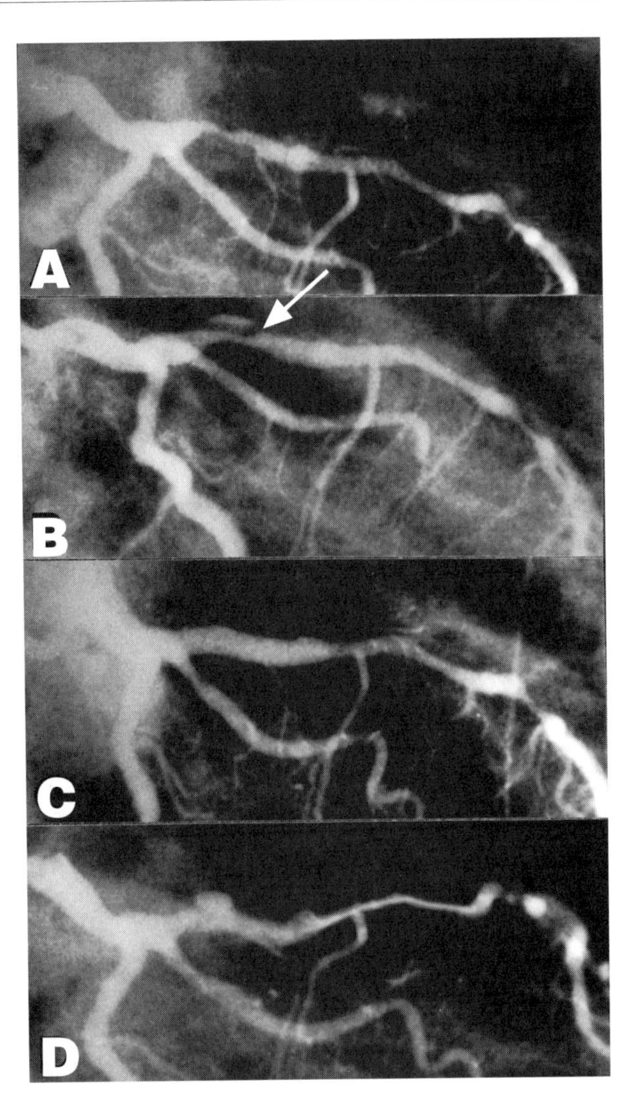

Figure 10.2 Aneurysm Formation after Angioplasty with Stent Implantation A severe stenosis of the proximal anterior descending artery (**a**) was treated with angioplasty resulting in a type C coronary dissection (**b**; arrow). Despite a good response to stent implantation (**c**) there was aneurysm formation at the 6 month angiogram (**d**).

DISCUSSION

Coronary Aneurysms

Coronary artery aneurysms may be congenital or acquired through atherosclerotic, inflammatory (Kawasaki's disease) or infectious (mycotic aneurysm) illnesses, or secondary to vascular trauma (angioplasty, atherectomy).[1] Coronary aneurysms are usually asymptomatic and not associated with adverse clinical consequences.[2] However, they may cause myocardial infarction due to thrombosis or distal embolization.[3] The coronary aneurysms which result from the trauma of intracoronary procedures have a distinct natural history compared to those observed in the pre-interventional period.[4]

Angioplasty-related Aneurysms

Post-angioplasty aneurysms may be divided into two types: early and late. The early aneurysms are recognized during or soon after coronary intervention and are thought to be contained perforations (pseudoaneurysms). Their prognosis is not benign and progressive enlargement and rupture have been described.[5,6] On the other hand, aneurysms which form late and are found at follow-up angiography (*CASE 10.2*) generally remain asymptomatic and follow a natural history closer to that of aneurysms in the pre-coronary intervention era.[7]

Definitions

Unfortunately there is no standardized definition of coronary artery aneurysms. Different definitions have been used, making the determination of the exact incidence of aneurysms after interventional procedures unknown. The Coronary Artery Surgery Study (CASS) definition of aneurysm is an arterial dilatation that exceeds 1.5 times the diameter of the normal adjacent vessel.[8] The incidence of aneurysm after angioplasty is 4-5%.[7,9] The incidence of aneurysm after atherectomy may be as high as 10%.[10] Although there was no apparent relation between the depth of the arterial resection as measured by presence of subintimal tissue, the presence of adventitia in a coronary atherectomy specimen may be an indicator of future aneurysm formation.

Aneurysms and Stents

Cardiologists have worried that stents might cause aneurysms since the earliest animal investigations.[11] It was hypothesized that as the coronary arteries move with the actively beating heart, vascular sheer forces, stress and strain would concentrate at the interface between the intima and the stent edges. A disrupted healing process could lead to gradual mural weakening and aneurysm formation. Although these latter phenomena did not occur in the small series of dogs studied, there was measurable thinning of the arterial media by 32 weeks post implant at the stented sites.[11] The thinning was most notable at the points of contact with the stent and was attributed to the reduction in overall wall stress provided by the immobile stent. Even though no aneurysms developed in these animal studies, occasional aneurysms are seen at follow-up in the segments of arteries receiving stents.[12]

Multicenter Studies

The exact incidence of coronary aneurysms after stent implantation is unknown. A substudy of the STRESS trial revealed that coronary aneurysms developed in 3.9% of stent patients compared to 7.1% of angioplasty patients.[13] It is unclear if the aneurysms reported are due to dissections and trauma prior to implantation or to the stent itself. Aneurysms occurred in 32% of patients receiving Gianturco-Roubin stents treated with colchicine and steroids.[14] While the aneurysms in this series were attributed to the use of anti-inflammatory agents, the concerns about increased medial atrophy caused by stents remain. Consequently, stents have traditionally been avoided in segments of vessels which already exhibit aneurysmal dilation.

Covered Stents

Some investigators have begun to evaluate stents prospectively to treat coronary aneurysms. Stephanadis et al[15]described the use of vein covered stents. Wong et al[16] repaired a post-atherectomy pseudoaneurysm using a Palmaz-Schatz biliary stent covered with a portion of a cephalic vein. The target vessel was protected by an internal mammary artery graft. Unfortunately, late follow-up angiography was not provided. It appears that the early concerns about stents causing aneurysms are being replaced with a new enthusiasm for stents used in the treatment of aneurysms.

SUMMARY

Preliminary evidence suggests that stents are no worse than angioplasty in causing aneurysms. When considering stent implantation in an aneurysm, it is important to remember that stent shortening will be significant when deployed with these large diameter segments and should be considered in device selection. Tapered balloons and short balloons are advised so that high pressure stent optimization can be performed without severe over dilatation of unaffected segments

References

1. Daoud AS, Pankin D, Tulgan H, et al. *Aneurysms of the coronary artery—report of ten cases and review of the literature.* Am J Cardiol 11:228 (1963).
2. Swaye PS, Fisher LD, Litwin P, et al. *Aneurysmal coronary artery disease.* Circulation 67:134-138 (1983).
3. Ebert PA, Peter RH, Gunnels JC, et al. *Resecting and grafting of coronary artery aneurysm.* Circulation 43:593 (1971).
4. Dralle JG, Turner C, Hsu J, Replogle RL. *Coronary artery aneurysms after angioplasty and atherectomy.* Ann Thorac Surg 59:1030-1035 (1995).
5. Garrand TF, Mintz GS, Popma JJ, et al. *Intravascular ultrasound diagnosis of a coronary artery pseudoaneurysm following percutaneous transluminal coronary angioplasty.* Am Heart J 125:882-884 (1993).
6. Van Suylen RJ, Serruys PW, Simpson JB, et al. *Delayed rupture of right coronary artery after directional atherectomy for bail out.* Am Heart J 121:914-916 (1991).
7. Bal ET, Plokker T, van den Berg EMJ, et al. *Predictability and prognosis of PTCA- induced coronary artery aneurysm.* Cathet Cardiovasc Diagn 22:85-88 (1991).
8. Robertson T, Fisher L. *Prognostic significance of coronary artery aneurysm and ectasia in the Coronary Artery Surgery Study (CASS) registry.* Prof Clin Biol Res 250:325-339 (1987).

9. Vassanelli C, Turri M, Morando G, et al. *Coronary arterial aneurysms after percutaneous transluminal coronary angioplasty—a not uncommon finding at elective follow-up angiography.* Int J Cardiol 22:151-156 (1989).

10. Bell MR, Garratt KN, Bresnahan JF, et al. *Relation of deep arterial resection and coronary artery aneurysms after directional coronary atherectomy.* J Am Coll Cardiol 20:1474-1481 (1992).

11. Schatz RA, Palmaz JC, Tio FO, et al. *Balloon-expandable intracoronary stents in the adult dog.* Circ 76:450-457 (1987).

12. Alfonso F, Hernandez R, Goicolea J, et al. *Coronary stenting for acute coronary dissection after coronary angioplasty: implications of residual dissection.* J Am Coll Cardiol 24:989-995 (1994).

13. Slota P, Fischman D, Savage M, et al. *Is coronary stent implantation associated with a higher-risk for coronary artery aneurysm formation than balloon angioplasty?* [abstr]. Circulation 92(suppl I):I-687 (1995).

14. Rab ST, King SB III, Roubin GS, et al. *Coronary aneurysms after stent placement: a suggestion of altered vessel wall healing in the presence of anti-inflammatory agents.* J Am Coll Cardiol 18:1524-1528 (1991).

15. Stephanadis C, Karayannakos P, Kallikazaros I, et al. *Transluminal vascular stenting using autologous vein grafts.* Eur Heart J 13[suppl]:260 (1992).

16. Wong SC, Kent KM, Mintz GS, et al. *Percutaneous transcatheter repair of a coronary aneurysm using a composite autologous cephalic vein-coated Palmaz-Schatz biliary stent.* Am J Cardiol 76:990-991 (1995).

CHAPTER 11

STENTS IN SAPHENOUS VEIN GRAFTS

CASE 11.1: Stents After Coronary Artery Bypass Graft Surgery

The patient is a 74 year old man with severe COPD who had an inferior wall myocardial infarction 21 years ago. Thirteen years ago he received four venous bypass grafts. He presented with progressive angina occurring over 15 days with minimal effort. Because of symptomatic peripheral vascular disease, he was referred directly for coronary angiography. The ejection fraction was 55% with akinesis of the inferior left ventricular wall. The native right coronary, first diagonal, and circumflex vessels were occluded proximally and the left anterior descending artery was occluded in its mid portion after providing septal collaterals to the posterior descending artery. The saphenous venous conduits to the right coronary and circumflex arteries were occluded. There were severe lesions in the remaining two grafts to the first obtuse marginal and left anterior descending artery (**Figure 11.1 a & e;** arrows). The patient was not considered a surgical candidate because of his age and underlying medical conditions (COPD, diabetes, hypertension). Primary stent implantation in both grafts as an alternative therapy was elected.

PROCEDURE 11.1

Because of the significant myocardium supplied by each of the remaining two grafts the procedure was staged, treating the more severe lesion in the graft to the obtuse marginal on the first day. The left anterior descending graft lesion was treated the following day.

The obtuse marginal graft lesion was long with the appearance of a large amount of athero-thrombotic bulk, factors associated with increased risk of thromboembolism (**Figure 11.1a**). The procedure was begun with a Transluminal Extraction Atherectomy (TEC) device followed by a long segment single Wallstent. A TEC guidewire was passed across the lesion into the distal obtuse marginal vessel. A 6 French TEC catheter was advanced at varying rates maintaining a constant flow of debris into the suction trap (**Figure 11.1b**). Next, a Wallstent was positioned so that the proximal and mid stent markers covered the diseased segment (**Figure 11.1c**). The stent membrane was withdrawn allowing release of the device and the region was post-dilated with a 4.5mm x 20mm balloon to 18 atm with no residual stenosis. The vascular sheaths were left in place and the patient remained anticoagulated until the following day.

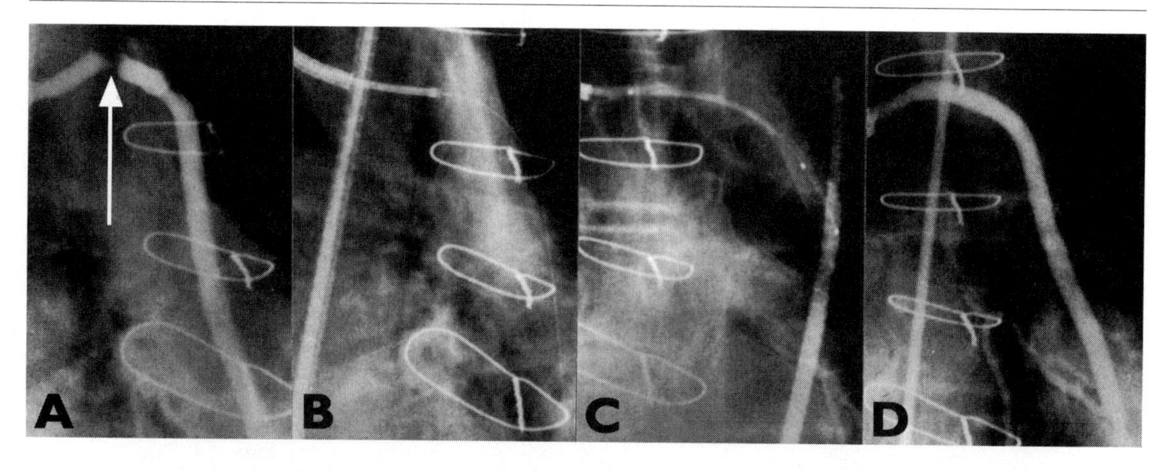

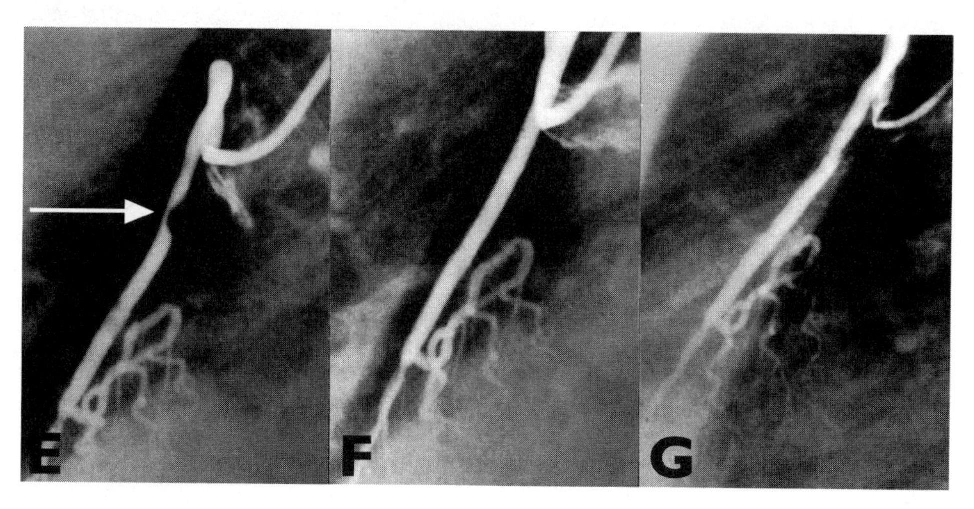

Figure 11.1 Stents and Saphenous Vein Grafts Severe lesions were located in the bypass grafts to the first obtuse marginal (**a**) and anterior descending (**e**) saphenous vein graft conduits. The obtuse marginal graft was debulked with TEC (**b**) and a Wallstent was deployed (**c**). The result obtained was maintained at 6-month angiography (**d**). The graft to the anterior descending artery (**e**) was also treated with implantation of a Wallstent (**f**) which had minor focal narrowing 6 months later (**g**).

The next day, an extra support guidewire was passed across the left anterior descending graft lesion into the apical left anterior descending artery segment (**Figure 11.1e**). The lesion was not predilated and a Wallstent was positioned to cover the diseased segment. The stent was released and post-dilated with a 4.0mm x 20mm balloon, again leaving no residual narrowing (**Figure 11.1f**). The patient became angina free and had no elevation of CPK during the hospitalization.

At 6-month follow-up, he remained angina free. An exercise test was stopped at 7 METS because of claudication without evidence of angina or electrocardiographic changes. Angiography revealed a good result in the obtuse marginal graft (**Figure 11.1d**) and a mild restenosis (40-50%) in the mid left anterior descending graft stent (**Figure 11.1g**). The patient has remained asymptomatic on medical therapy.

MATERIALS 11.1

DAY 1:	**Obtuse Marginal Graft**
Guiding Catheter:	Interventional Technologies FR 3.5 (10 F) TEC guiding catheter
Guidewires:	Interventional Technologies 0.014"x 300cm TEC guide wire
Atherotome:	Interventional Technologies TEC 2.0 mm coronary catheter (6F)
Balloons:	Schneider Bypass Spe``edy 4.5mm x 20mm
Stents:	Schneider Wallstent 5mm x 35mm (44mm length when deployed to 4.5mm)
DAY 2:	**LAD Graft**
Guiding Catheter:	Cook Lumax JR-4 8 French
Guidewires:	ACS Extra Support 0.014"x 300cm
Balloons:	Mansfield High Energy 4.0 x 20mm
Stents:	Schneider Wallstent 6mm x 23mm (>35mm length when deployed to 4.0mm)

CASE 11.2: Vein Graft Restenosis

The patient is a 70 year old who underwent 2-vessel bypass surgery 12 years earlier and had presented multiple times over the past 3 years with progressive disease of both the native vessels and of the saphenous vein graft to the right coronary artery. Because of severe left ventricular dysfunction and a stroke with

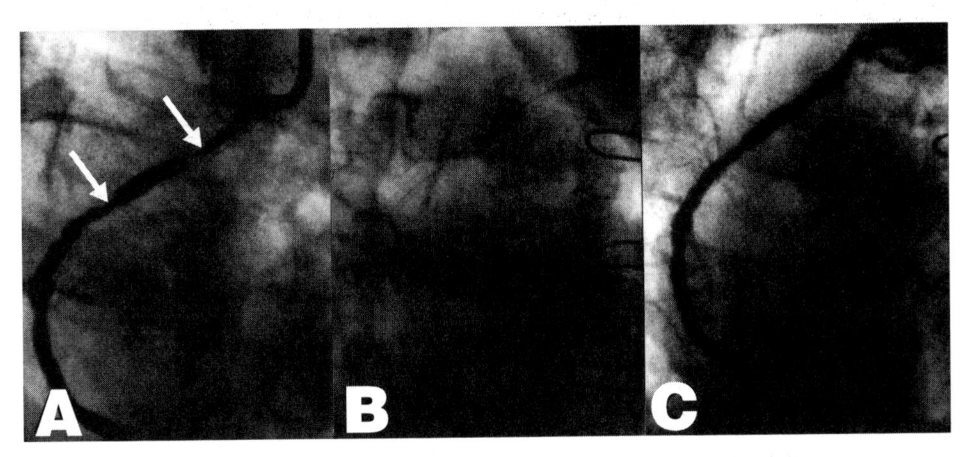

Figure 11.2 Stents and Saphenous Vein Grafts This restenotic graft to the right coronary artery already has a Wallstent implanted within a Palmaz-Schatz I stent (**a**) for prior disease. A laser catheter is noted debulking within the previous stents (**b**). The final result is seen in **c**.

residual hemiparesis, repeat coronary artery bypass graft operation was refused. He had received Palmaz-Schatz stents to proximal and distal segments of the right coronary graft 1 year earlier for refractory angina. Restenosis of the proximal stent resulted in refractory angina once again after 8 months. He had an implantation of a Wallstent within the proximal Palmaz-Schatz to improve the restenotic lumen. Balloon inflations to 20 atm were necessary to fully expand the fibrotic segment. Within 4 months of the second stenting, angina recurred due to a severe second restenosis in a diffuse pattern within the two stents (**Figure 11.2 a** arrows depict previous stents). As the patient remained symptomatic without a surgical option, he was referred for treatment of the in-stent restenosis.

PROCEDURE 11.2

Because of the extremely high pressures required on previous dilations and the diffuse nature of the restenosis, it was decided to ablate the lesion first with directional laser before proceeding with balloon dilation. Severe peripheral artery disease required using a brachial arterial access. An extra support guidewire was passed across the lesion into the native right coronary artery. The eccentric laser made 4 passes at a fluence of 60 mj/mm and a frequency of 30 repetitions per second. The resulting lumen (**Figure 11.2b**) was further dilated with a 3.5 x 35mm balloon to 18 atm (**Figure 11.2c**). The patient remains angina free.

MATERIALS 11.2

Guiding Catheter:	SciMed Mighty-Max MP-1 7 French
Guidewires:	ACS/Guidant Extra Support
Balloons:	USCI Samba Rely 3.5 x 20 mm
Stents:	None
Laser:	Spectranetics 2.0mm Vitesse E-II eccentric laser

DISCUSSION

Coronary Artery Bypass Grafting and Coronary Artery Disease Progression

Saphenous venous bypass segments begin a progressive degeneration immediately after surgery. Approximately 15-20% of venous bypass grafts are occluded by the end of the first post-operative year, most often due to technical problems during operation and thrombosis. Intimal proliferation and progressive atherosclerosis account for a rate of graft attrition of 2-4% per year.[1] Twelve percent of coronary artery bypass graft patients require an additional revascularization procedure after 5 years.[2] By 10 years, recurrent ischemia is present in 63% of patients.[3] In 76% of patients suffering a myocardial infarction after coronary artery bypass grafting, the culprit vessel will be a saphenous vein graft.[4] Since an increased morbidity/mortality rate and less effective relief of symptoms are associated with repeated coronary artery bypass graft procedures, alternate revascularization therapies are often preferred for these patients.[5,6]

Angioplasty Results for Saphenous Vein Grafts

There are important differences in the results of coronary angioplasty between vein grafts and the native coronary arteries. The absence of proximal tortuosity and side branches, the lower rate of dissection and the lower rate of acute occlusion (1.5% for saphenous vein graft vs. 5% for native vessels) make saphenous vein graft angioplasty seem less challenging than that of the native circulation.[7-9] However, severe fibrosis and increased elastic recoil are common and may require high pressure balloon inflations or lesion debulking. The tendency to produce vessel rupture may be greater in fibrotic vein grafts. The disparity of graft to target vessel size, the absence of multiple branch tributaries and the diffuse pattern of atherosclerosis in mature grafts is associated with a predisposition for thrombus formation. The amount of atheromatous material is often higher than in native vessels, and consequently, the rate of distal embolization and secondary infarction is proportionately higher. Embolization during saphenous vein graft angioplasty is associated with diffusely diseased segments, older lesions, thrombus, total occlusions, and eccentric or bulky lesions.[10-12] "No-reflow" reactions may occur during saphenous vein graft interventions in approximately 15% of patients.[13] Conventional angioplasty for saphenous vein graft disease is associated with reduced success, more frequent complications, and increased restenosis rates. While distal embolization may be limited to 5%,[14] angioplasty in grafts is associated with a 13% rate of non-Q myocardial infarction.[15] Saphenous vein graft disease is somewhat different from native vessels and the potential problems should be anticipated for prompt treatment.

Saphenous Vein Graft Restenosis after Angioplasty

Restenosis after balloon angioplasty in mature vein grafts ranges from 48-61%.[13,16-18] The restenosis rate after angioplasty in saphenous bypass grafts depends on both the age of the graft and the location of the stenosis (Table 11.1).[19]

These data demonstrate that while angioplasty of a distal anastomotic lesion within a year of surgery has a reasonable likelihood of long-term success, angioplasty of a proximal anastomotic segment of a degenerating 10 year-old graft has poor long-term success.

Alternative Percutaneous Techniques

Although one study reported that directional coronary atherectomy (DCA) provided similar efficacy to stents for vein graft disease,[20] DCA more typically is associated with an increased incidence of distal embolization (13%), increased periprocedural myocardial infarction, and no significant reduction in restenosis (46-63%) compared to angioplasty[14,21,22]

Table 11.1: Restenosis after Angioplasty in Bypass Grafts is Based on Time Since Surgery and on Location Within the Graft

TIME SINCE CABG	RESTENOSIS RATE AFTER PTCA (%)	
<6 months	32	
6-12 months	43	
1-5 years	61	
>5 years	64	
LOCATION OF SVG LESION	**RESTENOSIS RATE AFTER PTCA (%)**	**FIVE YEAR SURVIVAL (%)**
Proximal	68	67
Mid vein graft	61	72
Distal anastomotic	45	92

Adapted from Douglas JS Jr. Textbook of Interventional Cardiology, 2nd Ed. 1994 pp 339-354.

The TEC device was initially advocated for diffuse vein graft disease because of its ability to cut plaque and aspirate thrombus and atheromatous debris. However, TEC was associated with a 12% rate of distal embolization and high restenosis rates (69%) when applied to mature vein grafts.[23] Deferring balloon angioplasty after TEC until several weeks of anticoagulation have been completed may reduce the rate of distal embolization.[24] Nonetheless, this device appears to have a limited role except in the debulking of totally occluded, thrombosed segments.

Laser angioplasty has been used in the proximal vein graft anastomosis with high success and low complication rates.[25,26] Unfortunately, the restenosis rate remains high (57%).[27] Laser angioplasty is also plagued by high rates of distal embolization when applied to lesions in the body of bypass grafts.[28]

Stents for Saphenous Vein Grafts

The amount of elastic recoil in mature saphenous vein grafts and the need to scaffold large amounts of atheromatous material may account for the reported increased efficacy of stents for saphenous vein graft disease.[29] In contrast to angioplasty, the results of stent implantation are not so dependent upon the age of the conduit.[30,31] Stent implantation in vein grafts success rates of 97% appear more successful than native vessel stent deployment.[31] The residual lumen is larger, and there are lower rates of complications after stent implantation in mature vein grafts than after angioplasty, directional atherectomy or extraction atherectomy.[32] In addition, low subacute thrombosis (1%) and distal embolization (2%) rates suggest a particular advantage to stent implantation in vein grafts,[31-33] a result which may be due to a lower tendency for very large conduits to thrombose when stented compared to native vessels.

Saphenous Vein Graft Stents and Restenosis

The major advantage of stents in bypass graft therapy appears to be a reduction of restenosis. Restenosis rates after stenting of de novo graft lesions are about 20%, with an event-free survival at one year of 70-75%,[31,34] significantly better than any other percutaneous therapy for these lesions.[31,33-35] These results are being examined by a prospective randomized study of saphenous vein graft angioplasty vs stenting.[36] The major predictors of saphenous vein graft restenosis after stenting include restenotic lesions, small reference vessel size, diabetes mellitus, and residual percent stenosis. Importantly, saphenous vein graft age and the implantation of multiple stents are not predictive of restenosis.[31] However, the restenosis benefit in stented de novo grafts does not appear to extend to restenotic lesions, saphenous vein grafts of <3mm diameter, or ostial lesions.[34,37] Furthermore, although the 6-month restenosis rate after stenting of saphenous vein grafts may be as low as 17%, a 49% incidence of late revascularization by 2 years was reported and was attributed mainly to the progression of disease at other sites.[33] Unlike restenosis in native vessels, continuation of the restenotic process in the treated segment of vein grafts beyond a 6-month period has been suggested by the continued presence of reactive cells.[38]

Stent Designs for Saphenous Vein Graft Disease

There is a significant experience using Palmaz-Schatz,[31,39] Gianturco-Roubin,[40] Wiktor[41] and Wallstent[42] designs in vein graft lesions. Each design offers a particular advantage, such as extra radial support from the Palmaz-Schatz biliary design, flexibility and radiopacity with the Wiktor stent, and the ability to entrap friable graft material with the mesh design Wallstent. However, there is little comparative data among different types of stent.

The Palmaz biliary stent offers increased resistance to radial compressive force, increased radiopacity, and a greater expansion range (4-9mm vs 3-5mm) than the Palmaz-Schatz coronary stent (see **STENT REFERENCE CHART**). However, when compared in vein graft lesions, the two stents were not significantly different despite the theoretical advantages of the biliary stent.[43]

The Wiktor stent design, and possibly other coil designs in general, may not be well suited to lesions in the proximal graft anastomosis due to a tendency to unravel.[44] The relative incidence of embolization and restenosis of coil designs compared to more effective scaffolding designs will be addressed in ongoing trials. Whether different stent design features will confer special benefits in different types of graft lesions remains to be seen.

Technical Pearls

Certain technical points deserve emphasis when stenting patients with saphenous vein bypass graft lesions. Because of the significant rate of late progression of disease in degenerating vein grafts, the native vessels should be preferentially treated whenever possible. The long-term results of stenting short, occluded native segments will exceed the results in treating diffusely diseased graft segments.

Should less severely stenosed saphenous vein graft segments next to target lesions be treated? Since the late event rate in lesions of 40-50% may approach 40%, an aggressive treatment approach may be of value.[45]

Many vein graft lesions are far away from the guiding catheter. Have a sufficiently long balloon catheter to reach the stenosis. Balloon catheters with long shafts (140-150 cm), short guiding catheters (90 cm) or guiding catheter shortening maneuvers may be necessary to reach these distant lesions.[46]

The extra fibrosis of mature vein graft lesions often requires predilations of higher pressures than for native vessels. The operator should be prepared for such a contingency with an adequate predilation balloon. The extent of diseased segment predilatation should be limited to minimize distal embolization. Severe fibrosis occasionally may result in "slippage" of the balloon from the lesion. A long balloon will overcome this problem. High pressure angioplasty may rupture fibrotic, semi-inert saphenous vein graft segments. Every effort should be made to avoid oversizing balloons to the graft in ratios of greater than 1.1 to 1.2.

Finally, ReoPro (c7E3 Fab) may reduce the distal embolization rate by 5-7 fold during saphenous vein graft interventions in acute infarctions and may be useful in treating grafts with ominous angiographic characteristics.[47]

Special Considerations

While enthusiasm for stent implantation in vein grafts continues to increase, balloon angioplasty remains an excellent option for the treatment of distal anastomotic lesions, especially within the first post-operative year. Although acute success rates are impressive, percutaneous therapies of diffusely diseased grafts remain only palliative, not curative of the inevitable progression of disease elsewhere in the graft. Thus, repeat bypass surgery should remain the treatment of choice in patients with lesions characteristic of a poor percutaneous outcome. Multiple or bulky lesions and angiographic evidence of extensive thrombus are predictive of a poor outcome.[48] The frequency of distal embolization is directly related to the extent and severity of disease and thrombus.[49] Controversy exists regarding stents for ostial lesions. Restenosis after stent implantation has been reported from 16-60%.[34,50-52] The expected recurrence rate at the proximal anastomosis site remains unknown.

Treating Occluded Saphenous Vein Grafts

In situations in which the graft has become completely occluded, recanalization is frequently associated with poor outcomes. The low success rate and high rate of embolization and infarction in chronically occluded vein grafts have traditionally argued against treatment with conventional angioplasty.[53] Prolonged local urokinase infusions may recanalize a significant number of these grafts but at an increased cost of distal embolization, myocardial infarction, and abrupt closure in over 30% after adjunctive angioplasty.[54,55] The incidence of non-Q-wave infarction attributed to distal embolization and no-reflow may be reduced by intracoronary verapamil and by increasing the rate of urokinase infusion for chest pain or electrocardiographic changes.[56,57] The restenosis rate and one year event free survival after this technique are approximately 50%, a result which may be improved with post-lytic stent implantation.

SUMMARY

Preliminary results extended by ongoing prospective investigations and comparative trails among stent designs and techniques appear to support a preeminent role of stents in the treatment of diseased saphenous vein bypass grafts.

References

1. Bourassa MG, Enjalbert M, Campeau L, et al. *Progression of atherosclerosis in coronary arteries and bypass grafts: ten years later.* Am J Cardiol 53:102c-107 (1984).
2. Meeter KL, Van den Brand MJBM, Lubsen J, et al. *Incidence, risk and outcome of reintervention after aortocoronary bypass surgery.* Br Heart J 57:427-435 (1987).
3. Campeau L, Lesperance J, Hermann J, et al. *The relation of risk factors to the development of atherosclerosis of saphenous vein bypass grafts and the progression of disease in the native circulation: a study 10 years after aortocoronary bypass surgery.* N Engl J Med 31:1329-1332 (1984).
4. Grines CL, Booth DC, Nissen, et al. *Mechanism of acute myocardial infarction in patients with prior coronary artery bypass grafting and therapeutic implications.* Am J Cardiol 65:1292-1296 (1990).
5. Lytle BW, Loop FD, Cosgrove DM, et al. *Fifteen hundred coronary reoperations: results and determinants of early and late survival.* J Thorac Cardiovasc Surg 93:847-859 (1987).
6. Shaff HV, Orzulak TA, Gersh BJ, et al. *The morbidity and mortality of reoperation for coronary artery disease and analysis of late results with use of actuarial estimate of event-free interval.* J Thorac Cardiovasc Surg 85:508-515 (1983).
7. El Gamal M, Bonnier H, Michels R, et al. *Percutaneous transluminal angioplasty of stenosed aortocoronary bypass grafts.* Br Heart J 52:617-620 (1984).
8. Corbelli J, Franco I, Hollman J, et al. *Percutaneous transluminal coronary angioplasty after previous coronary artery bypass surgery.* Am J Cardiol 56:398-403 (1985).
9. Cote G, Myler RK, Stertzer SH, et al. *Percutaneous transluminal angioplasty of stenotic coronary artery bypass grafts: 5 year's experience.* J Am Coll Cardiol 9:8-17 (1987).
10. Liu MW, Douglas JS JR, Lembo NJ, et al. *Angiographic predictors of a rise in serum creatine kinase (distal embolization) after balloon angioplasty of saphenous vein coronary artery bypass grafts.* Am J Cardiol 72:514-517 (1993).

11. Altman D, Popma J, Hong M, et al. *CPK-MB elevation after angioplasty of saphenous vein grafts.* J Am Coll Cardiol 21(suppl A):232A (1993).

12. Lefkovits J, Holmes DR, Califf RM, et al. *Predictors and sequelae of distal embolization during saphenous vein graft intervention from the CAVEAT-II trial.* Circulation 92:734-740 (1995).

13. Platko WP, Hollman J, Whitlow PL, Franco I. *Percutaneous transluminal angioplasty of saphenous vein graft stenosis: long-term follow-up.* J Am Coll Cardiol 14:1645-1650 (1989).

14. Holmes DR, Topol EJ, Califf RM, et al. *A multicenter, randomized trial of coronary angioplasty versus directional atherectomy for patients with saphenous vein bypass graft lesions.* Circulation 91:1966-1974 (1995).

15. Douglas JS JR, Weintraub WS, Liberman HA, et al. *Update of saphenous graft (SVG) angioplasty: restenosis and longterm outcome.* Circulation 84(suppl II):II-249 (1991)

16. Douglas JS Jr, Gruentzig AR, King SB, et al. *Percutaneous transluminal coronary angioplasty in patients with prior coronary bypass surgery.* J Am Coll Cardiol 2:745-754 (1983).

17. Webb JG, Myler RK, Shaw RE, et al. *Coronary angioplasty after coronary bypass surgery: Initial results and late outcome in 422 patients.* J Am Coll Cardiol 16:812-820 (1990).

18. Reeves F, Bonan R, Cote G, et al. *Long-term angiographic follow-up after angioplasty of venous coronary bypass grafts.* Am Heart J 122:620-627 (1991).

19. Douglas JS Jr. *Percutaneous intervention in patients with prior coronary bypass surgery. In:* Topol EJ (ed) "Textbook of Interventional Cardiology, 2nd Edition. WB Saunders Co. 1994.

20. Pomerantz RM, Kuntz RE, Carrozza JP, et al. *Acute and long-term outcome of narrowed saphenous venous grafts treated by endoluminal stenting and directional atherectomy.* Am J Cardiol 70:161-167 (1992).

21. Hinohara T, Robertson GC, Selmon MR, et al. *Restenosis after directional coronary atherectomy.* J Am Coll Cardiol 20:623-632 (1992).

22. Cowley MJ, DiSciascio G. *Directional coronary atherectomy for saphenous vein graft disease.* Cathet Cardiovasc Diagn 1(suppl):10-16 (1993).

23. Safian RD, Grines CL, May MA, et al. *Clinical and angiographic results of transluminal extraction coronary atherectomy in saphenous vein bypass grafts.* Circulation 89:302-312 (1994).

24. Hong MK, Popma JJ, Pichard AD, et al. *The clinical significance of distal embolization after transluminal extraction atherectomy in diffusely diseased saphenous vein grafts.* Am Heart J 127:1496-1503 (1994).

25. Eigler NL, Weinstock B, Douglas JS, et al. *Excimer laser coronary angioplasty of aorto- ostial stenoses.* Circulation 88:2049-2057 (1993).

26. Bittl JA, Sanborn TA, Yardley DE, et al. *Predictors of outcome of percutaneous excimer laser coronary angioplasty of saphenous vein bypass graft lesions.* Am J Cardiol 74:144-148 (1994).

27. Untereker WJ, Palacios IF, Hartzler G, et al. *Excimer laser coronary angioplasty of saphenous vein grafts.* Circulation 86(suppl I):I-780 (1992).

28. Baumbach A, Bittl JA, Fleck E, et al. *Acute complications of excimer laser coronary angioplasty: a detailed analysis of multicenter results.* J Am Coll Cardiol 23:1305-1313 (1994).

29. Hong MK, Popma JJ, Leon MB, et al. *Vascular recoil in saphenous vein graft stenoses after investigational angioplasty [abstr].* J Am Coll Cardiol 19:263A (1992).

30. Abdelmeguid AE, Ellis S, Whitlow P, et al. *Lack of graft age dependency for success of directional coronary atherectomy and Palmaz-Schatz stenting.* J Am Coll Cardiol 21(suppl A):31A (1993).

31. Wong SC, Baim DS, Schatz RA, et al. *Immediate results and late outcomes after stent implantation in saphenous vein graft lesions: the multicenter U.S. Palmaz-Schatz stent experience.* J Am Coll Cardiol 26:704-712 (1995).

32. Leon MB, Ellis SG, Pichard AD, et al. *Stents may be the preferred treatment for focal aortocoronary vein graft disease.* Circulation 84(suppl II):II-249 (1991).

33. Piana RN, Moscucci M, Cohen DJ, et al. *Palmaz-Schatz stenting for treatment of focal vein graft stenosis: Immediate results and long term outcome.* J Am Coll Cardiol 23:1296-1304 (1994).

34. Fenton SH, Fischman DL, Savage MP, et al. *Long-Term angiographic and clinical outcome after implantation of balloon-expandable stents in aortocoronary saphenous vein grafts.* Am J Cardiol 74:1187-1191 (1994).

35. Pomerantz RM, Kuntz RE, Carrozza JP, et al. *Acute and long-term outcome of narrowed saphenous venous grafts treated by endoluminal stenting and directional atherectomy.* Am J Cardiol 70:161-167 (1992).

36. Douglas JS Jr, Savage MP, Bailey SR, et al. *Randomized trial of coronary stent and balloon angioplasty in the treatment of saphenous vein graft stenosis* [abstr]. J Am Coll Cardiol 27:178A (1996).

37. Wong SC, Hong MK, Popma JJ, et al. *Stent placement for the treatment of aorto-ostial saphenous vein graft lesions [abstr].* J Am Coll Cardiol 23:118A (1994).

38. van Beusekom HMM, van der Giessen WJ, van Suylen RJ, et al. *Histology after stenting of human saphenous vein bypass grafts: observations from surgically excised grafts 3 to 320 days after stent implantation.* J Am Coll Cardiol 21:45-54 (1993).

39. Leon MB, Ellis SG, Pichard AD, et al. *Balloon expandable stent implantation in saphenous vein grafts. In: Herrmann HC, Hirshfeld JW (eds). Clinical use of the Palmaz-Schatz balloon-expandable stent.* Mount Kisco, New York: Futura Publishing Company, 1993, pp.111-121.

40. Dorros G, Bates MC, Iyer S, et al. *The use of Gianturco-Roubin flexible metallic coronary stents in old saphenous vein grafts: in-hospital outcome and 7 day angiographic patency.* Eur Heart J 15:1456-1462 (1994).

41. Vaishnav S, Azia S, Layton C. *Clinical experience with the Wiktor stent in native coronary arteries and coronary bypass grafts.* Br Heart J 72:288-293 (1994).

42. Strauss BH, Serruys PW, Bertrand ME, et al. *Quantitative angiographic follow-up of the coronary Wallstent in native vessels and bypass grafts* (European experience-March 1986-March 1990). Am J Cardiol 69:475-481 (1992).

43. Wong SC, Popma JJ, Pichard AD, et al. *Comparison of clinical and angiographic outcomes after saphenous vein graft angioplasty using coronary versus 'biliary tubular slotted stents.* Circulation 91:339-350 (1995).

44. Chalet Y, Panes F, Chevalier B, et al. *Should we avoid ostial implants of Wiktor stents?* Cathet Cardiovasc Diagn 32:376-379 (1994).

45. Ellis SG, Brener SJ, DeLuca et al. *Late myocardial ischemic events after saphenous vein graft intervention— importance of initially "nonsignificant" vein graft lesions.* Am J Cardiol 79: 1460-1464 (1997)

46. Agarwal R, Kaul U, Jain P. *Technical considerations in deploying the sheathed Palmaz- Schatz stent in distal coronary artery and bypass graft lesions.* Cathet Cardiovasc Diagn 37:73-75(1996).

47. Challapalli RM, Eisenberg MJ, Sigmon K, Limberger J. *Platelet glycoprotein IIb/IIIa monoclonal antibody (c7E3) reduces distal embolization during percutaneous intervention of saphenous vein grafts.* Circulation 92(suppl I):I-607 (1995).

48. Liu MW, Douglas JS JR, King SB III, et al. *Angiographic predictors of coronary embolization in the PTCA of vein graft lesions.* Circulation 80(suppl II):II-172 (1989).

49. Lefkovits J, Holmes DR, Califf RM, et al. *Predictors and sequelae of distal embolization during saphenous vein graft intervention from the CAVEAT-II trial.* Circulation 92:734-740 (1995).

50. Nordrehaug JE, Priestley KA, Chronos NAF, et al. *Self expanding stents for the management of aorto-ostial stenoses in saphenous vein bypass grafts.* Br Heart J 72:285-287 (1994).

51. Rocha-Singh K, Morris N, Wong C, et al. *Coronary stenting for treatment of ostial stenoses of native coronary arteries or aortocoronary saphenous venous grafts.* Am J Cardiol 75:26-29 (1995).

52. Rechavia E, Litvack F, Macko G, et al. *Stent implantation of saphenous vein graft aorto- ostial lesions in patients with unstable ischemic syndromes: immediate angiographic results and long-term clinical outcome.* J Am Coll Cardiol 25:866-870 (1995).

53. deFeyter PJ, Serruys P, van den Brand M, et al. *Percutaneous transluminal angioplasty of a totally occluded bypass graft: A challenge that should be resisted.* Am J Cardiol 64:88-90 (1989).

54. Sievert H, Kohler KP, Kaltenbach M, Kober G. *Wiedereroffnung langstreckig verschlossener aortokoronarer venen-bypasses.* Deutsch Med Wochenschr 113:637-640 (1988).

55. Hartman JR, McKeever LS, Stamato NJ, et al. *Recanalization of chronically occluded aortocoronary saphenous vein bypass grafts by extended infusion of urokinase: Initial results and short term clinical follow-up.* J Am Coll Cardiol 18:1517-1523 (1991).

56. Cecena FA, Hoelzinger DH. *Transcatheter therapy of thrombotic-occlusive lesions in saphenous vein grafts.* Am J Cardiol 78:31-36 (1996).

57. Hartmann JR, McKeever LS, O'Neill WW, et al. *Recanalization of chronically occluded aortocoronary saphenous vein bypass grafts with long-term, low dose direct infusion of urokinase (ROBUST): a serial trail.* J Am Coll Cardiol 27:60-66 (1996).

58. Levine DJ, Sharaf Bl, Williams DO. *Late follow-up of patients with totally occluded saphenous vein bypass grafts treated by prolonged selective urokinase infusion [abstr].* J Am Coll Cardiol 19:292A (1992).

59. Denardo SJ, Morris NB, Rocha-Singh KJ, et al. *Safety and efficacy of extended urokinase infusion plus stent deployment for treatment of obstructed, older saphenous vein grafts.* Am J Cardiol 76:776-780 (1995).

60. Kramer B. *Optimal therapy for degenerated saphenous vein graft disease.* J Invas Cardiol 7:14D-20D (1995).

61. Wong SC, Popma JJ, Kent KM, et al. *Clinical experience with stent implantation in the treatment of saphenous vein graft lesions. J Interven Cardiol 7:565-573 (1994).*

CHAPTER 12

BAILOUT STENTING

CASE 12.1: Uncovered Residual Dissection

A 64 year old man had recurrent angina after a non-Q-wave myocardial infarction (peak CPK 325 IU/liter). Quantitative coronary angiography revealed a 90% non-calcified mid right coronary artery lesion (**Figure 12.1a**). Ad hoc angioplasty was then performed.

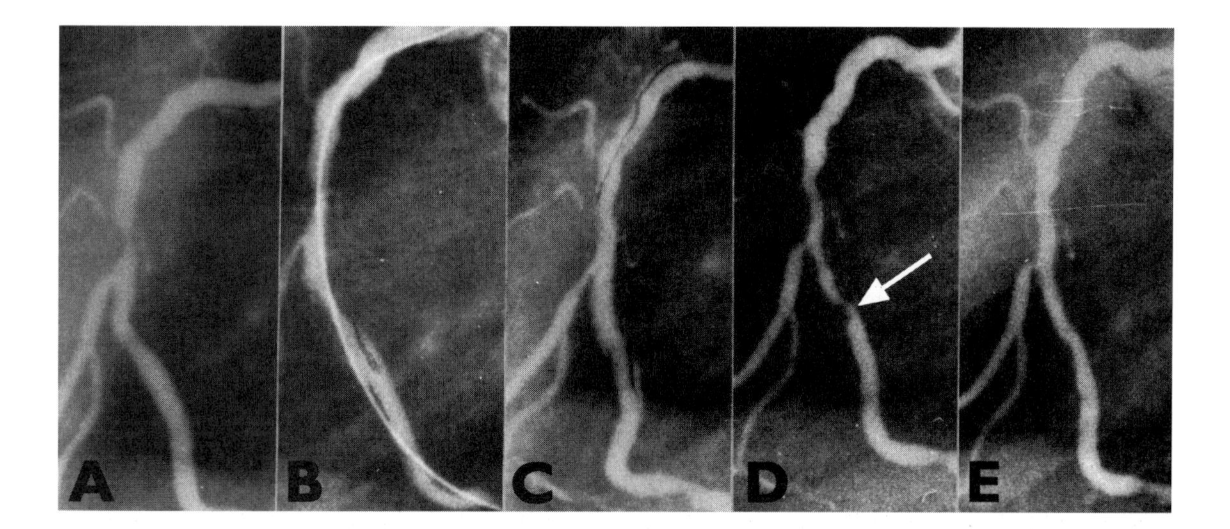

Figure 12.1 Restenosis of Uncovered Distal Dissection Angioplasty of this mid right coronary artery lesion (**a**) resulted in a type F dissection (**b**) which ultimately progressed to obstruction. A type B dissection distally was left untreated after stent implantation (**c**). At 6-month angiography, there was restenosis at the site of the untreated dissection (**d** arrow) which was treated with angioplasty. Angiography one year after the original procedure revealed a persistent good result (**e**).

PROCEDURE 12.1

Using a standard JR4 Judkins-shaped guiding catheter and a flexible exchange guidewire, the first balloon inflation (3mm balloon) was performed, producing a dissection distal to the dilation site. This dissection progressed with a spiral luminal defect with contrast filling outside the arterial lumen with TIMI grade 0 flow (NHLBI Dissection Grade F) (**Figure 12.1b**). A perfusion balloon was passed and inflated for 30 minutes providing improved flow but without significant improvement in the angiographic luminal filling defects. A Palmaz-Schatz stent was hand-mounted on the original balloon, passed distal to the original lesion site in the region of the most severe dissection, and implanted at 12 atm. Despite a persistent Grade B dissection distal to the stent (**Figure 12.1c**), normal flow resumed and the extraluminal contrast resolved. Excellent angiographic flow without ischemia was documented during a 20-minute observation period. It was elected not to place additional stents in the residual distal dissection. The patient had an uneventful recovery and was discharged several days later.

The patient was asymptomatic for 6 months. Angina returned with ischemia on exercise testing at 6 METS. Repeat angiography revealed an 80% restenotic lesion at the untreated dissection site distal to the stent (**Figure 12.1d**). Sequential 3.0mm balloon inflations at 14 atm resolved the narrowing to <20% residual stenosis. The patient was again discharged and remains asymptomatic. Angiography 12 months after the original procedure showed no evidence of a second restenosis (**Figure 12.1e**).

MATERIALS 12.1

Guiding Catheter:	Schneider Visiguide JR-4 8 French
Guide wires:	USCI Veriflex 0.014"x 300 cm
Balloons:	Schneider Speedy 3 x 20mm
	Schneider PCP Mainz 3 x 20mm (perfusion balloon)
Stents:	Johnson & Johnson P-S 153 (15mm)

CASE 12.2: Two Lumens after Stenting

A 63 year old man presented with recent onset of angina and an abnormal exercise test. There was no history of myocardial infarction. At cardiac catheterization, a subtotal distal occlusion of the right coronary artery with TIMI grade 1 flow was found.

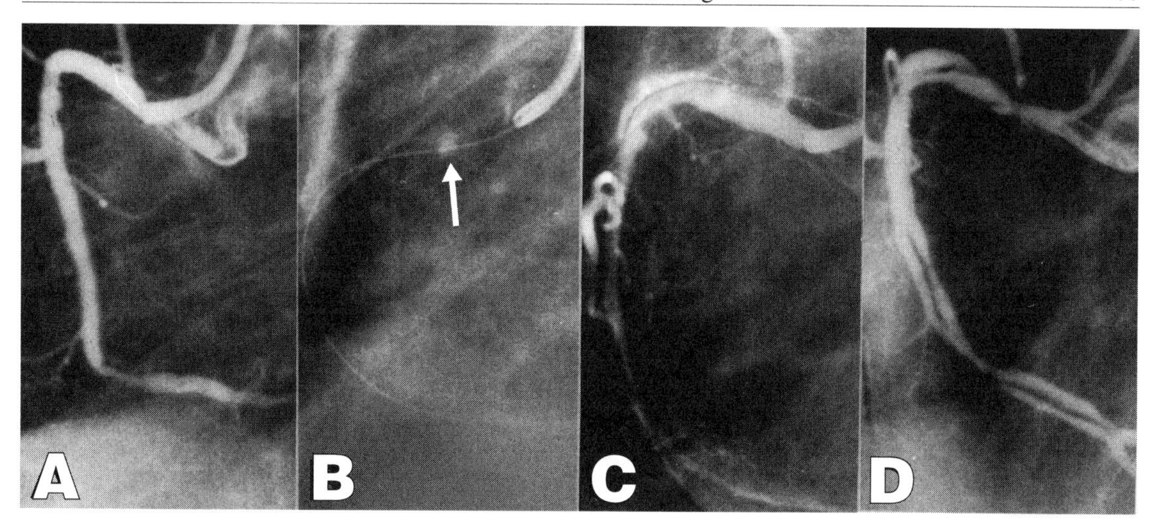

Figure 12.2 Stents and False Lumens The subtotal occlusion of this right coronary artery distally (**a**) was complicated by a Shepherd's crook curve in the proximal vessel. Guiding catheter trauma resulted in dissection and contrast staining of the coronary ostium (**b; arrow**). Despite treating the ostium with stent implantation, dissection persisted extending distally from just beyond the stent (**c**). At 6-month angiography, two lumens persisted with one beginning just after the stent and progressing into the posterolateral system, while the other started at the ostium and continued to the posterior descending artery (**d**).

PROCEDURE 12.2

Angioplasty required negotiation of an acutely angled proximal segment of the right coronary artery before reaching the distal subtotal occlusion (**Figure 12.2a**). The lesion was crossed with some difficulty using an 0.018" floppy guide wire. During dilation of the distal lesion, contrast staining of the ostia and proximal aorta (presumably due to guiding catheter trauma) was noted (**Figure 12.2b**). Further angiography demonstrated a severe dissection now extending from the coronary ostium to the crux. In an attempt to control the dissection, a Palmaz-Schatz I stent was implanted in the right coronary ostium. However, the dissection extended to the distal right coronary artery (**Figure 12.2c**). Despite the extensive dissection, the patient remained asymptomatic. It was elected to leave the suboptimal result rather than implanting additional stents into a potential false lumen.

At 6-month follow-up, the patient was asymptomatic with a negative treadmill test. Angiography revealed that the partial bailout had functioned better than anticipated. Two lumens were now present in the right coronary artery. The true lumen passed through the restenosed distal right coronary lesion into the posterior descending branch, while the false lumen beginning just after the stent (**Figure 12.2d**) extended parallel to the first, but diverged distally and filled the posterolateral system (**Figure 12.2d**). The patient was managed conservatively and remained asymptomatic with a negative exercise test one year after the initial procedure.

MATERIALS 12.2

Guiding Catheter:	Cook Lumax JR-4 8 French
Guide wires:	ACS high torque floppy 0.018"x 300cm
Balloons:	SciMed Cobra 3.5 x 20mm
Stents:	Johnson & Johnson PS 153

DISCUSSION

The definition of bailout stent implantation after angioplasty has included everything from the "touch-up" of vessels exhibiting residual stenosis or dissection to the rescue of acutely occluded vessels. Consequently, it is difficult to compare the results of different studies of bailout stenting because most studies contain different ratios of patients with complete occlusions or with suboptimal angiographic results. The likelihood of subsequent complications after bailout stent implantation varies considerably depending upon the percentage of acute occlusions included in each series. The decision when to implant a stent after angioplasty hinges upon the likelihood of acute occlusion. The predictors of acute occlusion after angioplasty also influence stent efficacy for procedural salvage. Certain clinical situations favor early stent implantation over prolonged angioplasty balloon inflations.

Abrupt Closure after Coronary Angioplasty

Abrupt closure is the major complication of the angioplasty resulting in myocardial infarction, emergent revascularization, and death. The incidence of acute closure after angioplasty has fallen markedly over the years as the technique has evolved. In the period between the two NHLBI registries (1979-1983 and 1985-1986), the rate of acute closure fell from 13.6% to 6.8%.[1,2] Pre-procedural factors which are predictive of acute coronary closure include unstable angina, female gender, stenosis length, location of the stenosis at a bend point of >45° or at a branch point, stenosis associated thrombus (filling defect or staining), other stenosis in the same vessel, recanalization of total occlusions, calcified lesions, right coronary artery location, and multivessel disease.[3-7] Peri-procedural factors predictive of acute closure include post-angioplasty percent stenosis, intimal tear or dissection, use of prolonged heparin infusion, and post-angioplasty pressure gradient >20mm Hg.[3]

Dissection Morphology and Acute Closure

The major mechanism by which angioplasty enlarges the arterial lumen is by dissection and disruption of the vessel. Early data suggested that this dissection is therapeutic and that without a visible dissection restenosis might be more frequent.[8] More recent analyses suggest that the presence of a visible dissection after angioplasty is unrelated to the incidence of restenosis.[9,56] However, some dissections are clearly problematic for acute occlusion. Waller et al[10] distinguished therapeutic from pathological dissections based on the extent of arterial disruption. Dissections limited to <50% of the vessel circumference and <1 cm in length pathologically were deemed therapeutic. Those dissections involving more of the circumference or length were termed complications.[10] A clinically useful system of describing dissections was applied in the NHLBI angioplasty registries (Appendix IV).[11] This dissection classification system is predictive of outcome. While low grade dissections (types A and B) result in a 3% incidence of major complications, more severe dissections (types C-F) are predictive of a 31% rate of acute closure.[12] Extra-luminal contrast and the absolute length of the dissection are the most important predictors of acute closure,[13] while complex dissections are generally accepted as harbingers of acute closure after angioplasty.[6] In the absence of any risk factors, acute occlusion occurs in about 2% of angioplasties, whereas in cases with three or more risk factors present (e.g. unstable angina, intracoronary thrombus, extreme age, long complex lesions, or diffuse disease), the risk of acute occlusion rises to 25%.[5]

Bailout Techniques for Angioplasty

Coronary bypass surgery was the original bailout technique for failed angioplasty. Urgent bypass surgery after angioplasty is associated with a 40% rate of myocardial infarction and a higher mortality rate than elective surgery.[14,15] Therefore, a number of alternatives have been proposed for rescue of failed angioplasty including thrombolysis,[16] prolonged inflations with oversized balloons,[17] perfusion balloons,[18] atherectomy,[19] radiofrequency thermal balloon,[20] and laser angioplasty.[21] However, no technique has rivaled the stent in the success rates after failed angioplasty.[22] Stenting for bailout of acute closure after angioplasty compared to prolonged balloon inflations reduces the 6-month rate of ischemic events.[23] In a study comparing bailout using Gianturco-Roubin stents with conventional bailout techniques of thrombolysis and prolonged balloon inflations, immediate treatment with a stent was associated with a lower incidence of myocardial infarction or emergent bypass surgery. In fact, thrombolytic therapy and prolonged balloon inflations were independently associated with increased risk of infarction compared to stent placement.[24] The ongoing studies comparing stent bailout with perfusion balloons and conventional angioplasty bailout techniques (Stent-by and TASC-II) are showing lower rates of myocardial infarction, re-intervention and, most importantly, restenosis (22% vs 50%) with stents.[25]

Complications After Bailout Procedures

Although early bailout experiences were associated with >90% success rates, the subacute thrombosis and its related complications reduced success to 75% by 30 days.[26,27] The incidence of subacute thrombosis (6-25%) is higher for bailout lesions than after elective stenting.[28-30] The frequency of subacute thrombosis correlates with the number of true acute occlusions included in each trial. Subacute closure has been associated with angiographically apparent thrombus[27] and with uncovered residual angiographic dissection.[29]

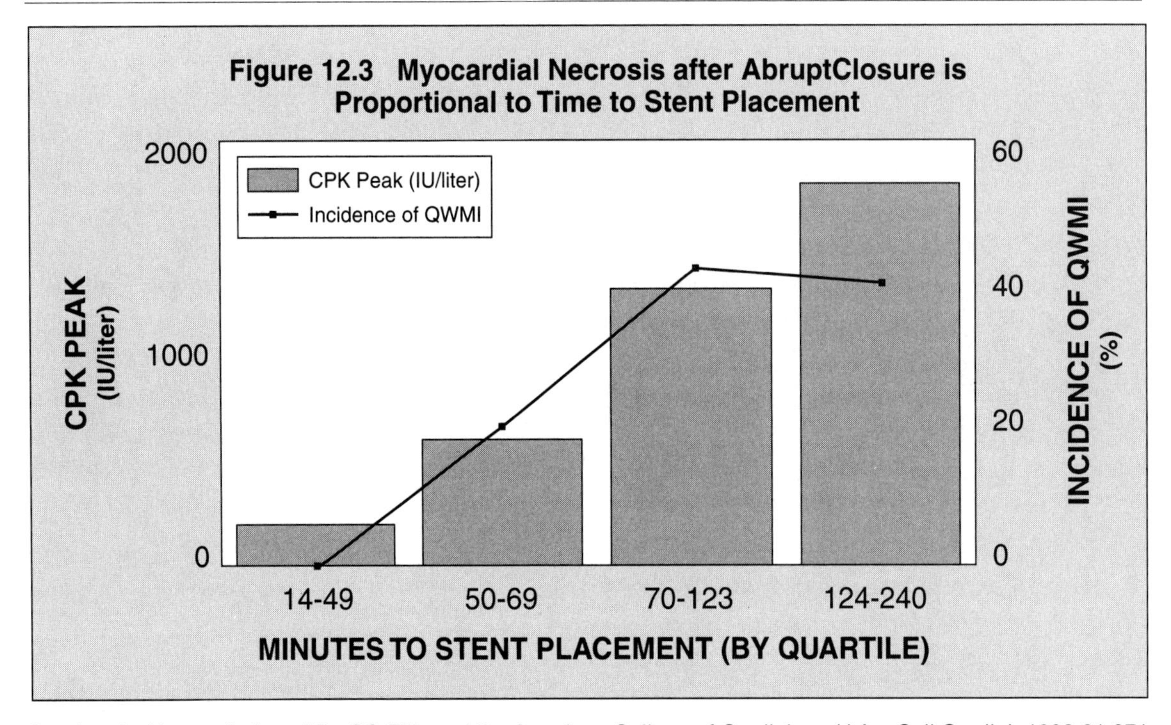

Reprinted with permission of Dr. SG Ellis and the American College of Cardiology (J Am Coll Cardiol: 1993;21;871

Figure 12.3 Myocardial Necrosis After Abrupt Closure is Proportional to the Time to Stent Placement. Delay after acute closure following angioplasty results in progressive myocardial necrosis in a proportional relation.

Restenosis is also more frequent after bailout stenting than after elective stenting, depending on the number of acute closures treated. Compared to restenosis rates of 20-30% after elective stenting, restenosis rates range from 39 to 53% after bailout implantation of both Palmaz-Schatz and Gianturco-Roubin stents.[27,29,31,32] When small vessels (<3.0mm in diameter) are stented for acute and threatened closure, the restenosis rates were especially high (66% in one study).[33]

The recent results of bailout stent implantation have been improved by implanting stents during the period of impending closure rather than waiting for acute closure after angioplasty.[34] Delay in bailout stenting has been repeatedly correlated with increased risk of ischemic complications.[24,35] Lincoff et al[24] demonstrated an increase in myocardial infarctions occurring when bailout stenting is delayed (**Figure 12.3**).

The use of aspirin and ticlopidine, instead of warfarin derivatives, after bailout for occlusive dissections may further reduce the incidence of complications.[36] Platelet receptor inhibitors (glycoprotein IIb/IIIa inhibitors) also reduced the cumulative complication rate (myocardial infarction, urgent revascularization, death, and major bleeding) at one month after bailout stenting from 49 to 31%.[37] Treatment with antiplatelet antibodies in the setting of complex angioplasty (EPIC and CAPTURE trials) is gaining popularity as reflected by their use in >40% of angioplasty in some centers currently. As high risk subsets of bailout patients are identified, the use of antiplatelet antibodies will be selectively applied to those patients with a significant risk of platelet-mediated occlusion despite restoration of flow with stents. Other features which may have improved bailout stent results include careful attention to angiographically visible thrombus and monitoring vessels in the laboratory for a period after successful stent implantation.[38]

Bailout and Stent Designs

Wallstents,[22] Palmaz-Schatz,[30,39] Gianturco-Roubin,[26] Strecker,[40,41] Wiktor,[42] and Micro[43] stents have all been demonstrated effective in bailout circumstances. Few comparative studies exist for different stents used for bailout procedures. Only one retrospective comparison between Palmaz-Schatz and Gianturco-Roubin results after bailout stenting is reported.[44] The Palmaz-Schatz stent had a better clinical outcome (15% vs 44% restenosis rate), a difference attributed to a significantly larger late loss after the Gianturco-Roubin stent. In another small trial of 65 patients, an initially better angiographic appearance after Palmaz-Schatz bailout stenting compared to the Wiktor stent was not associated with significant clinical benefit over the long-term.[45] The restenosis after Wiktor stents was not significantly worse than that after Palmaz-Schatz stents (38% vs 27%). However, the estimation of restenosis after implantation of very radiopaque stents such as the tantalum Wiktor stent may be difficult.[46] Given the differences in thrombogenicity and structural support inherent in the numerous stent designs, prospective evaluations for bailout of complicated angioplasty will be helpful.

Role of Residual Dissection

The importance of residual dissection after stent implantation for the bailout indication is controversial. Stents tack up intimal and medial flaps, thus, restoring lumen continuity and vessel geometry. It is generally thought that the total length of each dissection should be covered. However, in complicated bailout situations, it is often difficult to define the entire length of a dissection. Passing additional stents distally through proximally implanted stents to reach residual defects is not always straight forward or technically feasible. Furthermore, multiple stenting increases rates of both subacute occlusion and restenosis.[29,47-49] It is difficult to know if additional distal stents are truly necessary.

Some studies have suggested that residual dissections pose a significant increased risk of subacute occlusion and should always be stented.[35,50] Certainly, distal dissections compromising either the flow or the vascular lumen warrant aggressive intervention. However, data from one study indicated that the outcome of small residual dissections left uncovered by stents was benign if the dissection was stable without blood flow or lumen compromise.[51]

Intracoronary ultrasound imaging studies of dissection after angioplasty demonstrate that these tears do not predict restenosis.[52] Ultrasound has revealed a high incidence of angiographically invisible, small, marginal tears or pocket flaps after stent deployment as well. These dissections seem to have no clinical significance.[52,56] Between the extremes of these benign, small dissections and the dissections of higher NHLBI grades lies the point where further stent implantation is of value compared to its risk. On the one hand, a long dissection distal to a stent in a large diameter vessel subserving a large region of myocardium should probably receive further stenting. On the other hand, further stent implantations in a short dissection in a small (2.5mm) vessel distal to a stent may incur greater risk than benefit. Thus, the decisions for stenting small distal dissections are still best made on a case-by-case basis depending upon the clinical circumstances and operator experience.

Stents for Suboptimal Angioplasty Results

Apart from acute bailout situations, the approach to treatment of suboptimal angioplasty results is more straightforward. Suboptimal angioplasty refers to angioplasty resulting in residual dissection or in residual stenosis of >30%. A number of studies have shown that the presence of residual stenosis [3,13] and significant dissection[3,13,53] are predictive of a major complication after angioplasty. In light of the safety and procedural success rates of stent implantation, stents should be implanted for such suboptimal angioplasties in any vessel >3.0mm in size before, rather than after, an acute closure has occurred. With prompt and aggressive stent implantation after suboptimal and bailout angioplasties, there has been a striking reduction in the need for emergency coronary bypass procedures after percutaneous interventions.[54,55]

SUMMARY

Stents were successfully applied to bailout lesions six years before the reduction of restenosis was apparent. With the ability of interventionalists to categorize angioplasty results into low and high risk groups for acute closure, stent implantation in those lesions most at risk should be addressed before the complication of acute occlusion. While subacute closure and restenosis rates are increased after stent implantation for the bailout indication, the clinical benefit of effective rescue from an inadequate angioplasty result should be appreciated. The need for additional stenting of a residual dissection distal to the bailout stent remains to be clarified and currently are best handled on a case-by-case basis.

References

1. Cowley MJ, Dorros G, Kelsey S, et al. *Acute coronary events associated with percutaneous transluminal coronary angioplasty.* Am J Cardiol 53:12C-16C (1984).
2. Detre KM, Holmes DR Jr, Holubkov R, et al. *Incidence and consequences of periprocedural occlusion: the 1985-1986 NHLBI percutaneous transluminal angioplasty registry.* Circulation 82:739-750 (1991).
3. Ellis SG, Roubin GS, King SB III, et al. *Angiographic and clinical predictors of acute closure after native vessel coronary angioplasty.* Circulation 77:372-379 (1988).
4. Tenaglia AN, Fortin DF, Califf RM, et al. *Predicting the risk of abrupt vessel closure after angioplasty, results of a prospective, randomized trial.* Circulation 90:2258-2266 (1994).

5. de Feyter PJ, de Jaegere PPT, Serruys PW. *Incidence, predictors, and management of acute coronary occlusion after coronary angioplasty.* Am Heart J 127:643-651 (1994).

6. Tan K, Sulke N, Taub N, Sowton E. *Clinical and lesion morphologic determinants of coronary angioplasty success and complications: current experience.* J Am Coll Cardiol 25:855-865 (1995).

7. de Feyter PJ, van den Brand M, Jaarman G, et al. *Acute coronary artery occlusion during and after percutaneous transluminal coronary angioplasty: frequency, prediction, clinical course, management, and follow-up.* Circulation 83:927-936 (1991).

8. Leimgruber PP, Roubin GR, Anderson HV, et al. *Influence of intimal dissection on restenosis after successful coronary angioplasty.* Circulation 72:530-535 (1985).

9. Hermans WRM, Rensing BJ, Foley DP, et al. *Therapeutic dissection after successful coronary balloon angioplasty: no influence on restenosis or on clinical outcome in 693 patients.* J Am Coll Cardiol 20:767-780 (1992).

10. Waller BF, Orr CM, Pinkerton CA, et al. *Coronary balloon angioplasty dissections: "The good, the bad and the ugly."* J Am Coll Cardiol 20:701-706 (1992).

11. *Coronary artery angiographic changes after PTCA: manual for operations NHLBI PTCA registry,* 1985, pp 6-9.

12. Huber MS, Fishman MJ, Madison J, Mooney MR. *Use of morphologic classification to predict clinical outcome after dissection from coronary angioplasty.* Am J Cardiol 68:467-471 (1991).

13. Black AJR, Namay DL, Niederman AL, et al. *Tear or dissection after coronary angioplasty: morphologic correlates of an ischemic complication.* Circulation 79:1035-1042 (1989).

14. Cowley MJ, Dorros G, Kelsey SF, et al. *Emergency coronary bypass surgery after coronary angioplasty: the National Heart, Lung and Blood Institute's PTCA Registry experience.* Am J Cardiol 53:22C-26C (1984).

15. Connor AR, Vliestra RE, Schaff HV, et al. *Early and late results of coronary artery by- pass after failed angioplasty.* Thorac Cardiovasc Surg 96:191-197 (1988).

16. Gulba DC, Daniel WG, Simon R, et al. *Role of thrombolysis and thrombin in patients with acute coronary occlusion during percutaneous transluminal coronary angioplasty.* J Am Coll Cardiol 16:563-568 (1990).

17. Lincoff AM, Popma JJ, Ellis SG, et al. *Percutaneous support devices for high risk or complicated coronary angioplasty.* J Am Coll Cardiol 17:770-780 (1991).

18. van der Linden LP, Bakx ALM, Sedney MI, et al. *Prolonged dilation with an autoperfusion balloon catheter for refractory acute occlusion related to percutaneous transluminal coronary angioplasty.* J Am Coll Cardiol 22:1016-1023 (1993).

19. Lee TC, Hartzler GO, Rutherford BD, et al. *Removal of an occlusive coronary dissection flap by using an atherectomy catheter.* Cathet Cardiovasc Diagn 20:185-188 (1990).

20. Saito S, Arai H, Kim K, et al. *Initial clinical experiences with rescue unipolar radiofrequency thermal balloon angioplasty after abrupt or threatened vessel closure complicating elective conventional balloon coronary angioplasty.* J Am Coll Cardiol 24:1220-1228 (1994).

21. Jenkins RD, Spears JR. *Laser balloon angioplasty: a new approach to abrupt coronary occlusion and chronic restenosis.* Circulation 81(suppl IV):IV-101-IV-108 (1990).

22. Sigwart U, Urban P, Golf S, et al. *Emergency stenting for acute occlusion after coronary balloon angioplasty.* Circulation 78:1121-1127 (1988).

23. Meckel CR, Kjelsberg MA, Ahmed WH, et al. *Bailout stenting for abrupt closure during coronary angioplasty* [abstr]. Circulation 92 (suppl I):I-688 (1995).

24. Lincoff MA, Topol EJ, Chapekis AT, et al. *Intracoronary stenting compared with conventional therapy for abrupt vessel closure complicating coronary angioplasty: a matched case-control study.* J Am Coll Cardiol 21:866-875 (1993).

25. *Preliminary data presented by Haude, M (Stent-by) and Penn, I* (TASC II) Rotterdam, 1995.

26. Roubin GS, Cannon AD, Agrawal SK, et al. *Intracoronary stenting for acute and threatened closure complicating percutaneous transluminal PTCA.* Circulation 85:916-927 (1992).

27. Hermann HC, Buchbinder M, Clemen MW, et al. *Emergent use of balloon-expandable coronary artery stenting for failed percutaneous transluminal coronary angioplasty.* Circulation 86:812-819 (1992).

28. Nath FC, Muller DWM, Ellis SG, et al. *Thrombosis of a flexible coil coronary stent: frequency, predictors and clinical outcome.* J Am Coll Cardiol 21:622-627 (1993).

29. Foley JB, Brown RIG, Penn IM. *Thrombosis and restenosis after stenting in failed angioplasty: Comparison with elective stenting.* Am Heart J 128:12-20 (1994).

30. Schomig A, Kastrati A, Mudra H et al. *Four-year experience with Palmaz-Schatz stenting in coronary angioplasty complicated by dissection with threatened or present vessel closure.* Circulation 90:2716-2724 (1994).

31. Hearn JA, King SB III, Douglas JS, et al. *Clinical and angiographic outcomes after coronary artery stenting for acute or threatened closure after percutaneous transluminal coronary angioplasty: initial results with a balloon-expandable stainless steel design.* Circulation 88:2086-2096 (1993).

32. George BS, Voorhees WD III, Roubin GS, et al. *Multicenter investigation of coronary stenting to treat acute or threatened closure after percutaneous transluminal coronary angioplasty: clinical and angiographic outcomes.* J Am Coll Cardiol 22:135-143 (1993).

33. Chan CNS, Tan AT, Koh TH, et al. *Intracoronary stenting in the treatment of acute or threatened closure in angiographically small coronary arteries (<3.0 mm) complicating percutaneous transluminal coronary angioplasty.* Am J Cardiol 75:23-25 (1995).

34. Herrmann HC, Malosky SA, Guidera SA, et al. *Patient selection reduces thrombotic complications of emergent stenting for failed PTCA.* Cathet Cardiovascular Diagn 34:286-292 (1995).

35. Metz D, Urban P, Hoang V, et al. *Predicting ischemic complications after bailout stenting following failed coronary angioplasty.* Am J Cardiol 74:271-274 (1994).

36. Haase J, Reifart N, Baier T, et al. *Bail-out stenting (Palmaz-Schatz) without anticoagulation* [abstr]. Circulation 92(suppl I):I-795 (1995).

37. Zidar JP, Kruse KR, Thel MC, et al. *Integrelin for emergency coronary artery stenting* [abstr]. J Am Coll Cardiol 27(suppl A):138A (1996).

38. Herrmann HC, Hirshfeld JW. *Improving the results of bail-out stenting.* Cathet Cardiovasc Diagn 35:210 (1995).

39. Haude M, Erbel R, Straub U, et al. *Results of intracoronary stents for management of coronary dissection after balloon angioplasty.* Am J Cardiol 67:691-696 (1991).

40. Reifart N, Langer A, Storger H, et al. *Strecker stent as a bailout device following percutaneous transluminal PTCA.* J Interven Cardiol 5:79-83 (1992).

41. Hamm CW, Beythien C, Sievert H, et al. *Multicenter evaluation of the Strecker tantalum stent for acute coronary occlusion after angioplasty.* Am Heart J 129:423-429 (1995).

42. Vrolix M van der Kreiken T, Piessens J. *Wiktor stent for acute and threatened closure after PTCA: an update of the European registry.* Circulation 86(suppl I):I-987 (1992).

43. Ozaki Y, Keane D, Ruygrok P, et al. *Acute clinical and angiographic results with the new AVE micro coronary stent in bailout management.* Am J Cardiol 76:112-116 (1995).

44. Fernandez-Ortiz A, Goicolea J, Perez-Vizcayno M, et al. *Late clinical and angiographic outcome of bailout coronary stenting: a comparison study between Gianturco-Roubin and Palmaz-Schatz stents* [abstr]. J Am Coll Cardiol 27(suppl A):111A (1996).

45. Goy JJ, Eeckhout E, Stauffr JC, et al. *Emergency endoluminal stenting for abrupt vessel closure following coronary angioplasty: a randomized comparison of the Wiktor and Palmaz-Schatz stents.* Cathet Cardiovasc Diagn 34:128-132 (1995).

46. Vrolix M, Piesens J, and the European *Wiktor Stent Study Group. Usefulness of the Wiktor stent for treatment of threatened or acute closure complicating angioplasty.* Am J Cardiol 73:737-741 (1994).

47. Strauss BH, Serruys PW, de Scheerder IK, et al. *Relative risk analysis of angiographic predictors of restenosis within the coronary Wallstent.* Circulation 84:1636-1643 (1991).

48. Ellis SG, Savage M, Fischman D, et al. *Restenosis after placement of Palmaz-Schatz stents in native coronary arteries: initial results of a multicenter experience.* Circulation 86:1836-1844 (1992).

49. Kastrati A, Schomig A, Dietz R, et al. *Time course of restenosis during the first year after emergency coronary stenting.* Circulation 87:1498-1505 (1993).

50. Agrawal SK, Ho DSW, Liu MW, et al. *Predictors of thrombotic complications after placement of the flexible stent.* Am J Cardiol 73:1216-1219 (1994).

51. Alfonso F, Hernandez R, Goicolea J, et al. *Coronary stenting for acute coronary dissection after coronary angioplasty: implications of residual dissection.* J Am Coll Cardiol 24:989-995 (1994).

52. Metz JA, Mooney MR, Walter PD, et al. *Significance of edge tears in coronary stenting: initial observations from the STRUT registry* [abstr]. Circulation 92(suppl I):I-546 (1995).

53. Bredlau CE, Roubin GS, Leimgruber PP, et al. *In-hospital Morbidity and mortality in patients undergoing elective coronary angioplasty.* Circulation 72:1044-1052 (1985).

54. Scott NA, Weintraub WS, Carlin SF, et al. *Recent changes in the management and outcome of acute closure after percutaneous transluminal coronary angioplasty.* Am J Cardiol 71:1159-1163 (1993).

55. Stauffer JC, Eeckhout E, Vogt P, et al. *Stand-by versus stent-by during percutaneous transluminal coronary angioplasty.* Am Heart J 130:21-26 (1995).

56 Peters RJG, Kok WEM, DiMario C, et al. *Prediction of restenosis after coronary balloon angioplasty. Results of PICTURE (Post-Intra Coronary Treatment Ultrasound Result Evaluation), a prospective multi-center intracoronary ultrasound imaging study.* Circulation 95: 2254-2261 (1997)

CHAPTER 13

STENTING ANGLED ARTERIES

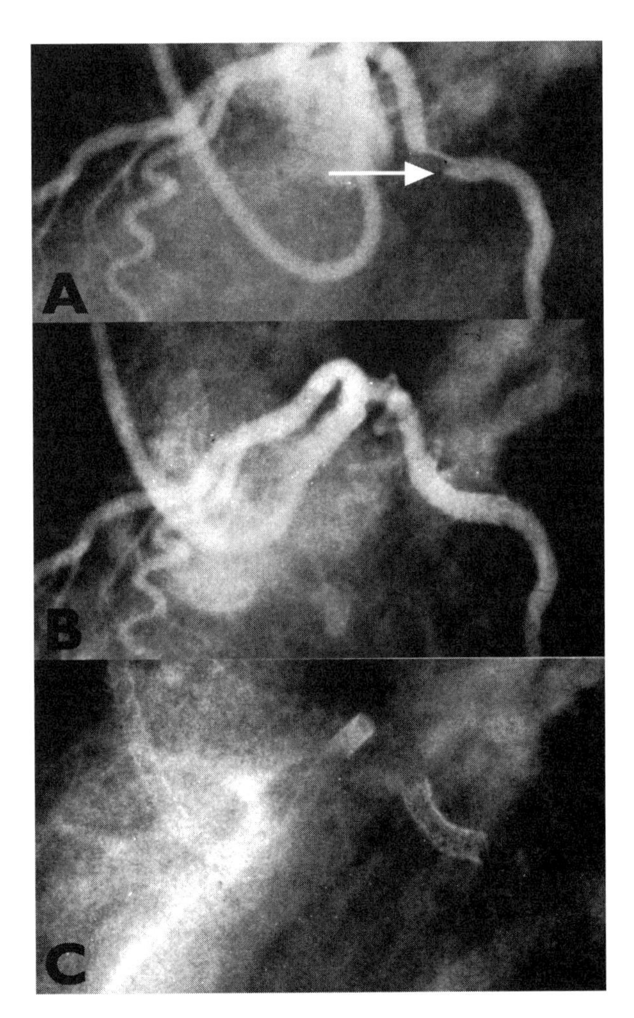

Figure 13.1 Tantalum for Curves This discrete mid circumflex lesion is situated on the vertex of a 90° angle without hinge motion (**a**). After treatment with a Cordis stent there was no residual stenosis (**b**). The radiopacity of tantalum is demonstrated in **c**.

CASE 13.1: Tantalum for Curves

A 63 year old woman had intermittent episodes of exertional chest pain for 8 years. An exercise test was positive during the first stage with ischemic ST changes inferolaterally. At angiography, a severe single discrete and concentric lesion of the mid circumflex was found, located at the vertex of a 90° bend (**Figure 13.1a** arrow). There was no marked change in the angle between systole and diastole. The patient underwent primary stent implantation.

PROCEDURE 13.1

There were two arterial curves involved in the approach to this lesion, one located at the ostium of the circumflex artery and another at the lesion site itself. A left Amplatz guide was selected to assist in passing the device through the first angulation. The lesion was crossed and predilated with a 3.0 mm balloon. A Cordis stent was selected because of its low crossing profile and flexibility (**Figure 13.2**). The stent easily passed to the angulated lesion site and was deployed at 8 atm. The deployment balloon was maintained in its position within the stent until final post deployment inflations of 10 and 12 atm produced the desired appearance of the

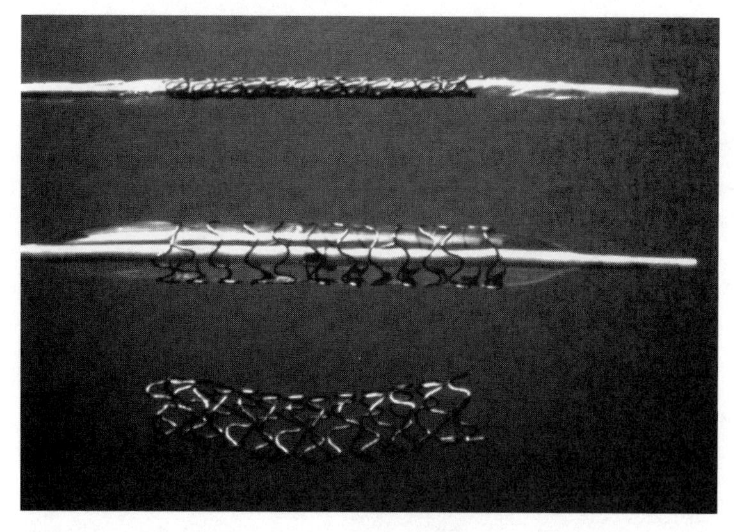

Figure 13.2 The Cordis Stent A single sinusoidal helical coil.

tantalum struts outside of the contrast-filled lumen with no residual narrowing (**Figure 13.1b**). The natural vessel curvature was well preserved as demonstrated by the unopacified image of this radiopaque stent (**Figure 13.1c**).

MATERIALS 13.1

Guiding Catheter:	Cook Lumax AL-1
Guide wires:	ACS/Guidant 0.014" x 300 cm Extra S'port
Balloons:	Schneider Goldie 3.0 x 20 mm
Stents:	Cordis 3.5 x 15 mm

CASE 13.2: Stenting a Curved Lesion

The patient, a 50 year old woman smoker with polycystic renal disease, had initiated dialysis for progressive renal failure 3 weeks ago. During dialyses she experienced angina with non-specific electrocardiographic changes inferiorly. Coronary angiography revealed a 69% mid right coronary lesion. Left ventricular function was normal (**Figures 13.3a**). Angina proved refractory to medical therapy. She was referred for angioplasty two weeks later.

PROCEDURE 13.2

In consideration of the increased restenosis risk of chronic dialysis patients, it was elected to proceed with primary stenting. Because of the lesion location on a curve distal to two severe curves, a stent with a low profile and ability to easily reach the lesion and to preserve the arterial morphology, was selected. The lesion was crossed with an extra support guidewire and predilated to 8 atm. A BARD XT **(Figure 4.8)** stent easily passed across the lesion and was positioned distal to the right ventricular branch using the radiopaque spine as a marker. The stent's dorsal spine was allowed to self-orient within the curve of the artery (**Figure 13.3b).** One inflation to 14 atm was sufficient to deploy the stent without a residual lesion (**Figure 13.3c**). The patient resumed dialyses and had no further angina over 5 months.

MATERIALS 13.2

Guiding Catheter:	Cook Lumax JR-4 8 French
Guide wires:	ACS/Guidant Extra Support 0.014"x 175cm
Balloons:	USCI/Bard Pronto Rely 3.5 x 20 mm
Stents:	Bard XT 16mm

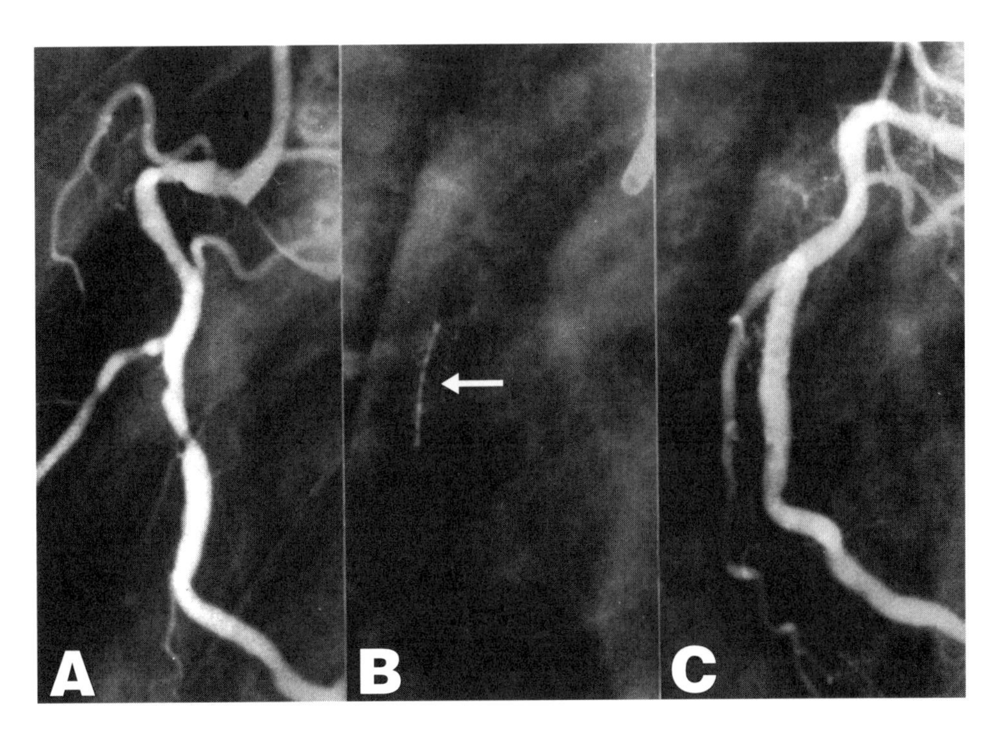

Figure 13.3 Vessel Tortuosity and Stents The mid right coronary artery stenosis (**a**) was 69% diameter narrowed. The Bard XT stent's dorsal spine self oriented in the curved segment (**b;** arrow), leaving no residual stenosis (**c**).

DISCUSSION

Risks of Angioplasty of Angulated Lesions

Atherosclerosis affects the coronary arteries in an uneven fashion with plaque formation occurring preferentially at bifurcations and curvatures, regions of low wall stress and reduced flow velocity.[1] Lesions at bend points of over 45° are present in one-third of angioplasties.[2-5] The angulation of coronary arteries is a demonstrated risk factor for reduced procedural success[2,6] and an increased complication rate[2,3] during angioplasty. For multivessel angioplasty, angulated lesions >60° are significant predictors of adverse events and provide prognostic information about procedural outcomes beyond that supplied by the standard AHA/ACC lesion classification system (see **Appendix III**)[7] The explanation for increased complications, and particularly for acute closures, at angulated sites is thought to be straightening of curved segments producing significant or complex intimal disruption or dissections.[4]

Angioplasty in angled segments (>45°) is also associated with an increased restenosis rate,[8] attributed both to the unique flow and shear stress associated with curved vessel segments. To some extent, the higher restenosis rate may , in part, be due to the reluctance of prudent operators to fully dilate these risky segments.[8,9] Angulation of the diseased arterial segment has also been shown to be a significant risk factor for complications in laser angioplasty,[10] rotational atherectomy,[11,12] and directional atherectomy.[13]

Special Considerations for Angled Segments

A number of special techniques may be applied to cope with the challenges of conventional angioplasty in curved vessel segments. Long balloons to cover the lesion and adjacent regions may diffuse the concentration of stress at the edges of the stenosis.[14] Short balloons may avoid the curve altogether in lesions not directly located on the angle. Non-compliant balloons of polyethylene teraphthalate (PET) may cause less straightening of angled arteries[2] and lower rates of dissection[15] than more compliant balloons, although little objective information exists to favor one material over another. In a study of the straightening forces generated by balloons of varying lengths and compliances, long and compliant balloons produced the least arterial straightening.[16] Special deflectable guidewires,[17,18] curved balloons,[19] and prolonged low pressure dilations with perfusion balloons,[20] all modifications of conventional angioplasty systems, have been reported to provide better results in these difficult segments.

Stents for Angled Lesions

The role of metallic stents in angulated coronary vessels remains unclear. Recent and ongoing stent trials have tended to exclude arterial segments with greater than 45° angulation.[21,22] This restriction was initially invoked because of concerns that rigid stents might not pass easily into angled segments. Consequently, the complication and restenosis rates of stents implanted in angled segments remains to be determined. The location of a lesion at an angle of >45° is an independent predictor of stent embolization or dislodgment

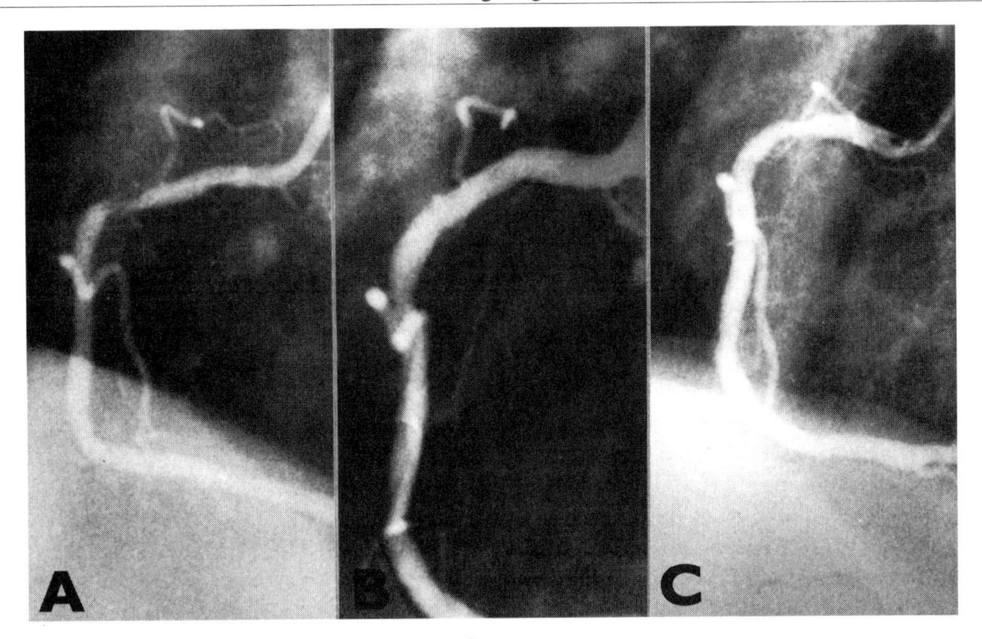

Figure 13.4 Arterial Angles Change After Stenting In this angiographic series a single 90° angle in the proximal right coronary artery (**a**) is changed by stent implantation into two 60° angles proximal and distal to the rigid stent (**b**). This type of stent induced morphological change did not result in restenosis (**c**).

during implantation.[23] The relative benefits of stents in curved compared to straight segments also requires examination. In one angioplasty study, lesions with "a high bending rate" showed less than normal amounts of recoil suggesting less elasticity on bend points.[24] The ability of stents to prevent recoil may be less important in angled lesion. How angled coronary segments will respond morphologically to the implantation of a rigid stent is unknown. In studies of risk factors for stent restenosis, the presence of a lesion on a bend point did not predict restenosis.[25,26] **Figure 13.4** shows a 90° angle in a right coronary artery transformed by stenting into two lesser angles. At 6 months, there appears to be no restenosis in such vessels. When measured before and after slotted tube stent implantation, most arterial angulations decrease by 10° after the procedure. Surprisingly, 10° of stented segments actually increase the degree of angulation after stent implantation, suggesting a heterogeneous response to the devices implanted. Increased contractility and arterial vasodilation may contribute to arterial angulation as much as the implantation of a rigid prosthesis.

Hinge Points

Hinge or kinking points are defined on segments in which the angulation changes over 15° during the cardiac cycle.[3,10] A hinge point lesion is demonstrated in **Figure 13.5** during diastole and systole. While the degree of angulation itself does not appear to be important, presence of a lesion on a "hinge point" is associated with significantly increased rates of restenosis.[26] When a dissection at a hinge site was stented,

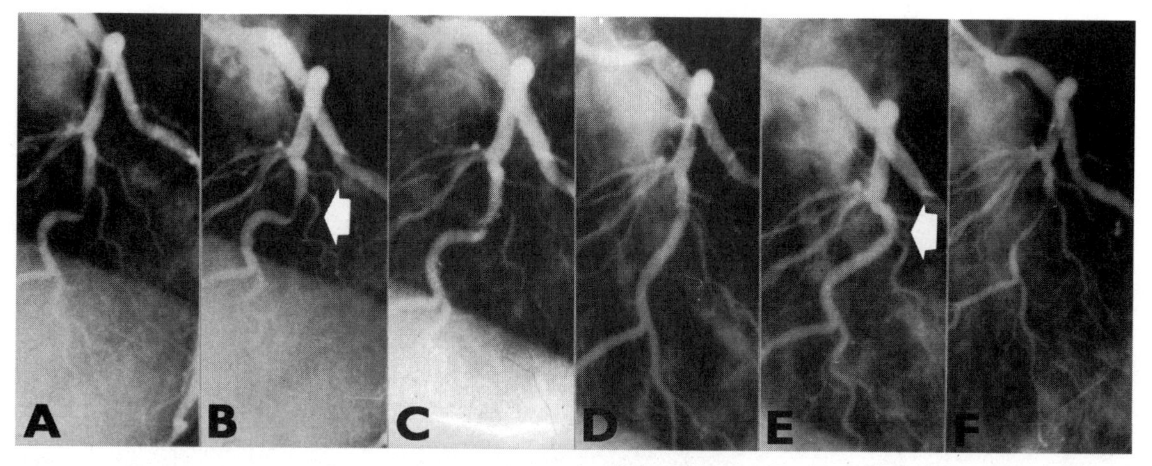

Figure 13.5 Arterial Hinge Motion The left anterior descending artery stenosis is present at a hinge point since the angle of the artery changes more than 15° between diastole (**a**) and systole (**b**; arrow). A dissection was produced by angioplasty at this site (**c**). Images **d & e** represent diastole and systole after stent implantation. When the stent was implanted, the hinge motion was increased and moved to the proximal stent site at the level of a small diagonal branch (**e**; arrow). Stent implantation at this hinge point was associated with restenosis 6 months later (**f**).

the hinge motion was transferred proximally (**Figure 13.5 d & e**) and resulted in restenosis at 6 months (**Figure 13.5f**). Hinge points presumably concentrate stress at the extremes of the rigid stents, theoretically inducing greater intimal reaction. When angulation and hinge motion were analyzed pre- and post-stent implantation, only implantation of the stent at a hinge point predicted increased restenosis (**Figure 13.6**).[26] It is unknown whether stents which are more axially compliant will have advantages in these segments. Stents which scaffold dissections while respecting the natural coronary morphology may reduce intimal stress associated with hinge point stents. To date there are no stent trials comparing different designs and the effects on angled segments.

SUMMARY

Endovascular stenting is being applied in increasingly complex anatomic situations. In some programs, over 50% of stents may be placed in arterial segments with angulations of over 45°.[26] Flexible stents demonstrate a major technical advantage over rigid stents in their ability to provide scaffolding while preserving the natural arterial contour. Whether these advantages translate into reduced restenosis rates is yet to be demonstrated.

While the degree of angulation itself does not appear to be important, presence of a lesion on a "hinge point" is associated with significantly increased rates of restenosis.[26]

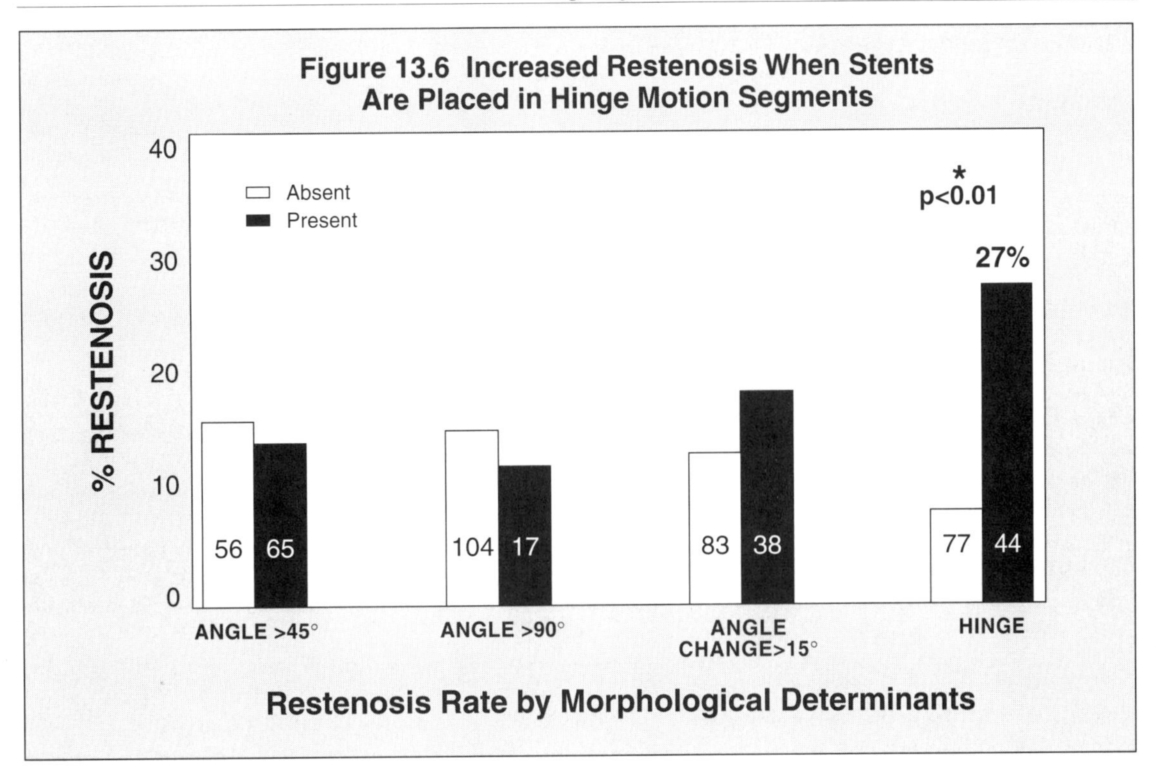

Figure 13.6 Increased Restenosis When Stents are Placed in Hinge Motion Segments The black bars represent the restenosis rate in lesions in which hinge morphology is present. The open bars represent the restenosis rate in lesions in which hinge morphology is not present. When angulation and hinge motion were analyzed pre and post stent implantation, only implantation of the stent at a hinge point predicted increased restenosis. Reprinted with permission from Exerpta Medica, Inc. (*Am J Cardiol* 1997;79:192).

References

1. Glagov S, Zarins C, Giddens DP, Ku DN. *Hemodynamics and atherosclerosis- insights and perspectives gained from studies of human arteries.* Arch Pathol Lab Med 112:1018-1031 (1988).
2. Ellis SG, Topol EJ. *Results of percutaneous transluminal coronary angioplasty of high- risk angulated stenoses.* Am J Cardiol 66:932-937 (1990).
3. Ellis SG, Roubin GS, King SB III, et al. *Angiographic and clinical predictors of acute closure after native vessel coronary angioplasty.* Circulation 77:372-379 (1988).
4. Ischinger T, Gruntzig AR, Meier B, Galan K. *Coronary dissection and total coronary occlusion associated with percutaneous transluminal coronary angioplasty: significance of initial angiographic morphology of coronary stenoses.* Circulation 77:372-379 (1986).
5. Ellis SG, Vandormael MG, Cowley MJ, et al. *Coronary morphologic and clinical determinants of procedural outcome with angioplasty for multivessel coronary disease—Implications for patient selection.* Circulation 82:1193-1202 (1990).
6. Detre K, Holubkov R, Kelsey S, et al. *The National Heart, Lung and Blood Institute Registry.* N Engl J Med 318:265-270 (1988).
7. Ellis SG, Vandormael MG, Cowley MJ, et al. *Coronary morphologic and clinical determinants of procedural outcome with angioplasty for multivessel coronary disease-implications for patient selection.* Circulation 82:1193-1202 (1990).
8. Ellis SG, Roubin GS, King SB III, et al. *Importance of stenosis morphology in the estimation of restenosis risk after elective percutaneous transluminal coronary angioplasty.* Am J Cardiol 63:30-34 (1989).
9. Ellis SG, Cowley MJ, Whitlow PL, et al. *Prospective case-control comparison of percutaneous transluminal coronary revascularization in patients with multivessel disease treated in 1986-87 versus 1991: improved in-hospital and 12-month results.* J Am Coll Cardiol 25:1137-1142 (1995).

10. Ghazzal ZMB, Hearn JA, Litvack F, et al. *Morphological predictors of acute complications after percutaneous excimer laser coronary angioplasty-results of a comprehensive angiographic analysis: importance of the eccentricity index.* Circulation 86:820-827 (1992).

11. Safian RD, Niazi KA, Strzlelecki M, et al. *Detailed angiographic analysis of high-speed mechanical rotational atherectomy in human coronary arteries.* Circulation 88:961-968 (1993).

12. Ellis SG, Popma JJ, Buchbinder M, et al. *Relation of clinical presentation, stenosis morphology and operator technique to the procedural results of rotational atherectomy and rotational atherectomy-facilitated angioplasty.* Circulation 89:882-892 (1994).

13. Ellis SG, DeCesare NB, Pinkerton CA, et al. *Relation of stenosis morphology and clinical presentation to the procedural results of directional coronary atherectomy.* Circulation 84:644-653 (1991).

14. Cannon DA, Roubin GS, Hearn JA, et al. *Acute angiographic and clinical results of long balloon percutaneous transluminal coronary angioplasty and adjuvant stenting for long narrowings.* Am J Cardiol 73:635-641 (1994).

15. Berry KJ, Drew TM, McKendall GR, et al. *Balloon material as a risk factor for coronary angioplasty procedural complications* [abstr]. Circulation 84(suppl II):II-130 (1991).

16. Barasch E, Conger JL, Kadipasaoglu KA, et al. *PTCA in angulated segments: effects of balloon material, balloon length, and inflation sequence on straightening forces in an in vitro model.* Cathet Cardiovasc Diag 39:207-212 (1996).

17. Myler RK, Tobis JM, Cumberland DC, et al. *A new flexible and deflectable tip guidewire for coronary angioplasty and other invasive and interventional procedures.* J Invas Cardiol 4:393-397 (1992).

18. Chandra P, Cribier A, Seth A. *Utility of pilot wire in angioplasty of tortuous and highly angulated coronary arteries.* Cathet Cardiovasc Diagn 37:268-270 (1996).

19. Vivekaphirat V, Zapala C, Foschi AE. *Clinical experience with the use of the angled- balloon dilatation catheter.* Cathet Cardiovasc Diagn 17:121-5 (1989).

20. Ohman EM, Marquis JF, Ricci DR, et al. *A randomized comparison of the effects of gradual prolonged versus standard primary balloon inflation on early and late outcome: results of a multicenter clinical trial.* Circulation 89:1118-1125 (1994).

21. *Benestent I and II procedure and protocol manuals.* Cardialysis, Rotterdam, The Netherlands, 1992, 1995.

22. Fischman DL, Leon MB, Baim DS, et al. *A randomized comparison of coronary-stent placement and balloon angioplasty in the treatment of coronary artery disease.* N Engl J Med 331:496-501 (1994).

23. Alfonso F, Martinez D, Hernandez R, et al. *Stent embolization during intracoronary stenting.* Am J Cardiol 78:833-835 (1996).

24. Rensing BJ, Hermans WR, Strauss BH, Serruys PW. *Regional differences in elastic recoil after percutaneous transluminal coronary angioplasty: a quantitative angiographic study.* J Am Coll Cardiol 17:34B-38B (1991).

25. Ellis SG, Savage M, Fischman D, et al. *Restenosis after placement of Palmaz-Schatz stents in native coronary arteries-initial results of a multicenter experience.* Circulation 86:1836-1844 (1992).

26. Phillips P, Alfonso F, Segovia J, et al. *The effects of rigid stents on angled coronary arteries.* Am J Cardiol 79: 191-193 (1997).

CHAPTER 14

STENTS FOR THROMBOTIC LESIONS

CASE 14.1: Platinum Implanted In Thrombus

A 67 year old man, former smoker with prior anterior myocardial infarction, had undergone angioplasty of the proximal left anterior descending artery with sequential Gianturco-Roubin I stenting for a suboptimal angiographic result 6 months earlier. He had also received ReoPro™.

He now presents with prolonged angina culminating in a non-Q-wave infarction. A new severe lesion in the proximal right coronary artery enveloped in thrombus was identified. The new right coronary lesion

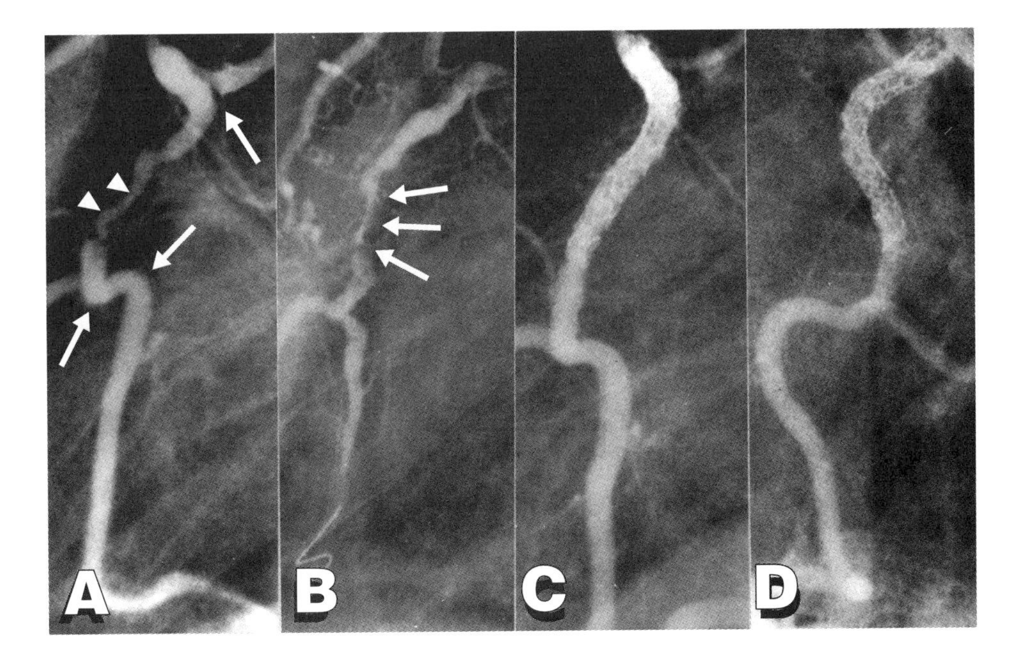

Figure 14.1 Platinum in Thrombus This right coronary artery lesion(**a**) is complicated by multiple arterial curves (arrows) and by the large amount of thrombus persisting after 4 days of heparinization (**a;** arrowheads). The thrombus is more apparent after guide wire passage (**b;** arrows). After implantation of an Angiostent, the thrombus was no longer apparent (**c**). In a lateral projection with only partial contrast filling the radiopacity of this platinum stent is appreciated. The preservation of native artery's curved morphology can be seen (**d**).

was also located among a series of curves (**Figure 14.1a** arrows). The stented proximal left anterior descending segment remained widely patent. The left ventricular ejection fraction was 77% with normal wall motion. Because of thrombus in the right coronary artery, the patient remained on heparin 4 days before returning to the laboratory for intervention.

PROCEDURE 14.1

The pre-procedural angiogram was minimally improved. A glycoprotein IIb/IIIa inhibitor was withheld because of the patient's prior exposure. Because platinum is one of the least thrombogenic materials used in stent construction, an Angiostent was considered (**Figure 14.2**). An extra support guidewire was passed across the heavily thrombus-laden right coronary lesion into the posterior descending branch (**Figure 14.1b**). Pre-dilation with a 3mm balloon required 8 atm before the lumen appeared acceptable. Because of the significant arterial tortuosity, lesion length, and persistent thrombus, a pre-mounted 3.5 x 35mm Angiostent was passed to the lesion site and deployed at 14 atm without difficulty (**Figure 14.1c**), preserving the native vessel morphology (**Figure 14.1d** lateral plane). The patient was discharged 2 days later without complications and remained asymptomatic at 4-month follow-up.

MATERIALS 14.1

Guiding Catheter:	Cook Lumax JR-4 8 French
Guidewires:	ACS Extra Support 0.014"x300cm
Balloons:	Schneider Goldie 3.0x20mm
	SciMed Cobra 18 3.5x20mm
Stents:	Angiostent 3.5x35mm

DISCUSSION[1]

Thrombus is prevalent in the coronary lesions of acute myocardial infarction,[2,3] unstable angina,[4] and chronic coronary occlusions.[5] It may be apparent angiographically as a rounded or globular contrast-lucent mass but it is often overlooked by contrast techniques.[6] Angioscopy is more accurate than angiography in identifying thrombus.[7,8] Intracoronary ultrasound, on the other hand, is unable to distinguish thrombus from arterial wall. While stents have generally been proscribed in the setting of thrombus because of concerns that the metallic foreign body would only incite further thrombosis, these devices have been applied with increasing success in clinical situations known to be associated with thrombosis. This fact, and the belief that the improved flow provided by stents would exceed their thrombus generating tendencies, has led to the application of stents in thrombus laden vessels such as that described in *CASE 14.1*.

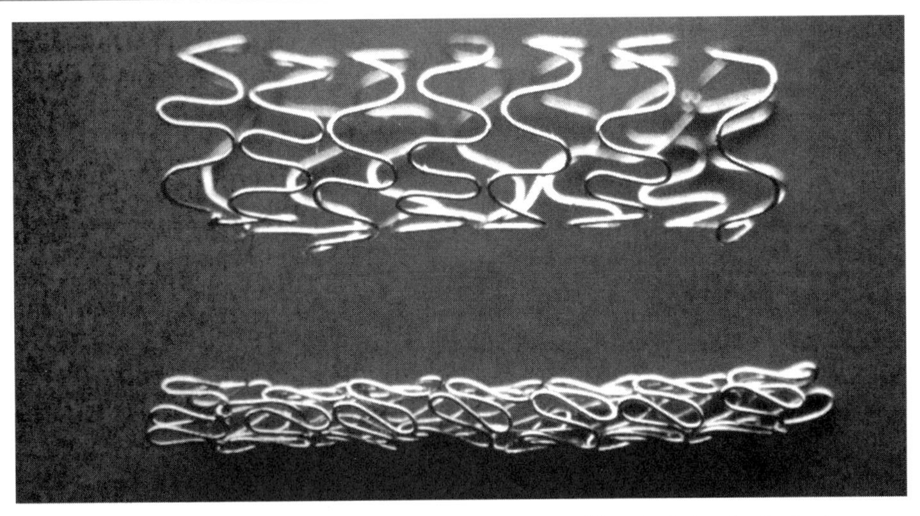

Figure 14.2 The Angiostent. Single wire sinusoidal shape with a single longitudinal spine

Thrombus and Angioplasty Complications

Intracoronary thrombus is an independent predictor of procedural complications after angioplasty.[9] The major complication associated with intracoronary stent implantation has been thrombotic occlusion. Previous studies have shown that the presence of thrombus angiographically is a risk factor for subsequent stent thrombosis.[10,11] Because of this, the angiographic appearance of thrombus has been an accepted contraindication to stent implantation from the very beginning of the technique. However, recent advances in stent implantation, including high-pressure deployment and aggressive antiplatelet therapies, have resulted in a marked reduction in the incidence of thrombotic occlusion after stenting.[12-14]

The coronary lesions of acute ischemic syndromes, unstable angina and acute myocardial infarction, are known to be thrombus-rich.[15,16] Stent implantation using traditional deployment techniques and antiplatelet therapy was associated with a higher incidence of subacute thrombosis in the setting of unstable angina.[17,18] Nonetheless, stent implantation as it is currently practiced may not be associated with a higher rate of adverse outcomes in unstable patients.[19] Stents are now implanted with high success and minimal complications even in the thrombus-laden setting of acute myocardial infarction.[20-22] In particular, recent subacute thrombosis rates in stented infarct vessels of 0 to 3% suggest that this setting is not associated with a significantly higher rate of thrombotic complications.

Totally occluded coronary arteries are also associated with significant thrombus. At angioscopy, red thrombus overlying an occlusive yellow plaque is the most frequent finding of these lesions.[23] Despite this, stents have met with increased success and minimal complications when used for total occlusions compared to angioplasty.[24-27] Preliminary results from prospective trials have also revealed a low rate of complications after stent implantation in these thrombus-laden lesions.[28,29] The rate of acute closure was significantly lower in the stent compared to the angioplasty group in one study.[29] Thus, in the clinical settings of acute ischemic syndromes or total occlusion, the association of thrombus has not resulted in adverse consequences after stenting.

Devices for Thrombus-Containing Lesions

Devices which attempt to prepare the thrombotic arterial substrate for subsequent angioplasty have been demonstrated effective. Transluminal extractional atherectomy has successfully been applied to coronary arterial and saphenous vein graft thrombi with approximately a 5% rate of distal embolization. The AngioJet rheolytic thrombectomy catheter or POSSIS device has been shown effective in preliminary trials of thrombus removal.[30] These two techniques attempt to remove thrombus before alleviating the stenosis and flow abnormalities which predispose to clot formation. It is unknown whether the prior treatment approach of the thrombotic lesion will prove more effective than direct angioplasty and endogenous fibrinolysis.

Reduced blood flow is a major constituent of thrombotic arterial occlusion, particularly after angioplasty. The regions of high shear stress caused by turbulence and residual stenosis after inadequate balloon dilation are pivotal in contributing to the development and maintenance of arterial thrombus.[31] The improved rheology provided by stent implantation is thought to exceed the tendency toward thrombosis caused by the stent material itself.[32] Kaul et al[33] successfully deployed Palmaz-Schatz stents into 12 thrombus-containing lesions without thrombotic complication. Romero et al[34] reviewed results of 51 thrombus-containing stented arteries and found a 34% restenosis rate in 51% of patients who were restudied. Alfonso et al[35] examined 86 stents implanted in thrombus and confirmed a high success rate without thrombotic complication. Furthermore, with 92% angiographic follow-up, there was a restenosis rate of 30% for stents placed in this setting.[35] These studies support a common conclusion that an optimally deployed stent is safe and effective therapy for thrombus-laden lesions.

Suggestions for Stenting Thrombotic Lesions

Thus, while early stent deployment guidelines cautioned strongly against placement in thrombotic situations, current dictums may be more relaxed. Stenting thrombus-rich lesions of unstable angina, acute myocardial infarction, and total coronary occlusion is not an absolute contraindication. Observational studies reveal an acceptable incidence of subacute closure and restenosis associated with the high level of angiographic success in thrombotic lesions. As reviewed in **Chapter 2,** ionic contrast media (e.g., Hexabrix) may also offer a theoretical advantage over nonionic contrast media in reducing thrombus propagation.

SUMMARY

Stenting should be considered for thrombotic lesions that remain inadequately treated by balloon angioplasty. The most common situation for stenting of thrombus-containing lesions is acute myocardial infarction. Stenting in lesions with copious amounts of thrombus may be limited and considerations to thrombolytic or rheolytic therapy prior to stent implantation should be made.

References

1. Alfonso F. Rodriguez P, Phillips P et al. *Clinical and angiographic implications of coronary stenting in thrombus-containing lesions.* J Am Coll Cardiol 29:725-733 (1997)
2. Dewood MA, Spores J, Notske R, et al. *Prevalence of total coronary occlusion during the early hours of transmural myocardial infarction.* N Engl J Med 303:897-902 (1980).
3. Davies MJ, Thomas A. *Thrombosis and acute coronary lesions in sudden cardiac ischemic death.* N Engl J Med 310:1137-1140 (1984).
4. Sherman TC, Litvack F, Grundfest W, et al. *Coronary angioscopy in patients with unstable angina pectoris.* N Engl J Med 315:913-919 (1986).
5. Alfonso F, Goicolea J, Hernandez R, et al. *Angioscopic findings during coronary angioplasty of coronary occlusions.* J Am Coll Cardiol 26:135-141 (1995).
6. Rehr R, Disciascio G, Vetrovec G, Cowley M. *Angiographic morphology of coronary artery stenoses in prolonged rest angina: evidence of intracoronary thrombosis.* J Am Coll Cardiol 14:1429-1437 (1989).
7. White CJ, Ramee SR, Collins TJ, et al. *Coronary angioscopy of abrupt occlusion after angioplasty.* J Am Coll Cardiol 25:1681-1684 (1995).
8. Teirstein PS, Schatz RA, DeNardo SJ, et al. *Angioscopic versus angiographic detection of thrombus during coronary interventional procedures.* Am J Cardiol 75:1083-1087 (1995).
9. Ferguson JJ, Barasch E, Wilson JM, et al. *The relation of clinical outcome to dissection and thrombosis formation during coronary angioplasty.* J Invas Cardiol 7:2-10 (1995).
10. Agrawal SK, Ho DSW, Liu MW, et al. *Predictors of thrombotic complications after placement of a flexible coil stent.* Am J Cardiol 73:1216-1219 (1994).
11. Nath FC, Muller DWM, Ellis SG, et al. *Thrombosis of a flexible coil coronary stent: frequency, predictors and clinical outcome.* J Am Coll Cardiol. 21:622-627 (1993).
12. Colombo A, Hall P, Nakamura S, et al. *Intracoronary stenting without anticoagulation accomplished with intravascular ultrasound guidance.* Circulation 91:1676-1688 (1995).
13. Morice, MC, Zemour G, Benvensite E, et al. *Intracoronary stenting without coumadin: one month results of a French multicenter study.* Cathet Cardiovasc Diagn 35:1-7 (1995).
14. Schomig A, Neumann FJ, Kastrati A, et al. *A randomized comparison of antiplatelet and anticoagulant therapy after the placement of coronary-artery stents.* N Engl J Med 334: 1084-1089 (1996).
15. Sherman TC, Litvack F, Grundfest W, et al. *Coronary angioscopy in patients with unstable angina pectoris.* N Engl J Med 315:913-919 (1986).
16. Mizuno K, Satomura K, Miyamoto A, et al. *Angioscopic evaluation of coronary-artery thrombi in acute coronary syndromes.* N Engl J Med 326:287-291 (1992).
17. Nath FC, Muller DWM, Ellis SG, et al. *Thrombosis of a flexible coil coronary stent: frequency, predictors and clinical outcome.* J Am Coll Cardiol. 21:622-627 (1993).
18. Haude M, Erbel R, Issa H, et al. *Subacute thrombotic complications after intracoronary implantations of Palmaz-Schatz stent.* Am Heart J 126:15-22 (1993).

19. Malowsky S, Hirshfeld J, Jermann H. *Comparison of results of coronary stenting in patients with unstable vs stable angina.* Cathet Cardiovasc Diagn 3:95-101 (1994).

20. LeFevre T, Morice MC, Karrillon G, et al. *Coronary stenting during acute myocardial infarction. Results from the stent without coumadin* French registry [abstr]. J Am Coll Cardiol 27:69A (1996).

21. Garcia-Cantu E, Spaulding C, Corcos T, et al. *Stent implantation in acute myocardial infarction.* Am J Cardiol 77:451-454 (1996).

22. Rodriguez AE, Fernandez M, Santaera O, et al. *Coronary stenting in patients undergoing percutaneous transluminal coronary angioplasty during acute myocardial infarction.* Am J Cardiol 77:685-689 (1996).

23. Alfonso F, Goicolea J, Hernandez R, et al. *Angioscopic findings during coronary angioplasty of coronary occlusions.* J Am Coll Cardiol 26:135-141 (1995).

24. Medina A, Melian F, Suarez de Lezo J, Pan M, et al. *Effectiveness of coronary stenting for the treatment of chronic total occlusion in angina pectoris.* Am J Cardiol 73:1222-1224 (1994).

25. Sato Y, Kimwa T, Nosaka H, Nobuyoshi M. Randomized *Comparison of balloon angioplasty (BA) versus coronary stent implantation (CS) for total occlusion (TO): preliminary results.* Circulation 92(suppl I):I-475 (1995).

26. Ooka M, Suzuki T, Yokoya K, Huyase M, Kojima A, Kato H, Tani T, Inada T. *Stenting after revascularization of chronic total occlusion* [abstr]. Circulation 92(suppl I):I-94 (1995).

27. Goldberg SL, Colombo A, Maiello L, Borrione M, Finci L, Almagor Y. *Intracoronary stent insertion after balloon angioplasty of chronic total occlusions.* J Am Coll Cardiol 26: 713-719 (1995).

28. Sines PA, Golf S, Myreng Y, et al. *Stenting in chronic coronary occlusion (SICCO): a randomized, controlled trial of adding stent implantation after successful angioplasty.* J Am Coll Cardiol 28:1444-1451 (1996)

29. Thomas M, Hancock J, Holmberg S, et al. *Coronary artery stenting following successful angioplasty for total occlusions: preliminary results of a randomized trial* [abstr]. J Am Coll Cardiol 27:153A (1996).

30. Rames SR, Kuntz RE, Schatz RA, et al. *Preliminary experience with the POSSIS coronary AngioJet rheolytic thrombectomy catheter in the VeGAS I pilot study* [abstr]. J Am Coll Cardiol 27:69A (1996).

31. Merino A, Cohen M, Badimon JI, et al. *Synergistic action of severe wall injury and shear forces on thrombus formation in arterial stenosis: definition of a thrombotic shear rate threshold.* J Am Coll Cardiol 24:1091-1094 (1994).

32. Grinstead WC, Raizner AE, Churchill DA, et al. *Intracoronary thrombosis prior to stenting: impact on angiographic success and clinical outcome* [abstr]. J Am Coll Cardiol 21:30A (1993).

33. Kaul U, Agarwal R, Jain P, Wasir H. *Safety and efficacy of intracoronary stenting for thrombus-containing lesions.* Am J Cardiol 77:425-427 (1996).

34. Romero M, Medina A, Suarez de Lezo J, et al. *Elective Palmaz-Schatz stent implantation in acute coronary syndromes induced by thrombus containing lesions* [abstr]. J Am Coll Cardiol 27:179A (1996).

35. Alfonso F, Rodrieguez P, Phillips P, et al. *Clinical and angiographic implications of coronary stenting in thrombus-containing lesions* [abstr]. J Am Coll Cardiol 29(suppl A):96A (1997).

CHAPTER 15

STENTS FOR LEFT MAIN DISEASE

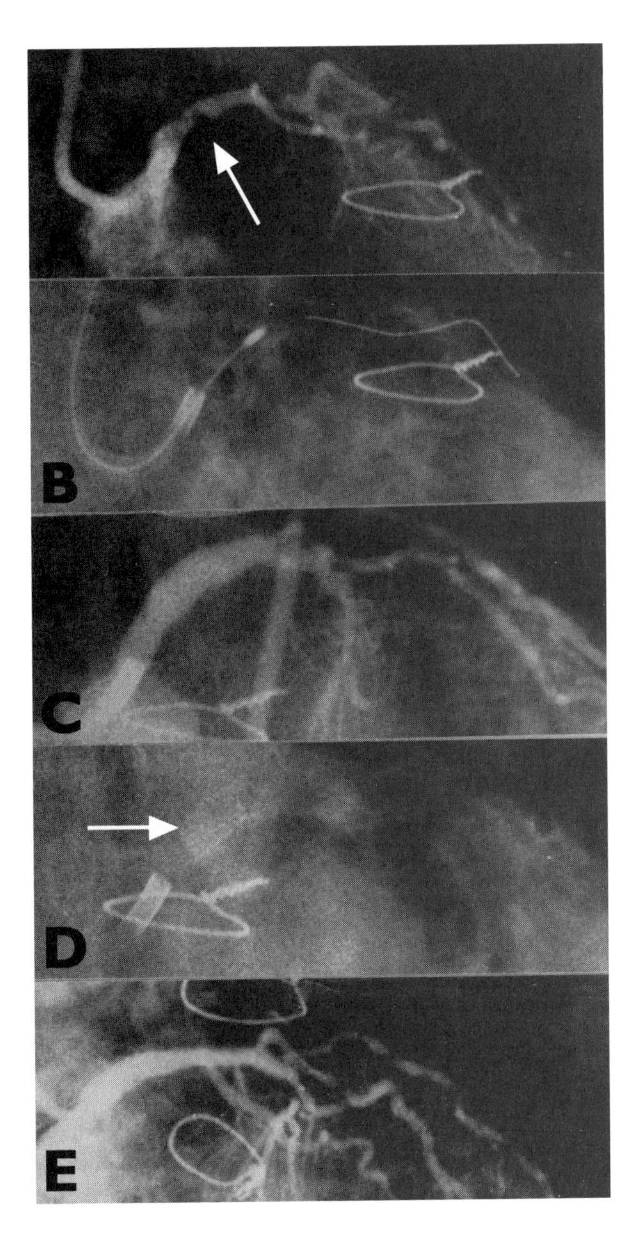

CASE 15.1: Left Main Stenting after Debulking

A 69 year old retired miller with hypertension, diabetes, polycystic kidney disease and chronic renal failure on peritoneal dialysis had undergone two-vessel coronary bypass surgery three years ago. He presented with unstable angina. At angiography, he had a patent internal thoracic artery conduit to the left anterior descending artery which filled the distal left anterior descending, but did not retrogradely fill two diagonals and a septal branch. There was a new 85% left main stenosis with severe calcification which compromised antegrade flow to these tributaries. The circumflex and right coronary arteries were occluded. There was a moderate stenosis in the proximal portion of the saphenous vein graft to the right coronary artery.

The patient was not considered a surgical candidate. When his unstable angina persisted with ischemic electrocardiographic changes over the anterolateral leads after optimizing medical therapy, a transcatheter remedy was requested.

Figure 15.1 Stenting the Left Main Trunk The heavy calcification in the severe lesion of the left main artery (**a;** arrow) was treated first by rotational atherectomy debulking (**b**). After stent implantation there was no residual stenosis (**c**). The biliary stent may be seen in an image without contrast (**d;** arrow). There 6 month angiogram revealed an enduring result (**e**).

PROCEDURE 15.1

The severity of the calcification of the left main was approached with rotational atherectomy using a 1.5mm burr (**Figures 15.1a** and **15.1b**). The 50% residual narrowing after rotablation was treated with a 10mm Palmaz-Schatz biliary stent (P-104). It was placed on a balloon catheter and carefully positioned in the left main artery with the guiding catheter withdrawn into the aorta. The stent was dilated to 20 atm leaving no residual stenosis (**Figure 15.1c**). The radiopaque biliary device is faintly visible in an image without contrast (**Figure 15.1 d**). During the 20 second stent dilatation, the patient's blood pressure remained stable. The patient became angina free and at angiography six months later, there was minimal diffuse left main coronary narrowing of 20% (**Figure 15.1 e**).

MATERIALS 15.1

Guiding Catheter:	8F JL-4 Cook
Guidewires:	Heart Technology Rotablator guide wire 0.09"x 325cm, ACS
	Hi- torque floppy 0.14"x 175 cm
Balloons:	SciMed Cobra 2.0 x 20 mm, 3.5 x 20 mm, 4.0 x 20mm
Stents:	Johnson & Johnson Biliary P 104

CASE 15.2: Stenting Leading to the Left Main Stenosis

A 50 year old man had undergone coronary bypass surgery at the age of 38, receiving a left internal mammary graft to the left anterior descending artery and a saphenous vein graft to the right coronary artery. Three years ago when severe anginal symptoms developed, the proximal left anterior descending stenosis was treated with balloon angioplasty. Six months ago, the patient had angina due to late restenosis or a new lesion of the proximal left anterior descending before the origin of large septal and diagonal tributaries. Because the left anterior descending was occluded in its mid portion, the intact internal mammary artery graft provided no flow to this region. Consequently, stent implantation to the proximal left anterior descending artery was performed. A distal dissection after placement of a Palmaz-Schatz stent was treated by passing an AVE Micro stent distally. **Figures 15.2 a & b** depict the left anterior descending coronary lesion prior to treatment and the Palmaz-Schatz and AVE Micro stents in place with the persistent distal dissection.

The patient tolerated the procedure without complications and again became asymptomatic. However, four months after the procedure, he again developed exertional angina. Angiography demonstrated a new stenosis of the left main segment (**Figure 15.2c**), presumably due to catheter trauma and/or a non-visualized dissection extending into the left main from the previous procedure. It was elected to proceed with stent implantation in the left main coronary artery.

PROCEDURE 15.2

The left main procedure was not felt to require extra hemodynamic support because of good left ventricular function and two patent saphenous vein grafts. A NIR stent (16mm) was chosen because of its high radial support. An extra support guidewire was passed across the left main lesion and into the distal left anterior descending vessel. The lesion was pre-dilated with a partly compliant 4mm balloon for 15 seconds at 4 atm. The NIR stent was positioned with the guiding catheter withdrawn from the ostium (**Figure 15.2d**). The stent was deployed with one 40 second inflation at 16 atm. The final result is shown in **Figure 15.2e**. The comparative radiopacity of three stainless steel stents (NIR, P-S Biliary, and AVE-Micro) can be seen in **Figure 15.2f**. The patient remains asymptomatic 3 months after the procedure.

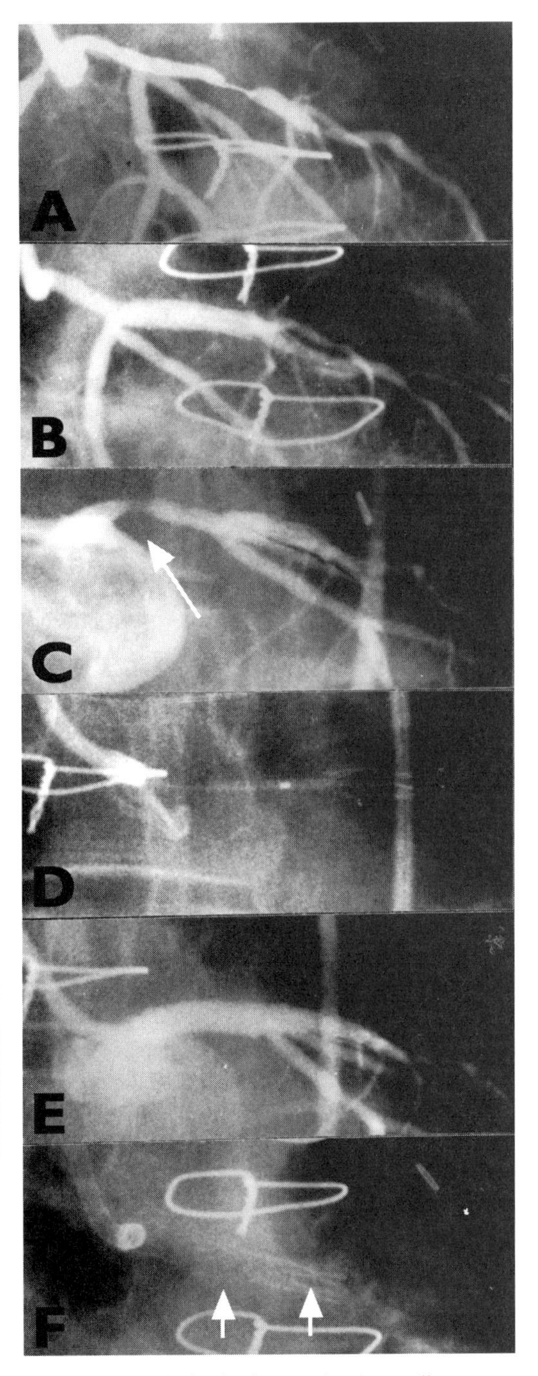

MATERIALS 15.2

Guiding Catheter:	Cook Lumax JL-4
Guide wires:	ACS Extra Support 0.014"
Balloons:	SciMed/Boston Scientific Viva 4.0 x 20 mm
Stents:	SciMed/Boston Scientific Rigid Flex NIR 16mm

Figure 15.2 Stenting Leading to Stenosis of the Left Main Trunk The severe lesion in the anterior descending artery (**a**) was treated first with a Palmaz-Schatz I stent. Dissection distally was partly treated by passing a Micro stent through the Palmaz-Schatz device leaving some distal dissection (**b**). Four months later a new stenosis of the left main (**c; arrow**) was treated with a Rigid-Flex (NIR) stent leaving no stenosis (**e**). Note that the guiding catheter is withdrawn into the ascending aorta during stent positioning (**d**). The final result is excellent (**e**). The relative radiopacity of the distal Micro then mid Palmaz-Schatz I and proximal Rigid-flex (NIR) stent is seen in an image without contrast injection (**f; arrows**).

DISCUSSION

Percutaneous revascularization for disease of the left main coronary artery remains controversial. Evidence is overwhelming that surgical therapy is superior to medical therapy. Any patient with significant left main coronary disease who is a candidate should be referred for surgery. Nonetheless, certain clinical circumstances accompanying left main lesions have, at times, supported a non-surgical approach. Given the shortcomings of angioplasty for left main coronary artery stenosis, the application of stents in this setting has appeal.

Indications for Left Main Coronary Angioplasty

Among the first five patients to undergo coronary angioplasty, Andreas Gruentzig dilated two left main coronary arteries.[1] Procedural difficulties and the early cardiac death of one of these two patients led Gruentzig to conclude that disease of the left coronary common trunk was a contraindication to angioplasty.[2] Traditional guidelines for angioplasty have considered angioplasty of the left main artery in the absence of a patent bypass graft ("unprotected left main") to be the single major contraindication.[3] Surgical mortality for patients with left main artery lesions and prior coronary bypass may exceed 20% .[4] Thus, recent reviews support angioplasty of the left main artery only under certain extenuating clinical circumstances.[5] In addition to cases protected by prior coronary bypass surgery, cases involving acute or subacute occlusion of the left main trunk requiring urgent revascularization and cases with coincident non-cardiac contraindications to surgery have been accepted as candidates for percutaneous revascularization. Aided by techniques of portable cardiopulmonary support, the incidence of angioplasty of the left main coronary has steadily increased. At the Clinique Pasteur in Toulouse, for example, left main coronary angioplasty had increased from one patient a year in 1989 to one patient a week in 1995.[4]

Results of Left Main Coronary Angioplasty

Reports of angioplasty of the left main coronary probably reflect a publication bias which favors positive results. Despite this bias, acute success rates of 90-95% followed by unfavorable long-term survival have been reported.[6,7] Elective, protected left main angioplasty cases have a 10% three-year mortality, while acute unprotected cases have been associated with a 70% three year mortality.[5] The hemodynamic support of intraaortic balloon counterpulsation and percutaneous cardiopulmonary bypass has improved the short term outcomes of these procedures, but has not resulted in a more favorable long-term prognosis.[8] Occasional reports suggesting improved 1-2 year survival over these original groups may be the result of technical advances, improved case selection, or may represent the aforementioned publication bias.[9,10] Despite reasonable acute success rates, these long-term failings have suggested that the restenosis rate of over 50% is the major obstacle to successful percutaneous left main revascularization.

Complications of Left Main Coronary Angioplasty

The aorta is 2-4mm thick at the origin of the left main artery. Thus, the left main ostium, contained within the wall of the aorta, contains more smooth muscle and elastic tissue than any other portion of the coronary system. There is frequently heavy calcification visible at this site further reducing the compliance of this region. These anatomic features produce considerable elastic recoil and may account for the increased restenosis and late failings of angioplasty of the left main coronary artery.[5,11] In addition, the major acute risk of angioplasty of the left main artery is vessel dissection and its dire consequences for this critical blood supply source.

To address the shortcomings of angioplasty for recoil and calcific lesion dissections, stenting has been applied successfully to left main artery lesions, first reported by Carlos Macaya and colleagues at Hospital Universitario San Carlos.[12] Three patients with unprotected left main artery disease received stents because of severe elastic recoil after angioplasty. All three were discharged without complication.[12] The Clinique Pasteur subsequently reported on 34 patients, one of whom had subacute thrombosis which was successfully treated.[13] At an average of 13 months follow-up, the restenosis rate was 13% including one sudden death. The results were felt to compare favorably with the risk of surgery in this group. In another report, 32 patients, 91% of whom had a protected left main vessel, had an 80% event-free survival at 6-month follow-up with no deaths.[14]

Special Considerations for Stenting

The success rates reported by groups with extensive experience reflect a respect for the procedural risks, as well as an appreciation of procedural techniques to reduce those risks. Cases with left coronary artery dominance, absence of collaterals or the protection of bypass grafts, reduced left ventricular function, or acute hemodynamic compromise have the highest risk for procedural morbidity and mortality. These patients also derive the greatest benefit from hemodynamic support during the procedure.

Several anatomic features may preclude stenting in the left main artery location. Disease in the ostia of the left anterior descending or circumflex arteries and severe angulation between the left main and the proximal circumflex prohibit stenting. Heavy calcification may require debulking with rotational atherectomy prior to stent implantation, as was performed in *Case 15.1.*

In addition to these pre-procedural considerations, special precautions need to be taken during the procedure. The guiding catheter must be kept in the aorta, non-selectively engaging the left main to allow maximal flow during catheter manipulations. Non-engagement of the ostium also prevents inflation of balloons of 4-5mm diameter within the guiding catheter. Balloons and stents must be positioned to avoid trauma to the ostia of the left anterior descending and circumflex arteries. Since the angioplasty balloons usually protrude proximally into the aorta, short balloons are favored for some of the shorter left main artery segments. The proximal end of the stent should be positioned so that a 1-2mm portion protrudes into the aorta, but ensuring complete scaffolding of the ostium. The final post-deployment balloon inflation should demonstrate the balloon positioned well proximal to the stent, ensuring that the stent struts are flared to the wall of the aorta.

After deployment of the stent, particular care must be taken not to damage these protruding struts during further catheter injections. One particularly helpful technique when positioning the guiding catheter for final images is to inflate the balloon to 1 atm within the stent with 1-2 mm protruding into the aorta. With the balloon inflated and protecting the stent struts, the guiding catheter is pulled over the balloon into position for final angiography. This encourages coaxial intubation of the stented ostium and minimizes stent trauma. Above all, one must pay continuous attention to the arterial blood pressure during balloon inflations. Immediate balloon deflation should occur when the systolic pressure drops below 80mmHg.

Clinical Conditions Associated with Poor Survival

Notwithstanding the current percutaneous technical progress, surgical therapy remains the method of first choice for any patient with disease of the left main who is a surgical candidate. Percutaneous remedies should remain uncommon in most centers. Many laboratories may first confront angioplasty or stenting of the left main trunk in the least favorable setting, such as acute myocardial infarction complicated by hemodynamic compromise. In this setting, knowing when a salvage procedure is futile is as important as any technical experience. Patients in shock presenting eight and nine hours after the onset of infarction associated with occlusion of the left main have been resuscitated by angioplasty of this vessel.[15] Survival in these cases was most dependent on the sufficiency of collaterals. No patient with left coronary dominance survived occlusion of the left main in this series. A retrospective review of the prognosis in patients with anterolateral infarction, shock and left main disease revealed a 94% mortality independent of surgical bypass, angioplasty, or medical treatment.[6] This non-randomized series suggested that these patients had suffered a fatal left ventricular injury by the time of admission and that conservative measures were advised. While this approach may not apply to patients who occlude their left main artery in a catheterization laboratory, no patient whose pain started more than 12 hours before catheterization survived. Thus, patients with both temporal and hemodynamic extremes of clinical presentation of left main coronary occlusion will benefit the least from percutaneous interventions.

SUMMARY

Although stenting for left main disease remains a therapy of last resort for this technique, clinical outcomes have often demonstrated good medium-term benefit. Decisions for stenting left main should consider concomitant medical conditions, suitability for bypass surgery, and future need for coronary revascularization.

References

1. Gruentzig AR. *Transluminal dilatation of coronary artery stenosis.* Lancet 1:263 (1978).
2. Gruentzig AR, Senning A, Siegenthaler WE. *Nonoperative dilatation of coronary-artery stenosis.* N Engl J Med 301:61-67 (1979).
3. *Guidelines for percutaneous transluminal coronary angioplasty: a report from the ACC/AHA task force.* Circulation 78:486-502 (1988).
4. Loop FD, Lytle BW, Cosgrove DM, et al. *Reoperation for coronary atherosclerosis: changing practice in 2509 consecutive patients.* Ann Surg 212:378-385 (1990).
5. Fajadet J, Brunel P, Jordan C, Cassagneau B, Marco JP. *Left main coronary stenting. Sixth complex coronary angioplasty course.* Clinique Pasteur, Toulouse, France, 1995.
6. O'Keefe JH, Hartzler GO, Rutherford BD, et al. *Left main coronary angioplasty: early and late results of 127 acute and elective procedures.* Am J Cardiol 64:144-147 (1989).
7. Stertzer SH, Myler RK, Insel H, et al. *Percutaneous transluminal coronary angioplasty in left main coronary stenosis: a five year appraisal.* Int J Cardiol 9:149-159 (1985).
8. Tommaso CL, Vogel JHK, Vogel RA. *Coronary angioplasty in high-risk patients with left main coronary stenosis: results from the National Registry of Elective Supported Angioplasty.* Cathet Cardiovasc Diagn 25:169-173 (1992).
9. Eldar M, Schulhoff N, Herz I, et al. *Results of percutaneous transluminal angioplasty of the left main coronary artery.* Am J Cardiol 68:255-256(1991).
10. Crowley ST, Morrison DA. *Percutaneous transluminal coronary angioplasty of the left main coronary artery in patients with rest angina.* Cathet Cardiovasc Diagn 33:103-107 (1994).
11. Simonton CA. *Lesion-specific technique considerations in directional coronary atherectomy.* Cathet Cardiovasc Diagn 1(suppl I):3-9 (1993).
12. Macaya C, Alfonso F, Iniguez A, Goicolea J, Hernandez R, Zarco P. *Stenting for elastic recoil during coronary angioplasty of the left main coronary artery.* Am J Cardiol 70:105-107 (1992).
13. Fajadet J, Brunel P, Jordan C, et al. *Is Stenting of left main coronary artery a reasonable procedure?* Circulation 92(Suppl I):I-74-75 (1995).
14. Lopez JL, Caputo RP, Kalon KL, et al. *Percutaneous treatment of left main coronary stenosis with new devices: acute results and intermediate term followup.* Circulation 92(suppl I):I-147 (1995).
15. Spiecker M, Erbel R, Rupprecht HJ, Meyer J. *Emergency angioplasty of totally occluded left main coronary artery in acute myocardial infarction and unstable angina pectoris-institutional experience and literature review.* Eur Heart J 15:602-607 (1994).
16. Quigley RL, Milano CA, Smith R, et al. *Prognosis and management of anterolateral myocardial infarction in patients with severe left main disease and cardiogenic shock: the left main shock syndrome.* Circulation 88[part 2]:65-70 (1993).

CHAPTER 16

STENT RETRIEVAL TECHNIQUES

CASE 16.1: Stent Embolization

A 63 year old man with a month of exertional angina presented with resting chest pain. Coronary angiography disclosed mild disease in the proximal left anterior descending artery and a critical lesion in the mid right coronary artery with ulceration and a visible large cleft (**Figure 16.1a**). There was a significant Shepherd's crook curve with a mild non-calcified lesion in the proximal right coronary artery.

PROCEDURE 16.1

The lesion was crossed with an extra support guidewire maintaining the tip pointed to the arterial wall opposite the plaque cleft. After dilation with a 3.0mm balloon, a type C dissection (**Figure 16.1b**) was

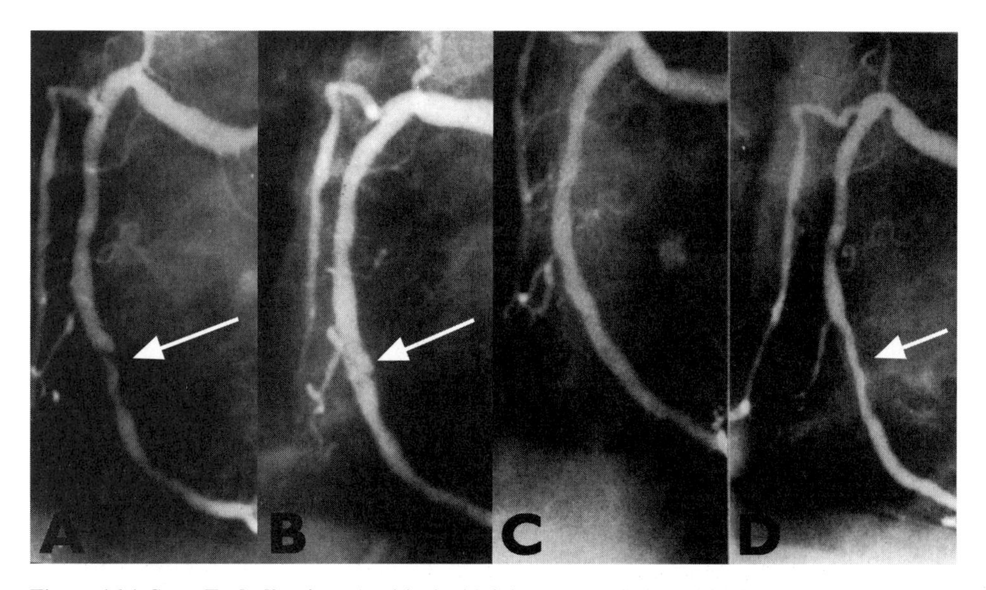

Figure 16.1 Stent Embolization A critical mid right coronary lesion with a large cleft (**a**) was distal to a Shepherd's crook arterial takeoff. Angioplasty resulted in a dissection (**b**) which was treated with stent implantation. The first stent was embolized into the profunda femora artery (see **Figure 16.2**) but the second stent resulted in a satisfactory result (**c**). At angiography 6 months later there was a 50% restenosis (**d**).

noted. It was elected to place a stent to reduce the risk of acute closure. A short stent (P-S 084) was chosen to facilitate passage through the proximal tortuous right coronary artery. The stent was crimped on the pre-deployment dilation balloon and passed to the Shepherd's crook where it could be neither advanced further nor withdrawn. During forceful withdrawal, the stent moved distally on the mounting balloon. As the system was pulled into the femoral artery sheath, the stent was sheared off and lodged in the mid profunda femora artery. The embolized stent can be seen in the profunda femora with and with-out contrast at the time of embolization (**Figure 16.2a & b**). Our attention returned to the right coronary dissection which was re-crossed with the guidewire. A 2 atm inflation was performed with the 3mm balloon to smooth any intimal disruption. A second P-S 084 was crimped on the balloon and this time with the guiding catheter seated deeply in the right coronary artery, the stent was passed to the dissection site and deployed. The final result revealed minimal residual stenosis (**Figure 16.1c**).

The patient remained symptom free at 6-month follow-up. Angiography revealed a 50% diffuse in-stent restenosis which was managed medically (**Figure 16.1d**). At follow-up 6 months later, the embolized stent was lodged in a small distal branch of the profunda femora (**Figure 16.2c**). The patient was without symptoms of peripheral arterial ischemia or angina one year after the procedure.

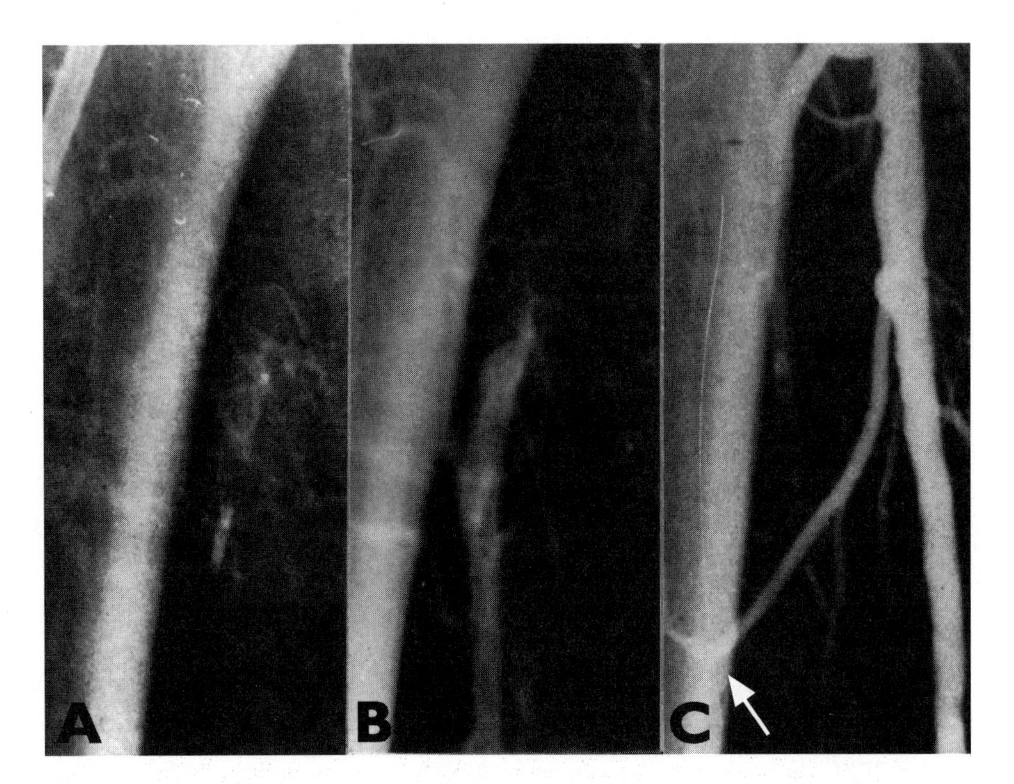

Figure 16.2 Stent Embolization The stent described in **Figure 16.1** slipped off of the guide wire during withdrawal into the femoral artery catheter and embolized into the profunda femora artery where it is seen with and without contrast (**a, b**). Six months later it could be seen lodged in a small distal branch (**c;** arrow).

MATERIALS 16.1

Guiding Catheter:	Schneider Guide-Zilla JR-4 8 French
Guidewires:	ACS/Guidant 0.014" x 300mm Extra Support
Balloons:	Schneider Goldie 3.0 x 20 mm
Stents:	Johnson & Johnson P-S 084 (2)

CASE 16.2: Stent Retrieval

A 54 year old man presented with one month of exertional angina progressing to intermittent rest angina associated with new anterior T-wave inversions. Coronary arteriography revealed a severe stenosis in the proximal left anterior descending artery at the origin of a large diagonal branch (**Figure 16.3a**). Because significant tortuosity of the iliac vessels made passage of the diagnostic catheters challenging, a radial artery approach was chosen for coronary angioplasty. There was minimal proximal left anterior descending tortuosity without calcification.

PROCEDURE 16.2

Using a soft tipped 6 French Amplatz guide catheter, the left anterior descending lesion was crossed with an extra support guidewire. Deep seating of the guiding catheter was necessary during balloon manipulations

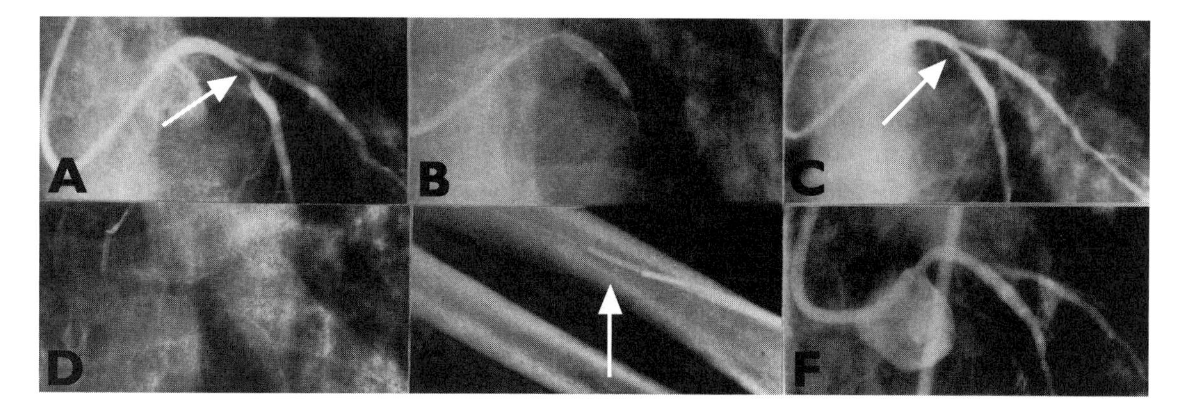

Figure 16.3 Stent Retrieval Using a radial artery approach, a proximal anterior descending artery lesion (**a;** arrow) required deep seating of the guiding catheter in order to pass a balloon to the lesion (**b**). A dissection resulted (**c;** arrow). A 15mm stent could not be passed to the dissection and became dislodged from its balloon. With the guiding catheter withdrawn into the ascending aorta the stent could be withdrawn from the left main artery and lassoed with a snare (**d**). The snare was withdrawn through the radial artery sheath (**e;** arrow). After two shorter stents were passed from the femoral approach, the lesion and dissection were well treated (**f**).

(**Figure 16.3a**). The large diagonal branch was protected with a separate stiff guidewire and, with considerable guiding catheter manipulation, a balloon was positioned and the left anterior descending lesion dilated (**Figure 16.3b**). The guiding catheter remained deep seated beyond the circumflex ostium so that the circumflex was not visualized throughout these maneuvers. A dissection from the initial balloon inflations (2 and 3 atm) resulted in TIMI 0-1 flow (**Figure 16.3c**). It was elected to stent the dissected segment using the 6 French angioplasty guiding catheter. A Palmaz-Schatz 153 stent was crimped on the angioplasty balloon and passed to the left main artery where the combination of a mild curve, distal intimal disruption and suboptimal guiding catheter support prevented further stent passage. On retraction, the stent had slipped off the balloon. The guidewire was extended and the guiding catheter-balloon-stent assembly withdrawn from the coronary artery. The stent was withdrawn from the left main into the ascending aorta where a snare was able to be passed around it (**Figure 16.3d**). The snare and stent were then withdrawn into the radial artery sheath (**Figure 16.3e**) and removed from the patient.

At this point, it was elected to proceed with two shorter stents using a stiffer 8 French Judkins-shaped guide via femoral access. The left anterior descending guidewire was left in place and a new extra support guidewire was passed across the dissected lesion. The original guidewire was withdrawn and a short stent (P-S 104) was easily passed to the target site and deployed. After the implantation of a second short stent proximally, there was no residual lesion or dissection in the left anterior descending or the diagonal branch (**Figure 16.3f**). The patient became angina free and was discharged on the fourth day post-procedure.

Angina recurred five months later. An angiogram at six months revealed a moderate (50%) diameter narrowing within the most proximal of the two stents and a new severe left main stenosis. This latter stenosis was attributed to procedural trauma of both the guiding catheter and the initially failed stent. The patient was referred for surgical revascularization

MATERIALS 16.2

Guiding Catheter:	Schneider Pink Power 6 French AL-1, Cordis 8 French JL-3.5
Guidewires:	ACS Extra Support 0.014"x 175cm, DOC extension, USCI Phantom 0.014"x 180mm
Balloons:	Schneider Goldie 3.0 x 20mm, 3.5 x 20mm
Stents:	Johnson & Johnson P-S 153(15mm), 104 (8mm) (2)
Snare:	Microvena Goose Neck Amplatz Snare 5mm x 120cm

DISCUSSION

Stent loss or embolization may occur during complex procedures. Stent deployment failure may result in stent dislodgment from the delivery balloon. **Figure 16.4** is a schematic of factors associated with stent deployment failure.

Stent Embolization

Stent embolization is defined as dislodgment of the stent from both the delivery balloon and the guide wire. It occurs most commonly with stents which are bare-mounted on balloons, a frequent practice in European centers. The use of bare-mounted biliary stents (Johnson & Johnson Interventional Systems, Warren NJ) and non-protected bailout stents (Cook) may also require application of various retrieval techniques. It should be noted that the problem of distal embolization is not obviated even with sheathed delivery systems. Deployment balloon rupture and "watermelon seed" slippage of balloons from within stents can result in dislodgment of a non-deployed stent.[2,3]

Lesions in the circumflex artery, lesions at angles >45°, and calcified lesions have been associated with stent dislodgment or embolization.[4]

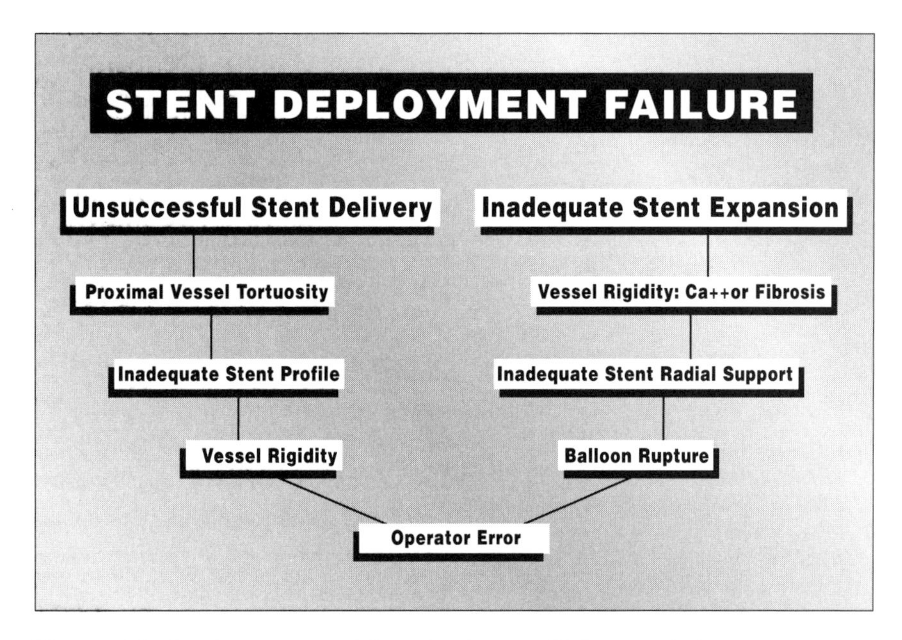

Figure 16.4 The Components of Stent Deployment Failure This figure diagrams the possible components of stent deployment failure. Reprinted with permission from Dr. LF Satler and John Wiley & Sons, Inc. (*Cathet Cardiovasc Diag* 1995;35:216).

Stent Deployment after Balloon Rupture

Keelan et al[2] have described a technique of partial stent deployment despite delivery balloon rupture. Withdrawal of the damaged balloon will often result in stent dislodgment in the proximal arterial segment. In order to avoid this complication the operators were able to partly deploy two stents using an automatic power injector. Using 50% contrast at a rate of 20cc/seconds over 0.25seconds and a pressure limit of 200-400 psi they found in each case that 1cc was injected before the pressure maximum was exceeded. The stents were sufficiently deployed with the damaged balloons to allow their removal. Stent optimization was then accomplished with intact balloons.

Stent Rescue: Snares, Loops, Forceps and Bioptomes

Using grasping devices, operators have been able to retrieve embolized stents from the arterial bed.[5,6] When no device is available, a snare may be fashioned from a 5 French multipurpose catheter into which both ends of a 0.014" exchange length (300cm) wire have been introduced.[7] These techniques require only pinning the stent between a surface and the operant device before capture and withdrawal. **Figure 16.5** demonstrates the method of stent retrieval with a snare. Although these retrieval devices are readily available, easy to apply, and have a high success rate, certain precautions need to be observed. First, these techniques require that the dislodged stent be located in a space sufficiently large to accommodate the rescuing device. Thus, anywhere distal to the coronary ostium is beyond reach. Second, the length of standard guiding catheters combined with a Touhey-Borst adapter exceeds the working length of these snares. Most common loops and snares of 110cm length require removal of the guiding catheter before there is sufficient snare length to reach stents outside of the guiding catheter. Finally, bioptomes and forceps must be used with obvious caution to avoid trauma to the arterial walls and to avoid severing of the distal guidewire.

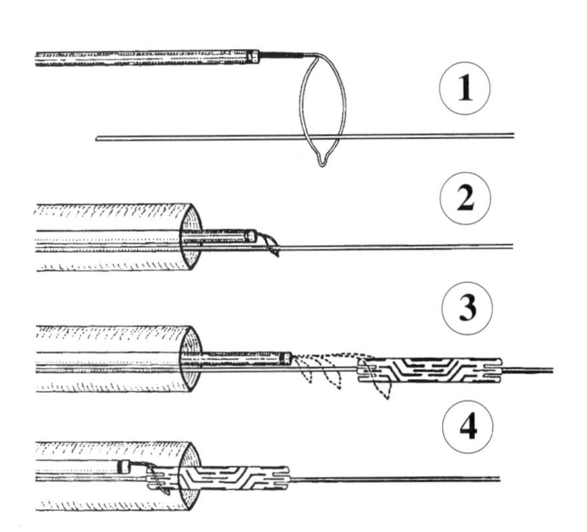

Figure 16.5 Stent Retrieval with a Snare The snare's loop is inserted into the guiding catheter over the guide wire (**1**). It is advanced through the distal catheter tip (**2**) until the stent is approached and lassoed (**3**). While the snare is held tightly withdrawn into its own sheath thus grasping the stent the entire apparatus is withdrawn (**4**). Reprinted with permission from Dr. Javier Goicolea, Clinica San Carlos, Madrid, Spain.

Balloon Embolectomy

Rozenman et al[8] have demonstrated effective removal of an unexpanded stent from a saphenous graft by passage of a second guide wire and 3mm balloon distal to the stent. After advancing the guiding catheter into the graft the distal 3mm balloon was inflated and withdrawn, thus capturing the stent between balloon and guiding catheter. The entire system was then withdrawn successfully resulting in effective embolectomy.

Mega-balloon Embolectomy

Cishek et al[9] successfully used a 9mm peripheral angioplasty balloon catheter to remove a stent in the ilio-femoral system. This large balloon was passed alongside the embolized stent and inflated to only 1 atm. Withdrawal of the balloon at this pressure caused the stent to become enveloped in the balloon's invaginations and allowed withdrawal into the femoral sheath. There was no arterial damage reported.

Double Wire Helix Technique

As previously applied to lost angioplasty device components, a technique involving two guidewires, has been successfully applied by Wong et al[8] to undeployed stents within the coronary arteries. The undeployed stent lying free within an artery remained on the original central guidewire. Using a new 175cm standard or extra support guidewire (a floppy wire will not work), the operator maneuvers the tip of this new wire through the stent struts and distal to the stent as far as possible. When capturing a Palmaz-Schatz stent in this way, a 0.014" guidewire must cross at the central articulation or at a partly deployed portion of the non-articulated versions. This is because the stent slots are only 0.012" apart and in the unexpanded state they will not accommodate a guidewire. After crossing the stent, the new guidewire is bound to the original guidewire by passing both of their distal ends through a steering device and tightening. Under fluoroscopy, the two wires are twisted clockwise 15-20 turns or until the wires are seen to respond within the coronary artery. Retraction of both wires together draws the guide deeply within the ostium if a proper stent capture has been accomplished. The guidewires and guiding catheter are withdrawn as a unit.

Partial Expansion Method

Another common method to recapture a stent involves passing a 1.5mm balloon within it and expanding the balloon. While this method occasionally succeeds, it may often only push the stent more distally on the guidewire.

Damaged Stents

Stents may be partially damaged while still in place on the delivery balloon more frequently than they are embolized or dislodged. This may occur due to unforeseen trauma of proximal lesions, calcification and tortuosity. A key technical point to remember is that a stent damaged by partial dislodgment may not re-enter the guiding catheter easily. It is desirable that the stent be sheathed by the guiding catheter before removal from the patient. To avoid the risk of cerebral embolization, the guiding catheter with the entire assembly of the protruding delivery balloon and stent should be withdrawn into the descending aorta before attempting to retract the delivery system into the catheter. While stent embolization is generally harmless, cerebral embolization should not be risked by unnecessary stent manipulations in the ascending aorta.[4]

SUMMARY

Obviously, the best approach is to never lose a stent in the first place. Significant vessel tortuosity, calcification, or mild stenoses proximal to the target lesion may contribute to stent dislodgment from its delivery balloon. The protective sheaths of stent delivery systems should not be withdrawn until the stent has been passed sufficiently distal to the lesion. Nonetheless, despite excellent technique and attention to underlying anatomy, stents will be displaced or misplaced in some unusual circumstances. In such a case, the techniques described above may prove useful to retrieve the stent or convert maldeployment to a successful placement.

References

1. Satler LF. *The frustrations of coronary stenting.* Cathet Cardiovasc Diag 35:216-217 (1995).
2. Keelan ET, Nunez BD, Berger PB, Holmes DR, Garrett KN. *Management of balloon rupture during rigid stent deployment.* Cathet Cardiovasc Diag 35:211-215 (1995).
3. Wong PHC. *Retrieval of undeployed intracoronary Palmaz-Schatz Stents.* Cathet Cardiovasc Diag 35:218-223 (1995).
4. Alfonso F, Martinez D, Hernandez R, et al. *Stent embolization during intracoronary stenting.* Am J Cardiol 78:833-835 (1996).
5. Foster-Smith KW, Garratt KN, Higaro ST, Holmes DR. *Retrieval techniques for managing flexible intracoronary stent misplacement.* Cathet Cardiovasc Diag 30:63-68 (1993).
6. Eeckhout E, Stauffer JC, Goy JJ. *Retrieval of migrated coronary stents by means of an alligator forceps catheter.* Cathet Cardiovasc Diag 30:166-168 (1993).
7. Pan M, Medina A, Romero M, Suarez de Lezo J, Hernandez E, Pavolic D, Melian F, Marrera J, Cabrera JA. *Peripheral stent recovery after failed intracoronary delivery.* Cathet Cardiovasc Diag 27:230-233 (1992).
8. Rozenman Y, Burstein M, Hasin Y, Gotsma MS. *Retrieval of occluding unexpanded Palmaz-Schatz stent from a saphenous aorto-coronary vein graft.* Cathet Cardiovasc Diag 34:159-161 (1995).
9. Cishek MB, Laslett L, Gershong G. *Balloon catheter retrieval of dislodged coronary artery stents: a novel technique.* Cathet Cardiovasc Diag 34:350-352 (1995).

CHAPTER 17

INTRAVASCULAR ULTRASOUND IMAGING (IVUS) FOR STENT OPTIMIZATION

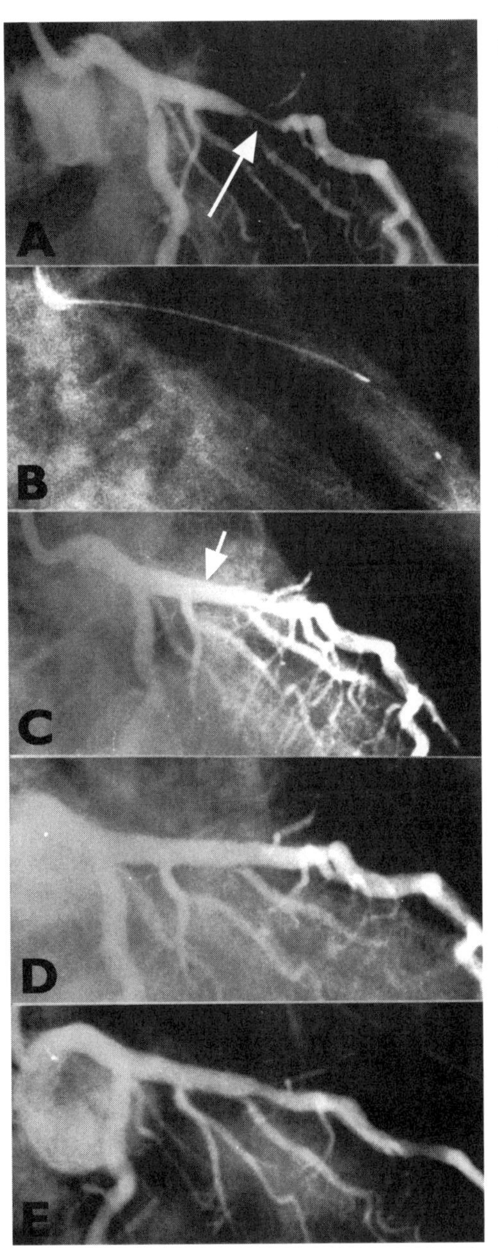

Figure 17.1 **Intracoronary Ultrasound of Dissection** A severe proximal left anterior descending lesion (**a;** arrow) was referred for angioplasty. Ultrasound catheter imaging was performed (**b**) (see **Figure 17.2**). A type C dissection developed after angioplasty (**c;** arrow) which responded to stent implantation (**d**). At 6 month follow up there was no restenosis (**e**).

CASE 17.1: IVUS and Arterial Dissection

A 52 year old man presented with recurrent angina after a non-Q-wave anteroseptal myocardial infarction with apeak CPK of 1070mg/d. Coronary angiography demonstrated a severe proximal left anterior descending stenosis (**Figure 17.1a**).

PROCEDURE 17.1

Angioplasty was performed with an extra support guidewire. For interest, IVUS evaluation was performed and revealed a reference vessel diameter of 3.9mm, a severe eccentric lesion, and a significant amount of deep calcium (240% arc) (**Figure 17.1b**). The acoustic signature of calcium, brighter than the adventitia with "echo drop-out" is apparent in **Figure 17.2a**.

Angioplasty with a 3.5mm balloon resulted in a type C dissection (**Figure 17.1c**). Despite prolonged low pressure balloon dilations, the dissection did not improve and, in fact, appeared more complex. Repeat IVUS evaluation showed a mobile flap of the dissection, also seen during contrast injections (**Figure 17.2 b & c**). A stent was passed and deployed. The dissection and original lesion were

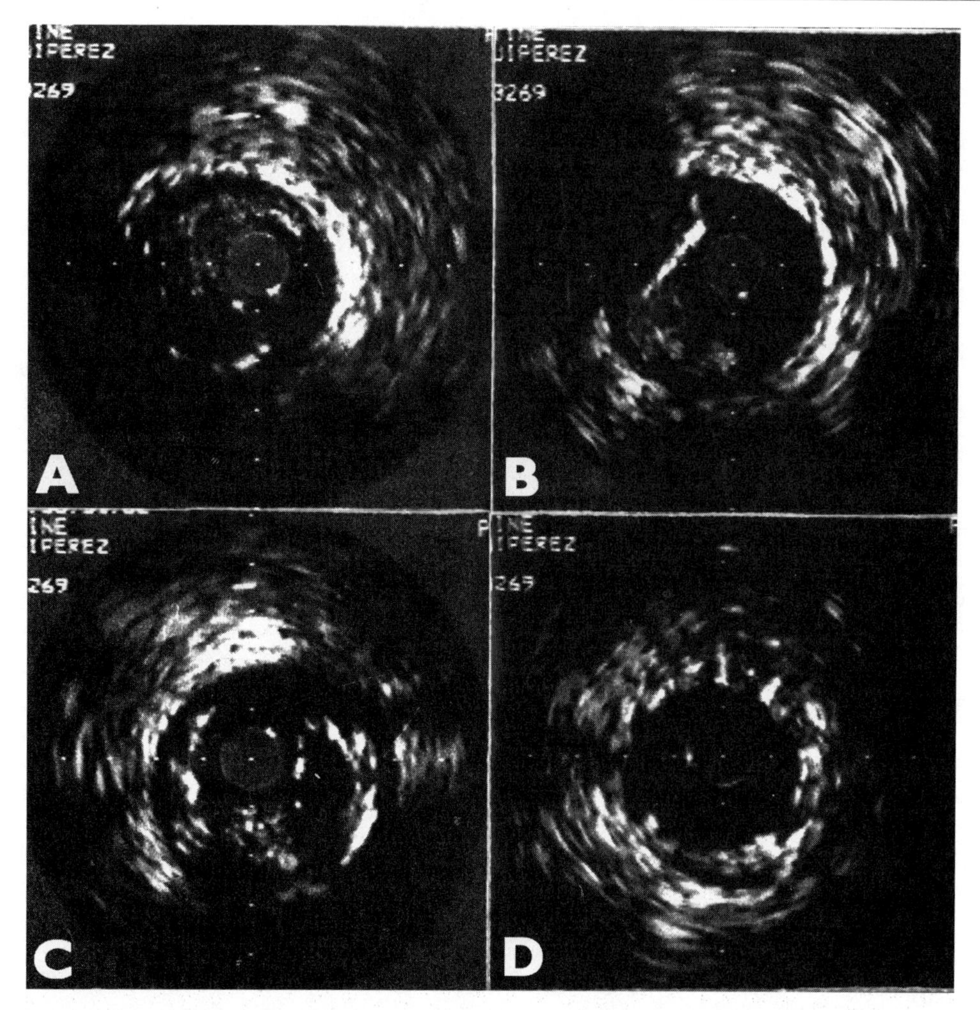

Figure 17.2 Intracoronary Ultrasound of Dissection. IVUS imaging of the artery in figure 17.1 reveals a surprising amount of deep calcium in an arc of 240% with typical "echo drop-out" at 6 to 9 o'clock (**a**). After angioplasty a mobile dissection is noted at 7 to 8 o'clock and then 4 to 6 o'clock (**b, c**). After stent implantation IVUS revealed resolution of the dissection and a symmetric apposition of the stent (**d**).

sealed leaving no residual obstruction (**Figure 17.1d**). After brief high pressure dilation with a 3.5 mm balloon to 12 atm, IVUS confirmed a satisfactory lumen (**Figure 17.2d**). The stented segment diameter was 3.5mm with complete apposition of the stent against the intima with a symmetry index of 0.89 (normal = 1.0). There was no evidence of dissection distally. No further dilations were performed.

The patient was asymptomatic after the procedure. Treadmill testing (12 METS) 6 months later was negative. Angiography revealed a 20% lesion in the proximal portion of the stent (**Figure 17.1e**). The patient remained asymptomatic and continues on medical therapy.

MATERIALS 17.1

Guiding Catheter:	Schneider Guide Zilla JL-4 8 French
Guidewires:	ACS Extra Support 0.014"x 175cm
Balloons:	USCI Pronto Rely 3.5 x 20mm, Schneider Speedino 3.5 x 9 mm
IVUS:	Mansfield Sonicath 3.5 French, 30 MHz on a Hewlett Packard Sonos System
Stents:	Johnson & Johnson P-S 154

CASE 17.2: IVUS and Intrastent Masses

A 37 year old man with multiple coronary artery disease risk factors had recurrent rest pain after a non-Q-wave inferior myocardial infarction. Angiography revealed a severe ulcerated lesion in the mid right coronary artery with associated thrombus (**Figure 17.3a**). The patient was treated with oral antiplatelet therapy and intravenous heparin and returned to the laboratory for angioplasty one week later.

PROCEDURE 17.2

Initial images of the target lesion revealed a complex lesion appearance with features of thrombus. After crossing the lesion with an extra support guidewire, 6 dilations were performed with a 3.5mm balloon to a maximum pressure of 12 atm for 120 seconds. The complex appearance of the lesion did not improve with a residual 50% diameter stenosis. A Gianturco-Roubin I stent was implanted across the affected site and post-dilated with a 4.0mm balloon (**Figure 17.4**). The majority of the lesion was well treated by this maneuver, but an amorphous contrast lucency was evident proximal to the coil stent. A 15mm Palmaz-Schatz stent was implanted at this site, resulting in a prominent lucency in the proximal portion of the Gianturco-Roubin stent which did not respond to post-stent dilations to 10 atm for 120 seconds (**Figure 17.3b**). A 3 French IVUS catheter was passed to the questionable site. A persistent dissection proximal to the Palmaz stent (**Figure 17.3c**) and an echo-dense mass intraluminally within the Gianturco-Roubin stent was identified (**Figure 17.3d**). During automated pull back of the IVUS catheter, a frond of dissected tissue or thrombus could be seen protruding between the overexpanded coils of the Gianturco-Roubin stent (**Figure 17.3e**). This density resolved at the point where the Palmaz-Schatz device scaffolded the opened coil device (**Figure 17.3f**). An additional half Palmaz-Schatz stent was implanted proximal to the first Palmaz-Schatz stent. The distal contrast lucencies resolved within the Gianturco-Roubin stent with a <10% residual narrowing in the target area (**Figure 17.3g**). Follow-up IVUS examination confirmed the resolution of intraluminal lucencies and masses. The patient became asymptomatic and was discharged after 48 hours on antiplatelet therapy.

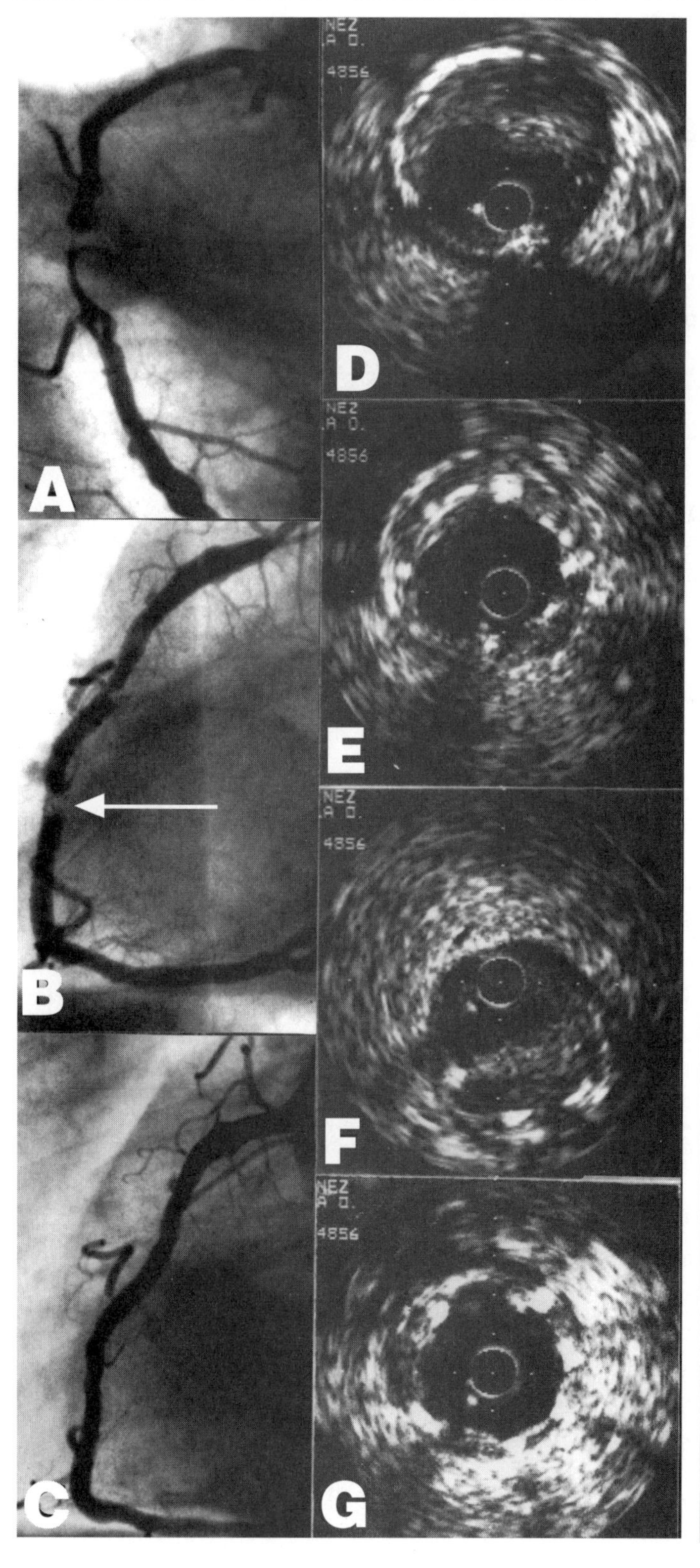

Figure 17.3 Intracoronary Ultrasound of Intrastent Masses (Left panels) A severe mid right coronary artery lesion was associated with thrombus (**a**). After deployment of Gianturco-Roubin I and Palmaz-Schatz II stents an amorphous mass remained within the proximal portion of the coil stent (**b;** arrow). IVUS evaluation revealed a frond of tissue or thrombus extruding between the over expanded coils of the Gianturco-Roubin stent which responded to implantation of an additional half Palmaz-Schatz stent in the proximal portion of the Gianturco-Roubin coil (**c**).

(Right panels) The IVUS image within the Gianturco-Roubin coil reveals an echo dense mass at 1 to 2 o'clock (**d**). Within the Palmaz-Schatz stent, there was no mass (**e**) except where it first apposed the coil stent (**f**). After further scaffolding of the coil stent with a half Palmaz-Schatz device there was no evidence of the mass (**g**). Note the well apposed struts of the slotted tube stent in **g**.

MATERIALS 17.2

Guiding Catheter:
- Cook Lumax JR-4 8 French

Guidewires:
- ACS/Guidant Extra Support 0.014"x 300cm

Balloons:
- Schneider Goldie 3.5 x 20 mm
- Schneider Spedino 4.0 x 20 mm

IVUS:
- 30 MHz Hewlett Packard Sonos System

Stents:
- Cook Gianturco-Roubin 4.0 x 20 mm
- Johnson & Johnson P-S 154 (15mm) 153 (15mm) used

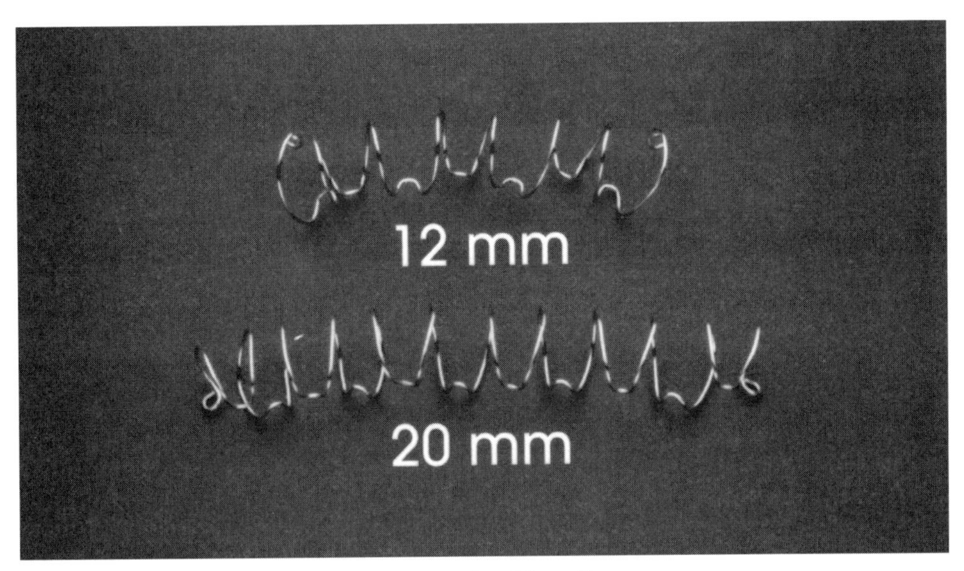

Figure 17.4 The Gianturco-Roubin I A flexible coil stent.

DISCUSSION

IVUS has been invaluable in the development of proper coronary stent deployment techniques. IVUS has been instrumental in planning an optimal interventional strategy[1] as well as in assessing and improving results after initial implantation.[2] Employing high pressure balloon inflations to optimize stent deployment was validated by IVUS and ultimately has been critical in facilitating the reduction of anticoagulant regimens after stenting.[3] IVUS-guided stent deployment has been associated with a low restenosis rate.[4] Despite the success of IVUS, an important question in most interventional laboratories remains: Is the routine application of IVUS to stent deployment a necessity or a luxury?

IVUS vs Angiographic Lumenology

Angiography is insufficient to reveal the underlying anatomy of a vessel. Anatomic detail is compromised by vessel foreshortening, oblique imaging axes, ostial locations, overlapping branches, and opaque catheters. IVUS can accurately delineate the underlying vascular anatomy and lesion severity. Lesion characteristics predisposing to complications or favoring alternate therapies may be more readily appreciated by IVUS.

Calcification predicts the length and severity of dissections at angioplasty,[6] as well as the failure of directional atherectomy[7] and the success of rotational atherectomy.[8] Lesion calcification is significantly underestimated by fluoroscopy when compared to IVUS examination.[5]

IVUS may reveal thrombus, eccentricity, dissection or distal lesions unsuspected by angiography, features vital to a successful intervention. When IVUS-acquired information such as this was applied in an organized study of interventional patients, the planned procedure was modified 40% of the time.[1]

An important use of an IVUS examination prior to stent implantation is the determination of the normal reference vessel diameter. The extent of underlying atherosclerosis is always more severe than revealed by angiography. Angiographically normal segments may have 35-50% of their cross-sectional area (CSA) occupied by plaque which is angiographically inapparent.[9,26] IVUS is ideally suited to identify the most normal segment for determination of reference diameters before stent deployment.

IVUS and Stent Deployment

Despite pre-procedural lesion and vessel information, the greatest procedural advantage of IVUS is confirming optimal stent deployment. Angiography does not demonstrate the geometry of complete stent expansion. This inadequacy led to early recommendations that stents should be routinely over-expanded by 10% angiographically.[10] With the exception of final minimal lumen diameter (MLD) correlating with post-procedural complications, angiography cannot predict subacute thrombosis. Unlike angiography, ultrasound criteria have been applied to assess the adequacy of stent deployment. These criteria include:

1. Symmetry of stent expansion: minor lumen diameter divided by the major perpendicular diameter (see **Figure 17.5**).
2. Apposition of stent to the vessel wall: absence of echo-free spaces between stent and vessel.
3. Adequate cross-sectional area ratios of stent-to-reference vessel segments.
4. Absence of persistent uncovered dissection.
5. Absence of inflow or outflow narrowings.

Although stents may seem optimally deployed by angiographic criteria, IVUS examination may reveal an inadequate stent deployment in over 80% of procedures.[2] Frequently stents may be inadequately or asymmetrically expanded with struts poorly apposed to the arterial wall despite an excellent angiographic appearance.[2,11] Suboptimal deployment occurred despite the routine use of a balloon 0.5mm larger than the QCA reference diameter. Seventy-five percent of these patients underwent further dilations based on ultrasound findings resulting in a 34% increase in the minimal stent cross-sectional area. The improvement in the stent cross-sectional area corresponded to an average increase of 0.5mm in the minimum lumen diameter by angiography. The stent angiographic diameter was mid way between the proximal and distal reference segment diameters. Interestingly, IVUS parameters are also imperfect. The IVUS symmetry index was not significantly improved and the cross-sectional area remained only 61-71%, the expected balloon cross-sectional area after optimal stent deployment.[11,27]

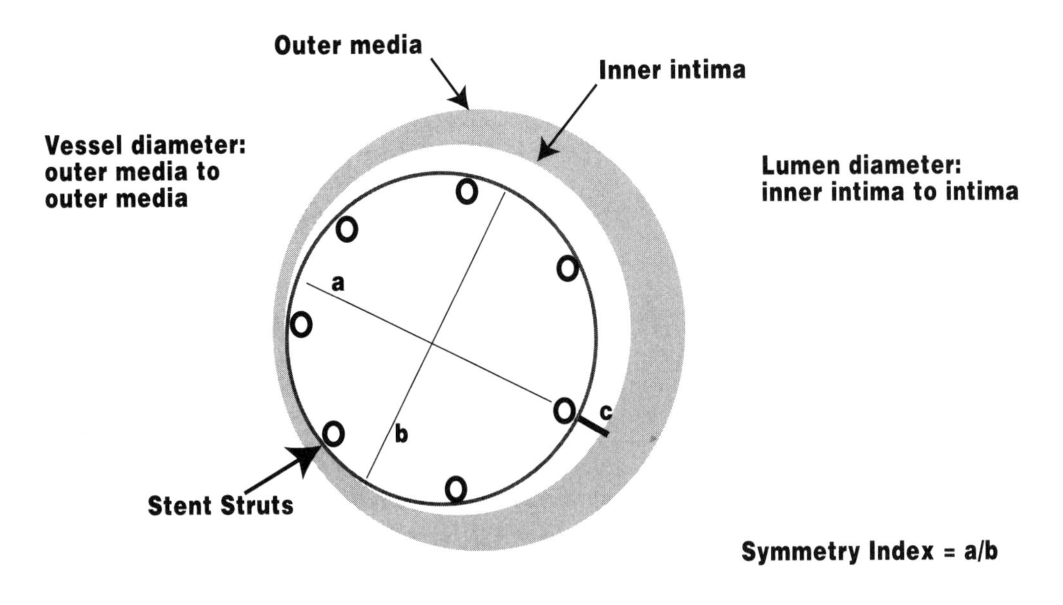

Figure 17.5 Intracoronary Ultrasound Measurements

IVUS-directed optimization of stent geometry resulted in strikingly low rates of subacute occlusion and strongly suggested that incomplete stent deployment, rather than the inherent thrombogenicity of the stent, resulted in stent occlusion. In conjunction with potent antiplatelet therapy, IVUS-guided stent deployment allowed the reduction in anticoagulant regimens prolonged hospitalization.[3] To achieve an acute and subacute occlusion rate <1%, Colombo et al[3] used balloons with a balloon-to-vessel ratio of 1.2:1 and an average inflation pressure of 15 atm to deploy stents. If IVUS confirmed adequate stent deployment, only antiplatelet agents were used post-procedure. The rate was significantly below the historic subacute occlusion rates of 3-4% in the STRESS[12] and Benestent[13] trials and argued strongly for IVUS-assisted stent implantation. Whether these excellent results can be obtained without IVUS using high pressure inflations and large balloons alone remains to be answered.

Antiplatelet Regimens and IVUS for Stenting

Antiplatelet agents and high balloon pressures, rather than the IVUS direction, may be of paramount importance in reducing subacute stent thrombosis. A French multicenter stent study which used intensive antiplatelet agents and deployment pressures of over 10 atm did not rely on IVUS criteria to achieve a subacute thrombosis rate of 1.2%.[14] In a retrospective review of high pressure (mean maximal pressure 15.8 atm) versus low pressure (mean maximal pressure of 6.9 atm) stent deployment techniques, homogeneous stent geometry and optimal stent expansion after high pressure stent deployment were not observed in all patients.[15] Of the low and high pressure groups, 43% and 17% had echo-free spaces between stent struts and vessel walls, suggesting inadequate stent deployment. However, this study was not designed to assess the benefits of IVUS-directed changes in therapy. It is not clear whether the echo-free spaces in the high pressure stent group are clinically significant or simply represent hypoechoic tissue surrounding a well deployed stent. The investigators noted that high pressure inflations did not uniformly prevent oblique struts, stent eccentricity, or persistent echo-free spaces, arguing against deployment without IVUS. Nonetheless, high pressure stent optimization without IVUS improved the symmetry index compared to the low pressure group.

High Pressure Stent Deployment and IVUS

When IVUS is performed after a priori high pressure stent inflation, the need for further balloon inflations was reduced from 88% to 40%.[2] Although QCA overestimates the final IVUS minimal luminal diameter after stenting, this discrepancy is decreased when high pressure inflations are used.[16] It is postulated that more radiopaque stents will help identify asymmetric or incomplete deployment. It was of interest that 12% of those undergoing IVUS-directed stent optimization did not receive a final IVUS evaluation to confirm the improved result.[11] Post-stent IVUS may be limited by ischemia, technical problems, or procedural time. In coil design stents, IVUS utility may be questioned when further high pressure or large balloon dilations can damage the stents.[16].

Risks of IVUS

The risks of IVUS-directed stent deployment are related to the IVUS catheter itself and to the large balloon, high pressure dilatations which may be indicated by the findings.[17] The clinical risks associated with the IVUS procedure were reported in a multicenter non-randomized registry of over 2,200 IVUS evaluations.[18] Acute procedural or major complications (including dissection, thrombus formation, embolism or significant arrhythmias) were attributed to IVUS in 1.9% of patients undergoing interventions. The complication rate from IVUS before the procedure, when the lumen is presumably the smallest, was only one-tenth the rate related to IVUS post-procedure. Coronary spasm remains the most frequent complication occurring in 2.9% of all IVUS evaluations.[17,18] The complication rate was not related to catheter size.

The risk of arterial rupture and distal dissection due to the repeated high pressure large balloon inflations that are indicated by a suboptimal IVUS result also needs to be considered. In the original series, one of 40 patients died as a consequence of repeated high pressure inflations, despite IVUS guidance during the procedure.[2] The 6-month clinical event and mortality (2.1%) rate was higher using IVUS directed optimization[3] than in the STRESS and BENESTENT trials.[4] Furthermore, as a result of IVUS findings, 40% of patients required multiple stents, a technique which may be associated with a higher restenosis rate.[4] Whether the trauma of over-aggressive stent optimization is responsible for worse clinical outcomes remains to be seen. When IVUS-guided selective balloon oversizing is applied to angioplasty without stents there does not appear to be any increase in serious complications.[26]

IVUS Image Interpretation

The reproducibility and reliability of single observer interpretation of IVUS examinations may not match that of the trials which recommend that ultrasound be used routinely for stent deployment. The reliability of a single observer compared to a panel interpretation of IVUS images was poor. Arterial ruptures were identified with a false positive rate of 43% and while 88% of dissections were identified, there was a 29% false positive rate.[19]

The variability of reference diameter determination by IVUS is sufficient to be of clinical concern.[20] IVUS measurements of reference diameter and percent lumen stenosis are consistently higher than angiographic measurements. Ultrasound detects the secondary enlargement or remodeling in response to plaque accumulation.[21] The vascular remodeling process, first described by Glagov,[22] maintains the vascular lumen, preserving normal blood flow characteristics until the plaque area approaches 30-40% of the vascular lumen area. The criteria for optimal stent deployment should incorporate vascular remodeling information. The most recent of the evolving criteria for optimal stent expansion include lumen cross-sectional areas greater than or equal to the distal reference lumen dimension.[3] This simplified criterion preserves the importance of leaving no stenosis within the stent that might affect outflow to the distal reference vessel.

IVUS Stent Trials

Results from the WEST (Western European Stent Trial) trial and AVID (Angiography Versus Intravascular Ultrasound Directed Stent Placement) trial will provide an objective assessment of the relative value and risks of IVUS-directed versus blinded high pressure stent optimization. Whether modified IVUS criteria will translate into a lower risk benefit relationship supporting routine application of IVUS for all stent implantations remains to be determined.

While three-dimensional IVUS reconstructions may improve IVUS variability, the current technology requires experienced IVUS reviewers in the catheterization laboratory to provide adequate guidance for coronary interventions. Excluding labor, the current costs of an IVUS examination using 15-30 minutes of additional laboratory time and $1000.00 per non-reusable IVUS catheters are considerable.[15]

SUMMARY

The greatest potential benefit of IVUS may be in reducing restenosis rates. A larger final minimal lumen cross-sectional area permits more room for intimal hypertrophy and hence a lower restenosis rate.[24] This "bigger is better" hypothesis (reviewed in Chapter 1) indicates that larger lumens, created by ultrasound guidance, will not only reduce the rates of subacute closure, but will also reduce restenosis. Preliminary data suggest a restenosis rate of 19% (14% for single stents) when IVUS optimization is applied aggressively.[4] Further studies will confirm the role of IVUS in stent optimization.

References

1. Mintz GS, Pichard AD, Kovach JA, et al. *Impact of preintervention intravascular ultrasound imaging on transcatheter treatment strategies in coronary artery disease.* Am J Cardiol 73:423-430 (1994).
2. Goldberg SL, Colombo A, Nakamura S, et al. *Benefit of intracoronary ultrasound in the deployment of Palmaz-Schatz stents.* J Am Coll Cardiol 24:996-1003 (1994).
3. Colombo A, Hall P, Nakamura S, et al. *Intracoronary stenting without anticoagulation accomplished with intravascular ultrasound guidance.* Circulation 91:1676-1688 (1995).
4. Hall P, Nakamura S, Maiello L, et al. *Clinical and angiographic outcome after Palmaz Schatz-stent implantation guided by intravascular ultrasound.* In: deFeyter PJ, Di Mario C, Serruys PW (ed): Quantitative Coronary Imaging. Barjestehl, Meeuwes & Co. Erasmus University Rotterdam (1995).
5. Mintz GS, Popma JJ, Pichard AD, et al. *Patterns of calcification in coronary artery disease— a statistical analysis of intravascular ultrasound and coronary angiography in 1155 lesions.* Circulation 91:1959-1965 (1995).
6. Fitzgerald P, Ports T, Yock P. *Contribution of localized calcium deposits to dissection after angioplasty: an observational study using intravascular ultrasound.* Circulation 86:64-70 (1992).
7. Popma JJ, Mintz GS, Satler LF, et al. *Clinical and angiographic outcome after directional atherectomy: a qualitative and quantitative analysis using coronary arteriography and intravascular ultrasound.* Am J Cardiol 72:55E-64E (1993).
8. Fitzgerald P, Stertzer s, Hidalgo B, et al. *Plaque characteristics affect lesion and vessel response to coronary atherectomy: an intravascular ultrasound study* [abstr]. J Am Coll Cardiol 23:323A (1994).
9. Tobis JM, Mallery J, Mahon D, et al. *Intravascular ultrasound imaging of human coronary arteries in vivo.* Circulation 83:913-926 (1991).
10. Schatz RA, Baim DS, Leon MB, et al. *Clinical experience with the Palmaz-Schatz coronary stent: initial results of a multicenter study.* Circulation 83:148-161 (1991).
11. Nakamura S, Colombo A, Gaglione A, et al. *Intracoronary ultrasound observations during stent implantation.* Circulation 89:2026-2034 (1994).
12. Fischman DL, Leon MB, Baim DS, et al. *A randomized comparison of coronary-stent placement and balloon angioplasty in the treatment of coronary artery disease.* N Engl J Med 331:496-501(1994).
13. Serruys PW, De Jaegere P, Kiemeneij F, et al. *A comparison of balloon-expandable-stent implantation with balloon angioplasty in patients with coronary artery disease.* N Engl J Med 331:489-495(1994).
14. Morice, MC, Zemour G, Benvensite E, et al. *Intracoronary stenting without coumadin: one month results of a French multicenter study.* Cathet Cardiovasc Diagn 35:1-7 (1995).
15. Gorge G, Haude M, Ge Junbo, et al. *Intravascular ultrasound after low and high inflation pressure coronary artery stent implantation.* J Am Coll Cardiol 26:725-730 (1995).
16. Blasini R, Schuhlen J, Mudra H, et al. *Angiographic overestimation of lumen size after coronary stent placement: impact of high pressure dilatation* [abstr]. Circulation 92:I-223 (1995).

16a. Werner GS, Schunemann S, Ferrari M, et al. *Comparison of slotted-tube and coil stents after high-pressure stent deployment by intravascular ultrasound* [abstr]. J Am Coll Cardiol 29(suppl A):275A (1997).

17. Alfonso F, Macaya C, Goicolea J, et al. *Angiographic changes induced by intracoronary ultrasound imaging before and after coronary ultrasound imaging before and after coronary angioplasty.* Am Heart J 124:877-880 (1993).

18. Hausmann D, Erbel R, Alibelli-Chermarin MJ, et al. *The safety of intracoronary ultrasound— a multicenter survey of 2207 examinations.* Circulation 91:623-630 (1995).

19. Kok WEM, Pasterkamp G, Di Mario C, and the PICTURE study group. *Analysis of vessel wall morphology after coronary balloon angioplasty in vivo: observer agreement in an intravascular ultrasound study.* In: deFeyter PJ, Di Mario C, Serruys PW (eds). Quantitative Coronary Imaging. Barjesteh, Meeuwes & Co. Erasmus University, Rotterdam (1995).

20. Kearney PK, Ramo P, Starkey IR, et al. *Assessment of the reproducibility of reference lumen quantitation with intravascular ultrasound in patients undergoing coronary stenting* [abstr]. Circulation 92:I-601 (1995).

21. Heermiller JB, Tenaglia AN, Kisslo KB, et al. *In vivo validation of compensatory enlargement of atherosclerotic coronary arteries.* Am J Cardiol 71:665-668 (1993).

22. Glagov S, Weisenberg BA, Zarins CK, et al. *Compensatory enlargement of human atherosclerotic coronary arteries.* N Engl J Med 316:1371-1375 (1987).

23. Hall P, Colombo A, Almagov Y, et al. *Preliminary experience with intravascular ultrasound guided Palmaz-Schatz coronary stenting: the acute and short term results on a consecutive series of patients.* J Interven Cardiol 7:141-159 (1994).

24. Kuntz RE, Safian RD, Carroza JP, et al. *The importance of acute luminal diameter in determining restenosis after coronary atherectomy or stenting* Circulation 86:1827-1835 (1992).

25. Kuntz RE, Gibson CM, Nobuyoshi M, Baim DS. *Generalized model of restenosis after conventional balloon angioplasty, stenting, and directional atherectomy.* J Am Coll Cardiol 21:15-25 (1993).

26. Stone GW, Hodgson JM, St. Goar FG, et al. *Improved procedural results of coronary angioplasty with intravascular ultrasound-guided balloon sizing - the CLOUT Pilot trial.* Circulation 95: 2044-2052 (1997)

27. Roberts D, Arthur A, Bellinger RL, et al. *The impact on coronary stent implantation of intravascular ultrasound guidance following "aggressive" angiographic stent implantation* [abstr]. J Am Coll Cardiol 29 (suppl A):275A (1997).

CHAPTER 18

RADIAL ARTERY ACCESS AND ANTICOAGULATION FOR STENTING

The Cost of Stenting

Given the current interest in curtailing health care costs, a new intervention must be compared against existing therapies by cost-efficiency analyses before it is accepted.[1,2] Even as stent implantation is being analyzed for cost-efficiency, the methods of implantation and the costs of the procedure are changing.

Extended hospital stays due to anticoagulation adjustments, increased vascular complications, and the stent itself have contributed to the high cost of this technology. The costs of stent implantation were significantly greater than for angioplasty from single center[3] or multicenter data.[4] The hospital stay in the stent group was over two days longer on average than after angioplasty, increasing the cost by almost $2,200. However, while the initial hospital costs were 30% higher, the reduced need for revascularization over the following year in the stent group reduced follow-up costs $1,400 per patient. Thus, at the end of one year, stent implantation is only $600- $800 more expensive per patient than angioplasty, according to a substudy of the STRESS trial using stent techniques of 1993 (large vascular access catheters and extensive anticoagulation regimens).[4,5] The cost of stenting per year of quality adjusted life expectancy is equal to that of many other accepted medical therapies using even 1993 stent techniques.

Rationale for Radial Artery Access for Stenting

The rate of major vascular complications after stenting using the femoral route with an aggressive anticoagulation protocol is much higher than after angioplasty. Major vascular complications after stent implantation occur in 16.8% compared to 6% after balloon angioplasty.[6] The high rate of vascular complications is the result of large catheter femoral access and the use of warfarin for anticoagulation. When stent implantation by the femoral route using a sheathed device was compared to the transradial bare stent technique, costs for the latter technique were 22% cheaper.[7]

Vascular access from the radial artery has been attractive for interventions because of the absence of nerves and veins near the access site[8] and ability to easily control bleeding. The miniaturization of both guiding catheters and angioplasty balloons made radial artery access a viable option for stenting.[9] Although early radial artery occlusion was present in 10% of patients, it was always asymptomatic with spontaneous restoration of flow occurring in 50% of the patients.[10] The feasibility of bailout stenting through a 6 French radial approach was demonstrated in 1993.[11] A 96% success rate could be obtained with this technique despite the occasional inadequate backup of standard Judkins and Amplatz-shaped catheters.[12]

Radial artery access has now matured with the use of long (23mm) sheaths to minimize vascular spasm and facilitate catheter manipulations. Deep intubation of soft-tipped 6 French guiding catheters provides good backup and excellent arterial opacification while minimizing contrast reflux. Removal of the radial sheath immediately after stent implantation is not associated with increased bleeding and may further reduce the rate of asymptomatic vascular occlusion.[13]

In a study where only patients whose radial artery could be cannulated were included, angioplasty procedure time, fluoroscopy time, the amount of contrast utilized, and the procedural success rate were identical to that of a group having angioplasty from the femoral approach. Access site complications were significantly less in the radial group. The length of hospital stay also averaged 1.5 days less than the femoral group.[13] The feasibility of outpatient stent placement by the radial route has been demonstrated in patients receiving warfarin anticoagulants with no complications in the first 24 hours.[14]

Drawbacks

The radial technique is not without its disadvantages. Only bare-mounted (i.e., no sheathed system) stents are sufficiently small to pass through 6 French catheters. Importantly, IVUS evaluation remains impossible through 6 French catheters due to the size of currently available IVUS catheters.

Role of Anticoagulation

Anticoagulation more than sheath size is associated with more vascular complications.[6] Vascular complications after atherectomy with >9 French sheaths were fewer than stenting with smaller sheaths but with an aggressive anticoagulation. Thus, the anticoagulation regimen is more important than the access site in reducing the costs associated with stent implantation. When comparing stenting with and without warfarin, total hospital costs were reduced 32% ($4,500) in the group receiving only antiplatelet agents.[15]

Warfarin-derivative anticoagulation after stent implantation is no longer required. There is increasing evidence that platelet aggregation and not thrombin formation plays the primary role in stent occlusion. Patients who are at the highest risk for subacute closure (thrombus containing lesions, residual dissections, acute infarctions) derive the greatest benefit from antiplatelet therapy compared to coumadin anticoagulation.[16] Cyclic flow variations in a thrombosing stent model suggest that periodic platelet thrombosis plays a central role in stent related thrombosis. Aspirin and heparin treatments alone are not sufficient to ablate cyclical flow variations suggesting a more potent platelet inhibitor is needed.[17,18] Ticlopidine, a potent antiplatelet agent, was added to aspirin resulting in the decline of warfarin-derived anticoagulation.[19] When stents are implanted with intracoronary ultrasound guidance and high pressure inflations, anticoagulation can be safely omitted from the post procedure management.[20] Non-randomized and subsequent prospective controlled studies comparing anticoagulant regimens suggest that the use of aggressive antiplatelet instead of traditional warfarin anticoagulation results in a significantly lower incidence of thrombotic complications even without the assistance of intracoronary ultrasound guidance.[21-24] Even in the setting of acute myocardial infarction, patients receiving only ticlopidine 500mg bid or ticlopidine and heparin after stenting have acceptable rates (1.3, 3, and 7.1%) of subacute occlusion.[25-27]

Further technical improvements such as antiplatelet glycoprotein IIb/IIIa antibody, heparin, or thrombolytic substances bound to stents may reduce stent thrombosis.[28,29]

Preliminary studies of small magnitude and limited power comparing aspirin alone with aspirin and ticlopidine have been conflicting. While some small studies suggest that aspirin alone may be as effective as aspirin and ticlopidine, other data show high thrombosis rates with aspirin alone. Since the current rate of subacute thrombosis hovers around 1%, it will take a large number of patients to demonstrate the superiority of one antiplatelet regimen over another. Furthermore, the STARS (STent Anticoagulation Regimen Study) which is evaluating optimal post stent antiplatelet therapies may have excluded the highest risk lesions where any antiplatelet benefit would have been most important. In the absence of scientific evidence and given the severe consequences of subacute stent thrombosis most interventionalists recommend the continued use of the broadest possible antiplatelet coverage. A number of lines of evidence support the importance of synergy between ticlopidine and aspirin.

Ticlopidine and aspirin together reduce the amount of thrombin generation after stent implantation compared to aspirin alone. A number of platelet aggregation inhibition studies have confirmed the importance of ticlopidine added to aspirin over aspirin alone. While the precise mechanism of this synergy remains under investigation, ticlopidine augments the inhibition of alpha degranulation of platelets as well as the inhibition of fibrinogen receptor activation compared to aspirin.[38,39] Recently short course (10-14 days) ticlopidine therapy has been validated. This short course allows for a maximum therapeutic benefit in reducing stent thrombosis while minimizing drug toxicities and has already become widely accepted.

SUMMARY

Evidence that well deployed stents can be managed without anticoagulation has led most centers to abandon the aggressive anticoagulation protocols which previously kept patients in the hospital for extended periods of time. At the same time, the risks of subacute occlusion and peripheral vascular complications and bleeding have been nearly eliminated.[21] Whether antiplatelet coverage without ticlopidine will be adequate to maintain these reduced levels of subacute thrombosis remains to be seen.

The advantages of radial artery access (reduced vascular complications and diminished bleeding) are offset by stent protocols which minimize anticoagulation after stent placement. Radial artery access is not favorable for procedures which require an exceptional amount of backup, pre-stent debulking with atherectomy, or devices. Nonetheless, radial artery access provides an important alternative access site for a majority of stent procedures.

References

1. Serruys PW, Strauss BH, van Beusekom HM, van der Giessen WJ. *Stenting of coronary arteries: has a modern Pandora's box been opened?* J Am Coll Cardiol 17:143B-154B (1991).
2. Leon MB, Wong SC. *Intracoronary stents: a breakthrough technology or just another small step?* Circulation 89:1323-1327 (1994).
3. Dick RJ, Popma JJ, Muller DW, et al. *In-hospital costs associated with new percutaneous coronary devices.* Am J Cardiol 68:879-885 (1991).
4. Cohen DJ, Krumholtz HM, Sukin CA, et al. *In-hospital and one-year economic outcomes after coronary stenting or balloon angioplasty—results from a randomized clinical trial.* Circulation 92:2480-2487 (1995).
5. Cohen DJ, Baim DS. *Coronary stenting: costly or cost-effective?* J Invas Cardiol 7 (Suppl A):36-42 (1995).
6. Moscucci M, Mansour KA, Kent C, et al. *Peripheral vascular complications of directional coronary atherectomy and stenting: predictors, management, and outcome.* Am J Cardiol 74:448-453 (1994).
7. Kiemeneij F, Hofland J, Laarman GJ, et al. *Comparison of costs between two modes of implantation of Palmaz-Schatz coronary stents: the transradial bare stent technique versus the transfemoral sheath protected stent technique.* Cathet Cardiovasc Diagn 35:301-308 (1995).
8. Campeau L. *Percutaneous radial artery approach for coronary angioplasty.* Cathet Cardiovasc Diagn 16:3-7 (1989).
9. Kiemeneij F, Laarman GJ, de Melker E. *Percutaneous radial artery entry for coronary angioplasty* [abstr]. Eur Heart Journal 14(suppl):289 (1993).
10. Stella P, Kiemeneij F, Laarman, et al. *Incidence and outcome of radial artery occlusion following transradial artery coronary angioplasty [abstr].* Circulation 92(suppl I):I-225 (1995).
11. Kiemeneij F, Laarman GJ. *Percutaneous transradial artery approach for coronary stent implantation.* Cathet Cardiovasc Diagn 30:173-176 (1993).
12. Kiemeneij F, Laarman GJ. *Bailout techniques for failed coronary angioplasty using 6 French guiding catheters.* Cathet Cardiovasc Diagn 32:359-366 (1994).
13. Mann JT III, Arrowood M, Cubeddu G. *PTCA using the right radial artery access site.* J Invasive Cardiol 7:142-147 (1995).
14. Kiemeneij F, Laarman GJ, Slagboom T, van der Wieken P. *Outpatient coronary stent implantation.* J Am Coll Cardiol 29: 323-327 (1997).

15. Goods CM, Ming WL, Iyer SS, et al. *A cost analysis of coronary stenting without anticoagulation versus stenting with anticoagulation using warfarin* [abstr]. Circulation 92 (suppl I):I-796. (1995).

16. Schömig A, Neumann FJ, WalterH, et al. *Coronary stent placement in patients with acute myocardial infarction: Comparison of clinical and angiographic outcome after randomization to antiplatet or anticoagulant therapy.* J Am Coll Cardiol 29: 28-34 (1997)

17. Aggarwqal RK, More RS, Ezekowitz MD, et al. *Stent-related thrombosis: assessment of effects of aspirin and heparin in a deep arterial injury, reduced flow model* [abstr]. Eur Heart J 16(suppl):12 (1995).

18. Gawaz M, Neumann F, Ott I, et al. *Platelet activation and coronary stent implantation: effect of antithrombotic therapy.* Circulation (In press, 1997).

19. Barragan P, Sainsous J, Silvestri M, et al. *Ticlopidine and subcutaneous heparin as an alternative regimen following coronary stenting.* Cathet Cardiovasc Diagn 31:133-138 (1994).

20. Colombo A, Hall P, Nakamura S, et al. *Intracoronary stenting without anticoagulation accomplished with intravascular ultrasound guidance.* Circulation 91:1676-1688 (1995).

21. Morice MC, Zemour G, Benveniste E, et al. *Intracoronary stenting without coumadin: one month results of a French multicenter study.* Cathet Cardiovasc Diagn 35:1-7 (1995).

22. Serruys PW, Emanuelsson H, van der Giesen W, et al. *Heparin-coated Palmaz-Schatz stents in human coronary arteries—early outcome of the Benestent-II pilot study.* Circulation 93:412-422 (1996).

23. Schomig A, Neumann FJ, Kastrati A, et al. *A randomized comparison of antiplatelet and anticoagulant therapy after the placement of coronary-artery stents.* N Engl J Med 334:1084-1089 (1996).

24. Karrillon GJ, Maurice MC, Benveniste E, et al. *Intracoronary stent implantation without ultrasound guidance and with replacement of conventional anticoagulation by antiplatelet therapy—30 day clinical outcome of the French Multicenter Registry.* Circulation 94:1519-1527 (1996).

25. Monassier JP, Elias J, Morice MC, et al. *Results of early (<24 h) and late (>24 h) implantation of coronary stents in acute myocardial infarction [abstr].* Eur Heart J 16 (suppl):12 (1995).

26. Verna E, Castigilioni B, Onofri M, et al. I*ntracoronary stenting of the infarct-related artery without anticoagulation in acute myocardial infarction* [abstr]. Eur Heart J 16 (suppl):12 (1995).

27. Levy G, Bouvagnet P, de Boisgelin X, et al. *Intracoronary stenting in direct infarct angioplasty: is it dangerous* [abstr]. Eur Heart J 16 (suppl):12 (1995).

28. Hardhammar PA, van Beusekom HMM, Emanuelsson HU, et al. *Reduction in thrombotic events with heparin-coated Palmaz-Schatz stents in normal porcine coronary arteries.* Circulation 93:423-430 (1996).

29. Aggarwal RK, Ireland DC, Ezekowitz MD, et al. *A platelet-targeted fibrinolytic agent: in vitro characterization and assessment of potential for reducing stent-related thrombosis* [abstr]. Eur Heart J 16 (suppl):12 (1995).

30. Hall P, Nakamura S, Maiello L, et al. A *randomized comparison of combined ticlopidine and aspirin therapy versus aspirin therapy alone after successful intravascular ultrasound-guided stent implantation.* Circulation 93:215-222 (1996).

31. Fernandez-Aviles F, Alonso J, Duran JM, et al. *Aspirin as the only antithrombotic therapy after coronary stenting guided by angiography: hospital stay and one and six months clinical and angiographic outcome* [abstr]. Circulation 94(suppl I):I-256 (1996).

32. Galli S, Trabattoni D, Loaldi A, et al. *Comparison of anticoagulation, combined ticlopidine and aspirin and aspirin alone therapy following coronary stenting* [abstr]. Circulation 94 (suppl I):I-684 (1996).

33. Machraoui A, Germing A, von Dryander S, et al. *Is the treatment regimen with coumadin plus aspirin or aspirin alone obsolete after high pressure coronary stenting? In-hospital and follow-up results of a randomized study [abstr].* Circulation 94(suppl I):I-256 (1996).

34. Leon MB, Baim DS, Gordon P, et al. *Clinical and angiographic results from the STent Anticoagulation Regimen Study (STARS)* [abstr]. Circulation 94(suppl I):I-685 (1996)

35. Colombo A. *Combined ticlopidine and aspirin versus aspirin therapy alone after stent implantation—Letter response.* Circulation 94:2994 (1996).

36. Gregorini L, Marco J, Fajadet J, et al. *Ticlopidine attenuates post-stent implantation thrombin generation [abstr].* J Am Coll Cardiol 27(suppl A):334-A (1996).

37. Darius H, Veit K, Rupprecht HJ, et al. *Synergistic inhibition of platelet aggregation by ticlopidine plus aspirin following intracoronary stent placement* [abstr]. Circulation 94 (suppl I):I-257 (1996).

38. Neumann FJ, Dickfeld TM, Gawaz M, et al. *Antiplatelet effect of ticlopidine in addition to aspirin after coronary stenting* [abstr]. Circulation 94(suppl I):I-684 (1996).

39. Rupprecht HJ, Darius H, Voigtlander T, et al. *Ticlopidine, aspirin or both after stent implantation [abstr]?* Circulation 94(suppl I):I-257 (1996).

40. Kataoka K, Sato Y, Ito H, Takatsu Y. Palmaz-Schatz stent *implantation with 10 days ticlopidine treatment* [abstr]. Circulation 94(suppl I):I-684 (1996).

41. Macaya C, Alfonso F, Iniguez A, Goicolea J, Hernandez R, Zarco P. *Stenting for elastic recoil during coronary angioplasty of the left main coronary artery.* Am J Cardiol 70:105-107 (1992).

42. Segovia J, Phillips P, Hernandez R, et al. *Restenosis after balloon angioplasty and coronary stenting of proximal left anterior descending lesions: a quantitative coronary analysis study* [abstr]. J Am Coll Cardiol 29(suppl A):497A (1997).

43. Ellis SG, Roubin GS, King SB III, et al. *Importance of stenosis morphology in the estimation of restenosis risk after elective percutaneous transluminal coronary angioplasty.* Am J Cardiol 63:30-34 (1989).

44. Dimas AP, Grigera F, Arora RR, et al. *Repeat coronary angioplasty as treatment for restenosis.* J Am Coll Cardiol 19:1310-1314 (1992).

45. Topol E, Ellis S Fishman J, et al. *Multicenter study of percutaneous transluminal angioplasty for right coronary artery ostial stenoses.* J Am Coll Cardiol 9:1214-1218 (1987).

46. Holmes DR, Vliestra RE, Smith GC. *Restenosis after percutaneous transluminal coronary angioplasty (PTCA):* a report from the PTCA registry of the National Heart, Lung and Blood institute. Am J Cardiol 53:77c-81c (1984).

47. Webb JG, Myler RK, Shaw RE, et al. *Coronary angioplasty after coronary bypass surgery: Initial results and late outcome in 422 patients.* J Am Coll Cardiol 16:812-820 (1990).

48. van Hout B. Cost-*Effectiveness of coronary stents in the Benestent study.* Second Thoraxcenter coronary stent course, Rotterdam, The Netherlands, December 14, 1995.

STENT GLOSSARY

ACUTE GAIN: The difference between minimal lumen diameter before and after an intervention.

ALLEN TEST: Used to confirm adequate collateral flow from the ulnar side before performing procedures such as stenting via the radial approach. This test is positive (normal) when, after compression of both radial and ulnar arteries sufficient to cause the hand to blanch, the normal color of the hand returns within 10 seconds after release of pressure over the ulnar artery.

ANGIOGRAPHIC-CLINICAL DISSOCIATION: Refers to the observation that better angiographic procedural results do not necessarily presage a better clinical outcome. The phenomenon is often used in reference to the CAVEAT trial, in which improved post-procedure result of atherectomy was associated with a poorer clinical outcome (increased rate of CPK rises and other clinical events) when compared to conventional angioplasty.[1]

APOPTOSIS: Apoptosis is the programmed, peaceful cell death without attendant necrosis or inflammation first hinted by Virchow (1859 necrobiosis). An example is the cell death and chromatolysis secondary to endovascular irradiation which does not result in the attraction of monocytes and lymphocytes and may thus reduce the intimal proliferation which causes restenosis.[2]

BAILOUT: Stent implantation under non-elective conditions is termed bailout stenting. Bailout criteria have been variously defined as acute closure, threatened closure, and suboptimal angioplasty result. Stents placed for bailout indications may have restenosis rates similar to those of elective stenting but the rate of acute closure and other complications is higher.

BATTERY EFFECT: The theoretical chemical reaction potentiated by placing two different metals of different potentials in proximity (e.g. a 216L stainless steel stent and its radiopaque markers of a different metal or stent brand A of one metal deployed inside stent brand B).

BUDDY WIRE: A buddy wire refers to a second guide wire passed parallel to and outside of the stent delivery system lumen in order to further straighten a tortuous vessel and facilitate stent passage. This wire is usually an extra support type or stiff wire.

BURST PRESSURE (minimal): The minimal burst pressure is the pressure below which 99.9% of angioplasty balloons will not rupture.

COMPLIANCE (Balloon): A balloon's compliance reflects its stretchability and is measured as the change in balloon diameter per atmosphere of inflation pressure. Compliant balloon materials such as POC (polyolefin copolymer) stretch 0.095mm/atmosphere applied pressure. Noncompliant balloon materials such as PET (polyethylene terephthalate) increase 0.010mm/atmosphere. Noncompliant balloons have higher burst pressures, and are associated with more conformability and less creep.[3] (See below).

COMPLIANCE TEST: A method to check the compliance of a lesion using balloon inflation within a suspect lesion prior to deciding upon optimal therapy. If the lesion effectively dilates at less than a given pressure, it is deemed safe to proceed directly to stent implantation (i.e., the compliance test has been passed). However, if the lesion does not dilate within a given pressure, a debulking procedure (Rotablator, atherectomy or laser angioplasty) is performed.

CONFORMABILITY(balloon): Refers to the ability of a balloon to adapt to the shape of a vessel. In angled coronary vessels noncompliant and more conformable balloons produce less straightening force within the artery and result in better angiographic results.[4]

CREEP (balloon): The tendency of an angioplasty balloon to enlarge after sequential inflations at the same pressure.

DECALCIFICATION: Decalcification is the Rotablator enthusiast's term for applying rotational atherectomy to heavily calcified lesions as a method of debulking before definitive therapy with balloon or stent.

DECREMENTAL DIAMETER BALLOON: A tapered balloon provides a decrease in diameter over its length to accommodate long and tapered lesions with a lower incidence of dissection.[5]

DIMPLE: Refers to a persistent defect in a dilating balloon's contour at full expansion suggesting that a hard plaque has yet to yield to dilatation. This is a common observation just before a higher pressure or larger balloon dilation leads to a dissection requiring stent placement and may be an indicator that a debulking procedure is needed.

DISTENSION FORCE: The force required to distend or dilate a stent ex-vivo usually expressed in atmospheres. Radial force is the force the stent continues to exert in a radial or outward direction after deployment.[6]

ECCENTRICITY INDEX (symmetry index): An intravascular ultrasound derived measurement of optimal stent deployment equal to the smallest stent diameter (minimal diameter) divided by the stent diameter perpendicular to it (major diameter). An eccentricity index of greater than 0.7 is generally acceptable.

EFFICIENCY INDEX: The ratio of the final lumen diameter to the final balloon diameter. It normalizes the final lumen diameter by balloon size and is an index of the "efficiency" of balloon mediated dilation.[7] It is used in determining elastic recoil and assessing facilitated angioplasty.

ELASTIC RECOIL: The difference between the diameter of the maximally inflated balloon and the resulting arterial minimal lumen diameter. Elastic recoil represents the immediate loss in lumen diameter upon balloon deflation.[8]

ENDOLUMINAL GRAFTING: The application of synthetic (e.g. polytetrafluoroethylene) or allograft (e.g. cephalic or saphenous vein) material to the internal lumen of an artery by stent apposition for the purpose of treating and sealing aneurysms, pseudoaneurysms, and fistulae.

FACILITATED ANGIOPLASTY: Also called "debulking and dilating," facilitated angioplasty refers to the improvement in post procedure dimensions for lesions treated with ablative or debulking techniques followed by adjunctive angioplasty.[9] See **SYNERGY**.

FOLDING ARTIFACT/ PSEUDO-SPASM/
ACCORDION EFFECT/INTUSSUSCEPTION: Also termed wrinkles (Chapter 9), these terms describe the lucencies and false lesions caused by stiff guide wires and rigid stents in curved arterial segments. The hallmark of this artifact is its occurrence as a perpendicular filling defect extending inward from the outer curve of a straightened segment often untouched by balloon dilations.[10]

GLAGOVIAN BALANCE: Glagov described the compensatory enlargement of the total vessel area by vascular remodeling in order to compensate for plaque growth encroaching on the arterial lumen.[11] This mechanism fails when the plaque burden exceeds 40% of the vascular area. The Glagovian balance is the relationship between vascular enlargement by remodeling and lumen encroachment (by plaque) or enlargement (by transcatheter techniques).

INHIBITION THEORY: The restenosis concept that neointimal proliferation is held in check by an active inhibitory function of the arterial media.

INITIAL LUMEN GAIN: The difference between minimal lumen diameter before and after an intervention.

INJURY SCORE: A pathological measure of arterial damage produced by an arterial intervention. The injury score is proportional to the amount of reactive intimal hypertrophy which results during restenosis.[12] The injury score has also been used to predict arterial injury at stent implantation by an index of balloon/artery ratio and maximal inflation pressure.[13]

LARGE LUMEN HYPOTHESIS: The belief that the size of the minimal luminal diameter — not the method by which it is achieved — predicts restenosis.[14] This "bigger is better" concept is widely accepted but as yet unproved. It is challenged by the finding of "angiographic-clinical dissociation" after atherectomy (see above).

LATE LUMEN LOSS: The difference between minimal lumen diameter immediately after intervention and that found at angiography 6 months later. Late loss averages 0.5mm after PTCA and 0.9mm after stenting.[15]

LOSS INDEX: The ratio between late lumen loss and initial lumen gain is the loss index which is proposed as a marker of the hyperplastic response to injury. The late loss index is greater after stenting than after angioplasty.

LOW PUNCTURE: Arterial punctures which are performed more than 3 cm below the inguinal ligament enter the superficial femoral artery and increase the risk of bleeding or the formation of arteriovenous fistulae and pseudoaneurysms. Fluoroscopic visualization of arterial entry superior to the inferior border of the femoral head helps to ensure a safe arterial entry.[16]

LUMENOGRAM: The intravascular image of the coronary arterial lumen afforded during contrast injection or with IVUS. Angiographic techniques provide a "projection image" of the lumen as opposed to an assessment of the cross-section of the vascular wall by IVUS.

MARGINAL TEAR (POCKET FLAP): A small dissection at the proximal or distal extremes of a stent deployed at high pressure. It is noted upon IVUS inspection after high pressure stent deployment where the protrusion of intima is attributed to the shear force effects of the deployment balloon. These may be entirely invisible at angiography.[17]

MEAN INJURY SCORE: A pathological measure of arterial damage produced by an arterial intervention. The injury score is proportional to the amount of reactive intimal hypertrophy which results during restenosis.[18] The injury score has also been used to predict arterial injury at stent implantation by an index of balloon/artery ratio and maximal inflation pressure.[19]

MELON SEEDING OR WATERMELON SEED SLIPPAGE: The sliding of an angioplasty balloon distal or proximal to a fibrotic lesion is graphically termed "melon seeding". More common in old vein grafts and ostial segments. Slippage is diminished by the use of long balloons.

OCULOSTENOTIC REFLEX: A hypothetical reflex of interventional cardiologists when viewing the angiographic appearance of a coronary artery lesion. The reflex causes balloon inflation or stent placement, generally bypassing the cerebral cortex (i.e., ischemia assessment). This reflex is generally cited in the clinical situation where a lesion seems to "need treatment" without documented ischemia or symptoms.

OPTIMAL ATHERECTOMY: This second generation approach of maximizing post treatment lumen diameter by more aggressive tissue removal and adjunctive balloon dilation. This technique may provide "stent-like" restenosis rates of 30% rather than the angioplasty-like rates of 50% which the CAVEAT trial produced.

PASSIVATION: The change in an arterial surface from one that supports platelet deposition to one that does not (i.e. after treatment with GP IIb/IIIa inhibitors).[21]

PATCHY RED REACTION: The angioscopic finding of red thrombus at sites of stent strut intersection early after implantation.

PINCUSHION DISTORTION: The selective magnification of objects in the perimeter of an angiographic image field due to the inherent geometric distortions of the technique. This may be corrected by use of a centimeter grid for analysis off line and is the reason for sizing arteries for stents in the center of the angiographic field.

PLASTICALLY DEFORMABLE: A property of a material (e.g. stents) to be deformed continuously and permanently without rupture.

POCKET FLAP (MARGINAL OR EDGE TEAR): A small dissection at the proximal or distal extremes of a stent deployed at high pressure. It is noted upon ICUS inspection after high pressure stent deployment where the protrusion of intima seen is attributed to the shear force effects of the deployment balloon. It may be entirely invisible at angiography.[15]

POPPING PRESSURE: The inflation pressure at which the angioplasty balloon becomes fully inflated.[22] See **COMPLIANCE TEST**.

PROVISIONAL STENTING: The practice of stenting only suboptimal angioplasty results.

PSEUDOLESION: See **FOLDING ARTIFACT**.

PSEUDO-RECOIL: The suggestion of stent recoil or compression at follow-up angiography due to incomplete dilatation at the time of original implantation.

PSEUDO-REGRESSION: The restenotic process involves not only the lesion site but also the reference vessel proximal and distal to the lesion. When there is more rapid loss of the reference vessel lumen than the lesion site there can appear to be regression of the lesion stenosis or pseudo-regression when in fact there has been no change or even progression.[23]

RELATIVE EXPANSION: A quantitative angiography term equal to minimum stent diameter divided by the average of the proximal and distal reference diameters.

REMODELING: A chronic compensatory arterial dilation which occurs in response to plaque accumulation and which maintains coronary flow until 30-40% of the lumen has become occupied by plaque.[24]

RESTENOSIS: The combined biologic healing processes (proliferative, thrombotic or remodeling derived) resulting in a renarrowing of the lumen after a transcatheter procedure.[25] Restenosis is often defined in a binary fashion to facilitate studies and by continuous terms to more accurately reflect the process. Percent stenosis 50% at follow-up angiography is the binary definition most often used. A 0.72mm loss in minimal luminal diameter or late loss of > 50% of the initial gain are other binary definitions used. The continuous definitions of residual minimal luminal diameter at control angiography or follow-up percentage stenosis may be more useful.

RHEOLYTIC THROMBECTOMY: Lysis of thrombus by dynamic fluid devices such as with the POSSIS device.

SCAFFOLDING: Scaffolding is defined as a platform used to provide support, but when used in stenting describes any force applied to support the vascular lumen.

SKI RAMP TECHNIC: It is often difficult to pass a balloon for high pressure inflations within the proximal portion of a deployed stent on a curve. This is usually due to the nose of the balloon engaging the stent wall eccentrically or non-axially. In order to facilitate coaxial entry of the balloon within the deployed stent a stiff guide wire may be shaped so that a bend in the wire directs the balloon tip into the center of the stent lumen thus facilitating passage. This wire configuration resembles a ski ramp thus giving rise to the name of this technique.[26]

SNOWPLOW EFFECT: When a plow leaves a mound of snow across intersecting roads, it resembles (in concept) the effect of an angioplasty balloon opening trunk lesions by pushing plaque across the intersecting branches.

STENT JAIL: The phenomenon of leaving a coronary artery side branch inaccessible to further interventions by placing a stent across its ostium.

STENT SYNERGY: The sequential use of a primary ablative device (Rotablator, directional atherectomy, laser ablation, extraction catheter) with adjunctive stenting in order to increase safety and improve acute and late angiographic results. The term is generally applied in the debulking of ostial or trunk lesions and for lesions with thrombus or excessive calcium. In the broader sense device synergy applies to the use of any series of devices for the same objective.[27]

STRETCH: Lesion stretch during balloon inflation is the difference between the actual diameter of the maximally inflated balloon and the minimal lumen diameter before the intervention. Lesion stretch is a function of plaque compliance.

SYMMETRY INDEX: See ECCENTRICITY INDEX

TOTAL VASCULAR RECONSTRUCTION: The application of stents to diffusely diseased vessels and to lesions of over 20mm length.

UNDER-OVER TECHNIC: The practice of under-sizing the predilatation balloon to minimize dissection and embolization risk while over-sizing the post stent deployment or touch-up balloon to maximize mean luminal diameter.

WIRE EXIT: A euphemism for perforations which occur during recanalization of total occlusions. The term has been used most often during work with laser wires.

REFERENCES

1. Bittl JA. Directional coronary atherectomy versus balloon angioplasty. N Engl J Med 329;273-274(1993).
2. Isner JM, Kearney M, Bortman S, Passeri J. Apoptosis in human atherosclerosis and restenosis. Circulation 91:2703-2711 (1995).
3. Safian RD, Hoffman MA, Almany S, et al. Comparison of coronary angioplasty with compliant and noncompliant balloons (The Angioplasty Compliance Trial). Am J Cardiol 76:518-520 (1995).

4. Ellis SG, Topol EJ. Results of percutaneous transluminal coronary angioplasty of high-risk angulated stenoses. Am J Cardiol 66:932-937 (1990).
5. Vidya S, Baker HA, Vemuri DN, et al. Effectiveness of decremental diameter balloon catheters (tapered balloon). Am J Cardiol 69:188-193 (1992).
6. Rensing BJ, Hermans WRM, Vos J, et al. Angiographic risk factors of luminal narrowing after coronary balloon angioplasty using balloon measurements to reflect stretch and elastic recoil at the dilatation site. Am J Cardiol 69:584-591 (1992).
7. Safian RD, Freed M, Lichtenbrg A, et al. Are residual stenoses after excimer laser angioplasty and coronary atherectomy due to inefficient or small devices? Comparison with balloon angioplasty. J Am Coll Cardiol 22:1628-1634 (1993).
8. Rensing BJ, Hermans WRM, Vos J, et al. Angiographic risk factors of luminal narrowing after coronary balloon angioplasty using balloon measurements to reflect stretch and elastic recoil at the dilatation site. Am J Cardiol 69:584-591 (1992).
9. Safian RD, Freed M, Reddy V, et al. Do excimer laser angioplasty and rotational atherectomy facilitate balloon angioplasty? Implications for lesion-specific coronary intervention. J Am Coll Cardiol 27:552-559 (1996).
10. Tenaglia AN, Tcheng JE, Phillips HR, Stack RS: Creation of pseudo narrowing during coronary angioplasty. Am J Cardiol 67:658-659 (1991).
11. Glagov S, Weisenberg E, Zarins CK, et al. Compensatory enlargement of human atherosclerotic coronary arteries. N Eng J Med 316:1371-1375 (1987).
12. Schwartz R, Huber KC, Murphy JG, et al. Restenosis and the proportional neointimal response to coronary artery injury: Results in a porcine model. J Am Coll Cardiol 19:267-274 (1992).
13. Mehran R, Mintz GS, Pichard AD, et al. Impact of vessel wall injury on in-stent restenosis: a serial quantitative angiographic and IVUS [abstract]. Circulation 94 (suppl I):I-262 (1996).
14. Kuntz RE, Gibson CM, Nobuyoshi M, Baim DS. Generalized model of restenosis after conventional balloon angioplasty, stenting, and directional atherectomy. J Am Coll Cardiol 21:15-25 (1993).
15. Kuntz RE, Gibson CM, Nobuyoshi M, Baim DS. Generalized model of restenosis after conventional balloon angioplasty, stenting , and directional atherectomy. J Am Coll Cardiol 1993; 21:15-25.
16. Kim D, Orron DE, Skillman JJ, et al: Role of superficial femoral artery puncture in the development of pseudoaneurysm and arteriovenous fistula complicating percutaneous femoral cardiac catheterization. Cathet Cardiovasc Diagn 25:91-97 (1992).
17. Metz JA, Mooney MR, Walter PD, et al. Significance of edge tears in coronary stenting: Initial observations from the STRUT registry [abstract]. Circulation 92 (suppl I):I-546 (1995).
18. Schwartz R, Huber KC, Murphy JG, et al. Restenosis and the proportional neointimal response to coronary artery injury: Results in a porcine model. J Am Coll Cardiol 19:267-274 (1992).
19. Mehran R, Mintz GS, Pichard AD, et al. Impact of vessel wall injury on in-stent restenosis: a serial quantitative angiographic and IVUS [abstract]. Circulation 94 (suppl I):I-262 (1996).
20. Nakamura S, Hall P, Maiello L, Colombo A. Techniques for Palmaz-Schatz stent deployment in lesions with a large side branch. Cathet Cardiovasc Diagn 34:353-361 (1995).
21. Topol EJ. Novel Antithrombotic Approaches to Coronary Disease. Am J Cardiol 75:27B-33B (1995).
22. Hirshfeld JW, Schwartz JS, Jugo R, et al (the M-HEART investigators): Restenosis After Coronary Angioplasty: A Multivariate Statistical Model to relate Lesion and Procedure Variables to Restenosis. J Am Coll Cardiol 18:647-656 (1991).
23. Vos J, de Feyter PJ, Simoons ML, et al. Retardation and arrest of progression or regression of coronary artery disease: a review. Prog Cardiovasc Dis 6:435-454 (1993).
24. Glagov S, Weisenberg BA, Zarins CK, et al. Compensatory enlargement of human atherosclerotic coronary arteries. N Engl J Med 316:1371-1375 (1987).
25. Serruys PW, Foley DP, Kirkeeide RL, King SB III. Restenosis revisited: Insights provided by quantitative coronary angiography. Am Heart J 126:1243-1267 (1993).
26. Tierstein P. "Coronary Interventions: 1996" Course La Jolla, October, 1996.
27. Pichard AD, Mintz GS, Kent KM, et al. Transcatheter device synergy: Preliminary experience with adjunct direction atherectomy following rotational atherectomy in treating calcific coronary artery disease. J Am Coll Cardiol 21:227A (1993).

APPENDIX I

CANADIAN CARDIOVASCULAR SOCIETY CLASSIFICATION[1]

CLASS 0: Free of exertional angina
CLASS 1: No angina at ordinary physical activity
CLASS 2: Angina causing slight limitation of ordinary activity
CLASS 3: Angina causing marked limitation of ordinary activity
CLASS 4: Inability to carry on any physical activity without anginal discomfort

1. Campeau L. Letters to the editor: Grading of angina pectoris. Circulation 1976;54:522.

APPENDIX II

BRAUNWALD UNSTABLE ANGINA SCORE[1]

ANGINA SEVERITY	CLINICAL CIRCUMSTANCES		
	Secondary to a non-cardiac condition (anemia, etc.)	Primary unstable angina	Within 2 weeks of MI
I. New onset of severe or accelerated angina without rest pain	IA	IB	IC
II. Angina at rest within the past month but not within 48 hrs	IIA	IIB	IIC
III. Angina at rest within 48 hrs	IIIA	IIIB	IIIC

1. Braunwald E. Unstable angina: A classification. Circulation 1989;80:410-414.

APPENDIX III

ACC/AHA CLASSIFICATION OF LESION TYPE FOR PREDICTION OF ANGIOPLASTY RISK[1,2]

TYPE A LESIONS (>85% Success, Low Risk)	
Discrete	Non-ostial
Little or no calcification	Nonangulated segment (<45°)
Concentric	No major branch involvement
Less than totally occlusive	Smooth contour
Readily accessible	No thrombus
TYPE B LESIONS (60-85% Success, Moderate Risk)	
B_1 characteristic	Moderate tortuosity of proximal vessel
B_2 characteristic	Ostial
Tubular (10-20mm in length)	Moderately angulated (45°-90°)
Moderate to heavy calcification	Bifurcation lesions requiring double wires
Eccentric	Irregular contour
Total occlusions < 3 months old	Some thrombus present
TYPE C LESIONS (<60% Success, High Risk)	
Diffuse (>20mm)	Inability to protect major side branches
Total occlusion >3 months old	Extremely angulated segments
Excessive tortuosity of proximal vessel	Degenerated vein grafts with friable lesions

1. Ryan TJ, Faxon DP, Gunnar RM, et al. Guidelines for percutaneous transluminal coronary angioplasty: A report of the American College of Cardiology/American Heart Association Task Force on Assessment of Diagnostic and Therapeutic Cardiovascular Procedures (Subcommittee on Percutaneous Transluminal Coronary Angioplasty). J Am Coll Cardiol 1988;12:529-545 and J Am Coll Cardiol 1993;22:2033-2054.
2. Ellis S, Vandormael M, Cowley M, et al. Coronary morphologic and clinical determinants of procedural outcome with angioplasty for multivessel coronary artery disease. Implications for patient selection. Circulation 1990;82:1193-1202.

APPENDIX IV

NHLBI CORONARY ARTERY DISSECTION CLASSIFICATION[1,2]

A. Radiolucent areas within the lumen without the persistence of contrast
B. Parallel tracts or double lumen with minimal to no persistence of contrast
C. Contrast outside lumen persisting after dye clears from the lumen
D. Spiral luminal filling defects often with staining of the vessel
E. New persistent filling defects
F. Any dissection leading to total occlusion

1. Coronary Artery Angiographic Changes after PTCA: Manual of Operations NHLBI PTCA Registry, 1985:6-9.
2. Huber MS, Fishman MJ, Madison J, Mooney MR. Use of morphologic classification to predict clinical outcome after dissection from coronary angioplasty. Am J Cardiol 1991;68:467-471.

APPENDIX V

TIMI CLASSIFICATION[1]

Grade 0: No perfusion.

Grade 1: Penetration with minimal perfusion. Contrast fails to opacify the entire bed distal to the stenosis for the duration of the cine run.

Grade 2: Partial perfusion. Contrast opacifies the entire coronary bed distal to the stenosis. However, the rate of entry and/or clearance is slower in the coronary bed distal to the obstruction than in comparable areas not perfused by the dilated vessel.

Grade 3: Complete perfusion. Filling and clearance of contrast equally rapid in the coronary bed distal to stenosis as in other coronary beds.

1. TIMI Study Group. Thrombolysis in myocardial infarction (TIMI) trial. N Eng J Med 1985;312:932-936.

APPENDIX VI

RADIAL ARTERY ACCESS FOR INTERVENTIONS

Pre-procedure: Allen test for patency of ulnar arterial supply to hand. Nifedipine sublingually to prevent radial artery spasm (optional).

Procedure: Arterial puncture with 22g radial artery catheterization set (Arrow Internation, Reading, PA), 21g Cook arterial cannulation set (Cook, Bloomington, Indiana), or standard 18g thin-walled needle. Puncture 1 cm proximal to styloid process. To prevent arterial spasm/thrombosis: lidocaine 2% (2 ml), nitroglycerin 0.2 mg (optional), heparin 10,000 units (required)

Guidewire Choices: 0.025" 260 cm length J-wire; 0.025" Terumo guide wire (Terumo Medical Corp., Somerset, NJ)

Sheath: 23 cm length (e.g., Daig arterial sheath; Daig Corp., Minnetonka, MN) preferred to prevent artery spasm.

Guiding Catheter Options

Left Anterior Decending Artery:	6 French Voda Curve 6 French Kimi Curve
Left Circumflex Coronary Artery:	6 French Voda Curve 6 French Kimi Curve 6 French Left Amplatz Curve
Right Coronary Artery:	6 French Kimi Curve 6 French Multipurpose 6 French Left Amplatz Curve
Vein Grafts:	6 French Multipurpose 6 French Amplatz Curve

Post-Procedure

Immediate sheath removal with occlusive compression for a minimum of 30 minutes. Pressure dressing and wrist immobilization with splint and/or sling for 24 hours.

1. Kiemeneij F, Laarman GJ. Percutaneous transradial artery approach for coronary Palmaz-Schatz stent implantation. Am Heart J 1994:128;167-174.
2. Mann JT III, Arrowood M, Cubeddu G. PTCA using the right radial artery access site. J Invasive Cardiol 1995:7;142-147.

APPENDIX VII

STENT DESIGN COMPENDIUM

Stent Radiopaque Marker Key

######	Indicates slotted tube or other stent material of high surface area
/////////	Indicates coil or other stent material of low surface area
■	Indicates radiopaque marker
____	Indicates stent spine
....	Indicates balloon material without markers

ACCUFLEX STENT

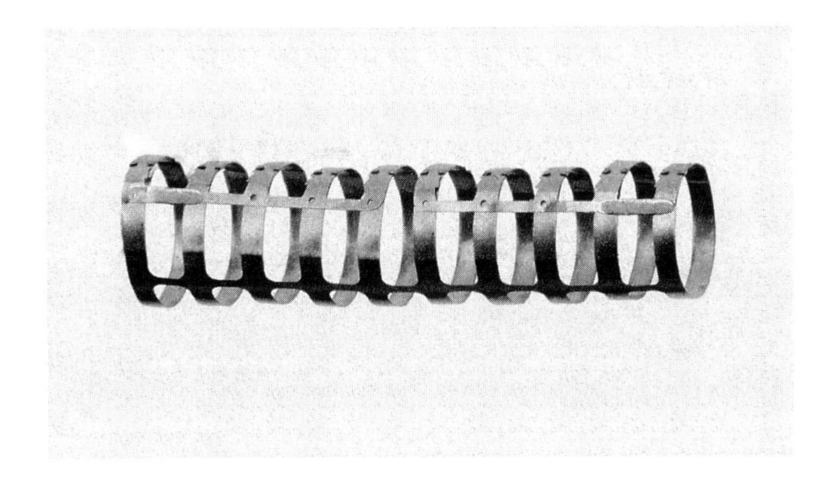

Manufacturer: Navius Corp.
Description: Multiple ratchetting radial bands on a twin backbone

Technical Specifications

Material:	316 L stainless steel
Surface Area After Expansion (%):	37.5%
Strut Thickness/Wire Diameter (mm):	0.025 mm
Lengths Available (mm):	8, 16 mm
Shortening After Delivery (%):	0%
Diameters Available (mm):	2.0-4.0 mm
Recoil (%):	0%
Profile Before Delivery:	1.27-1.52 mm
Ferromagnetic:	no

Delivery Specifications

Delivery System: Balloon expandable; pre-mounted on a balloon without sheath.

Minimum Guiding Catheter Lumen:	.064"
Radiopacity of Stent:	low (but highly opaque gold markers at ends)
Marker Positions:	■#####■
Deployment Pressure:	3-6 atm
Further Balloon Expansion:	to maximize stent size

Distinctive Features

Innovative lock-out or ratchetting design provides for very thin material construction, allowing distal passage into small (2.5 mm) vessels. Radial hoop strength is exceptional, resulting in no recoil after deployment.

ANGIOSTENT

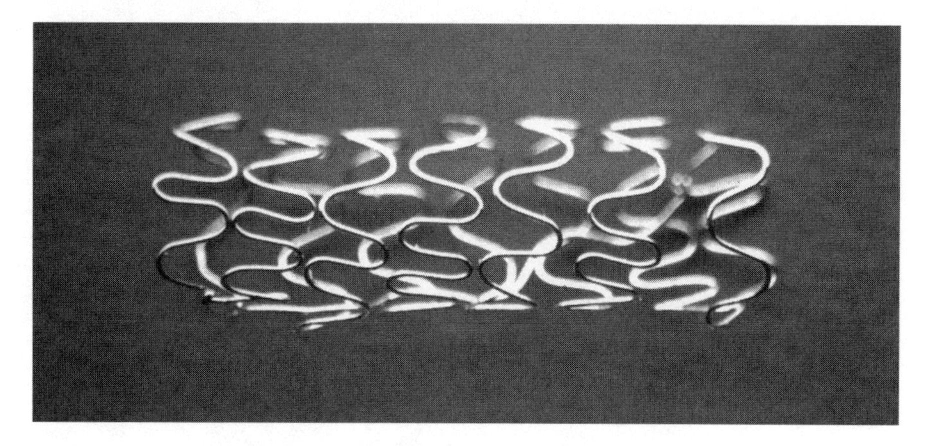

Manufacturer: AngioDynamics, E-Z-EM Inc.
Description: Single-wire sinusoidal shape with a longitudinal spine

Technical Specifications

Material:	90% platinum, 10% iridium
Surface Area After Expansion (%):	10-12%
Strut Thickness/Wire Diameter (mm):	0.127 mm
Lengths Available (mm):	15, 25, 35 mm
Shortening After Delivery (%):	<5% up to 5mm
Diameters Available (mm):	3.0, 3.5, 4.0, 5.0, 6.0 mm
Recoil (%):	7%
Profile Before Delivery:	5 french delivery system
Ferromagnetic:	no

Delivery Specifications

Delivery System: Balloon expandable; pre-mounted on a balloon with sheath.

Minimum Guiding Catheter Lumen:	0.084"
Radiopacity of Stent:	high
Marker Positions:	■#####■; additional marker on sheath
Deployment Pressure:	8-12 atm
Further Balloon Expansion:	as needed with noncompliant deployment balloon

Distinctive Features

Extremely flexible and very radiopaque provides for good positioning in tortuous vessels. Platinum is less thrombogenic than stainless steel, which may provide an advantage in thrombotic lesions.

BE STENT

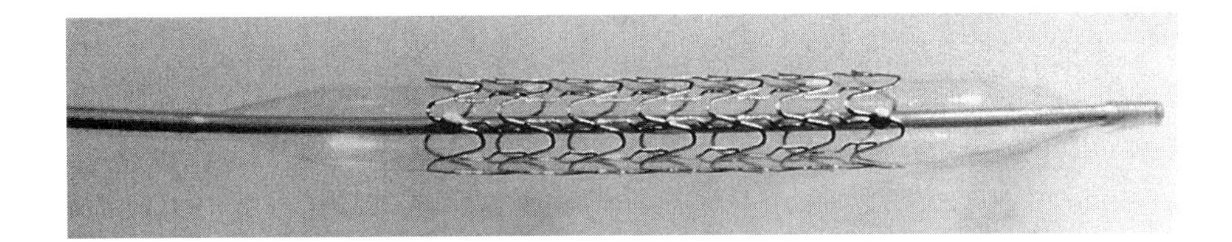

Manufacturer: InStent/Medtronic, Inc.
Description: Serpentine balloon expandable stent. Hepamed surface (hydrogel with covalently bonded heparin) version under development.

Technical Specifications

Material:	316 L stainless steel
Surface Area After Expansion (%):	11-18%
Strut Thickness/Wire Diameter (mm):	0.075-0.11 mm
Lengths Available (mm):	8, 15, 25 mm (35 mm under development)
Shortening After Delivery (%):	0%
Diameters Available (mm):	2.5-3.0 mm (small), 3.0-5.5 mm (large)
Recoil (%):	minimal (< 3%)
Profile Before Delivery:	< 1.0 mm
Ferromagnetic:	no

Delivery Specifications

Delivery System: Free stent is delivered onto balloon of choice using a mounting tool (provided), and is then hand-crimped. Premounted rapid exchange system (beStent Artist) is available outside the US. Over-the-wire system (beStent Rival) under investigation.

Minimum Guiding Catheter Lumen:	6F
Radiopacity of Stent:	low, but there are gold end markers
Marker Positions:	■#####■
Deployment Pressure:	8 atm
Further Balloon Expansion:	as indicated clinically, 10-14 atm is recommended

Distinctive Features

Serpentine strut design with orthogonal "rotating junctions" allows homogeneous stress distribution and no shortening upon expansion. Orthogonal locking mechanism provides good resistance to radial compression. Low crimped profile and high flexibility provide ease of passage through tortuous segments. Zero shortening design and radiopaque markers facilitate precise placement, making this design especially suitable for ostial locations, avoiding side branches, and tandem stenting.

BIOTRONIK (TENSUM) STENT

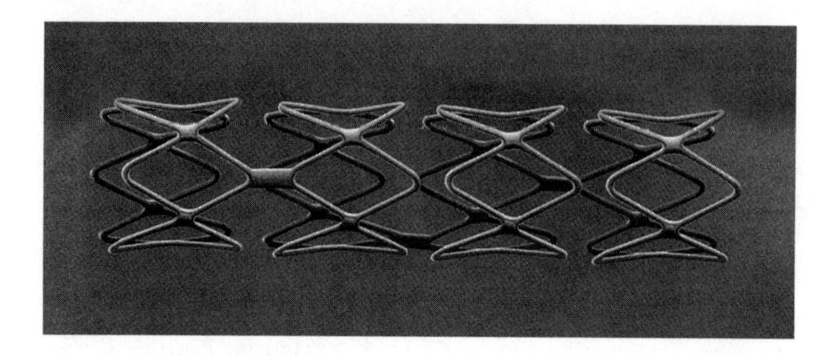

Manufacturer: Biotronic, Inc.
Description: Slotted tube with two articulations

Technical Specifications

Material:	Tantalum with silicon carbide
Surface Area After Expansion (%):	13%at 4.0 mm diameter
Strut Thickness/Wire Diameter (mm):	0.08 mm
Lengths Available (mm):	9, 14, 19 mm
Shortening After Delivery (%):	7%
Diameters Available (mm):	2.5 - 4.0 mm
Recoil (%):	5%
Profile Before Delivery:	1 mm crimped
Ferromagnetic:	no

Delivery Specifications

Delivery System: Balloon expandable; free mounted on balloon of choice or pre-mounted on a rapid exchange catheter system

Minimum Guiding Catheter Lumen:	0.064"
Radiopacity of Stent:	high
Marker Positions:	Stent is radiopaque
Deployment Pressure:	8 atm
Further Balloon Expansion:	not recommended above 4.0 mm

Distinctive Features

High radiopacity and flexibility allow easy passage through tortuous vessels and good access into side branches. Should not be placed in vein grafts > 4.0 mm in diameter. The space left between the articulated stent segments provides less than complete scaffolding and may allow plaque to prolapse into the arterial lumen.

CARDIOCOIL STENT

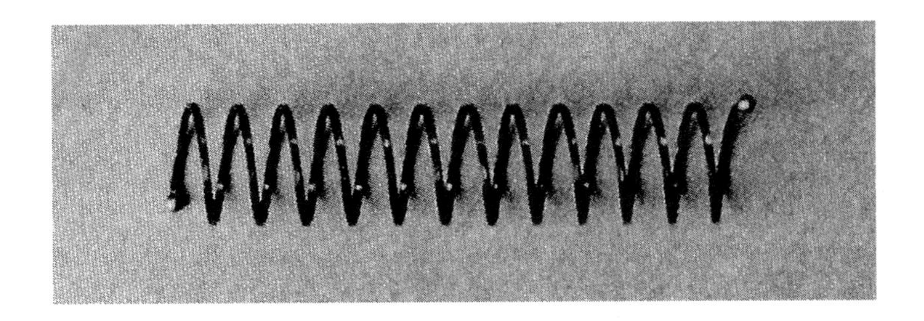

Manufacturer: Instent / Medtronic
Description: Self-expanding spiral coil with two terminal balls

Technical Specifications

Material:	Nitinol (nickle-titanium alloy)
Surface Area After expansion (%):	8-15 %
Strut Thickness/Wire Diameter (mm):	0.15 mm
Lengths Available (mm):	15, 40 mm
Shortening After Delivery (%):	24-32%
Diameters Available (mm):	3.0, 3.5, 4.0, 4.5, 5.0 mm
Recoil (%):	none
Profile Before Delivery:	1.59 mm
Ferromagnetic:	no

Delivery Specifications

Delivery System: Self expandable upon release of the holding strings--pre mounted on a balloon without sheath.

Minimum Guiding Catheter Lumen:	0.072" (up to 4 mm size)
Radiopacity of Stent:	moderate
Marker Positions:	■///////■/// (Radiopaque markers denote final stent location)
Deployment Pressure:	self expandable
Further Balloon Expansion:	recommended if stent is not fully opened

Distinctive Features

Good radiopacity and radial strength may be useful in ostial lesions. This stent will not expand beyond its nominal size; adequate sizing is essential. Side branches accesible to angioplasty through stent coils. It is important to watch for unexpanded coils within non-compliant portions of lesions. This gradually self-expanding stent may decrease deep wall injury to the artery, potentially reducing neointimal hyperplasia.

CORDIS STENT

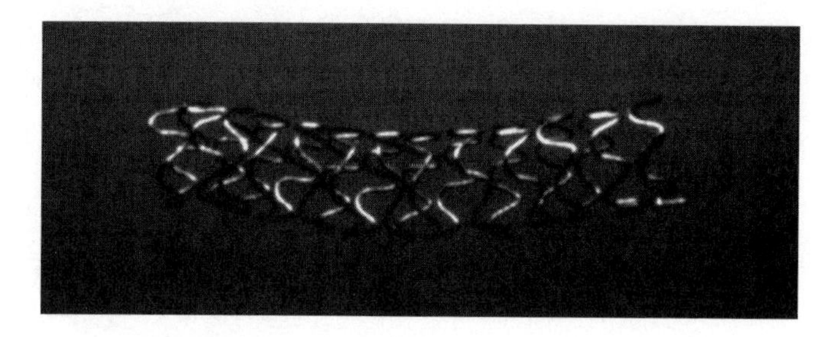

Manufacturer: Cordis, Inc.
Description: Single sinusoidal helical coil

Technical Specifications

Material:	Tantalum
Surface Area After Expansion (%):	15 %
Strut Thickness/Wire Diameter (mm):	0.125 mm
Lengths Available (mm):	15 mm
Shortening After Delivery (%):	10%
Diameters Available (mm):	3.0, 3.5, 4.0 mm
Recoil (%):	<10%
Profile Before Delivery:	1.50 mm
Ferromagnetic:	no

Delivery Specifications

Delivery System: Balloon expandable; pre-mounted on a balloon without sheath.

Minimum Guiding Catheter Lumen:	0.072"
Radiopacity of Stent:	high
Marker Positions:	////■////
Deployment Pressure:	8 atm
Further Balloon Expansion:	Use deployment balloon until the stent appears to sit outside the arterial lumen. Recrossing stent with a separate balloon is not advised.

Distinctive Features

Good radiopacity and excellent flexibility make this a good stent for tortuous segments. Side branches may be accessed but the stent in the trunk vessel. It is important to use a stent 1.15 times larger than the reference vessel with this device. Extra-support and stiffer guidewires should be avoided since wire bias will direct the uncovered stent coils against the arterial wall inhibiting passage. Unlike stents with greater scaffolding, the best results will be obtained by aggressive angioplasty before stent deployment. Coil stents will not improve a poor angioplasty result.

CROSSFLEX STENT

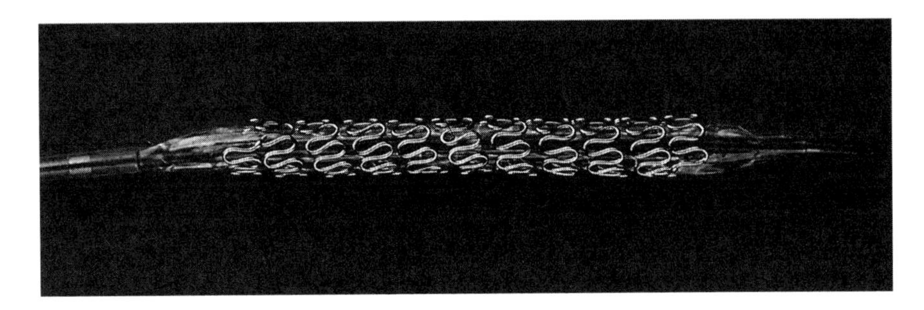

Manufacturer:	Cordis/Johnson & Johnson
Description:	Single sinusoidal helical coil

Technical Specifications

Material:	316 L stainless steel
Surface Area After Expansion (%):	15 %
Strut Thickness/Wire Diameter (mm):	0.152 mm
Lengths Available (mm):	15 mm
Shortening After Delivery (%):	N/A
Diameters Available (mm):	3.0, 3.5, 4.0 mm
Recoil (%):	minimal
Profile Before Delivery:	~ 4F (~ 0.60")
Ferromagnetic:	no

Delivery Specifications

Delivery System: Balloon expandable; pre-mounted on a balloon without sheath. Over-the-wire and rapid exchange systems available.

Minimum Guiding Catheter Lumen:	0.074" (3.5, 4.0 mm); 0.064" (3.0 mm)
Radiopacity of Stent:	moderate
Marker Positions:	////■////
Deployment Pressure:	10 atm
Further Balloon Expansion:	yes

Distinctive Features

Excellent trackability and conformability. Especially useful for sidebranches, distal lesions, and for smaller tortuous vessels.

CROWN (Palmaz-Schatz) STENT

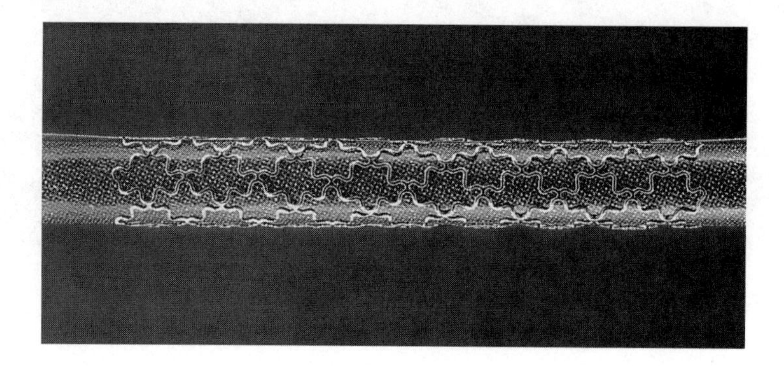

Manufacturer: Cordis, Inc.
Description: Continuous sinusoidally slotted tube

Technical Specifications

Material:	316 L stainless steel
Surface Area After Expansion (%):	<20 %
Strut Thickness/Wire Diameter (mm):	0.068 mm
Lengths Available (mm):	15, 22, 30 mm
Shortening After Delivery (%):	7-10%
Diameters Available (mm):	3.0, 3.5, 4.0 mm
Recoil (%):	minimal
Profile Before Delivery:	1.4 mm
Ferromagnetic:	no

Delivery Specifications

Delivery System: Balloon expandable; pre-mounted on a high pressure, non-compliant, sticky balloon without sheath.

Minimum Guiding Catheter Lumen:	6, 7 F guide
Radiopacity of Stent:	low
Marker Positions:	■######■
Deployment Pressure:	6 atm
Further Balloon Expansion:	as needed with deployment balloon.

Distinctive Features

More flexible than the earlier Palmaz-Schatz iterations with preservation of good scaffolding features. The sinusoidal longitudinal design allows better passage through angulated segments and better access to side branches.

ENFORCER STENT

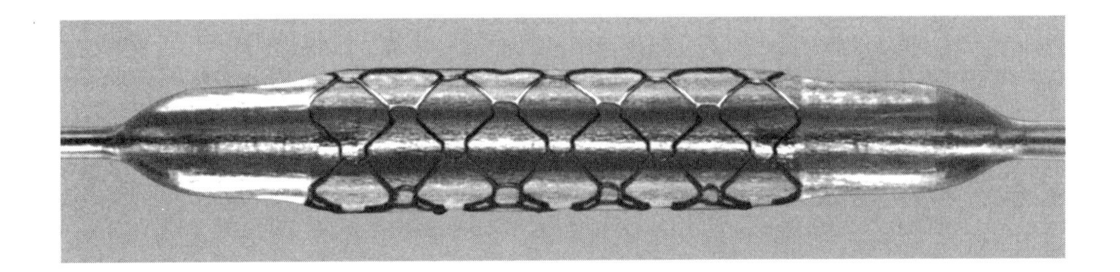

Manufacturer: CardioVascular Dynamics, Inc.
Description: Uniform cellular mesh

Technical Specifications

Material:	316 L stainless steel
Surface Area After Expansion (%):	10-12 %
Strut Thickness/Wire Diameter (mm):	0.09 mm
Lengths Available (mm):	17, 27 mm
Shortening After Delivery (%):	12% for 3.5 mm
Diameters Available (mm):	3.0, 3.5, 4.0 mm
Recoil (%):	< 5%
Profile Before Delivery:	self-mounted
Ferromagnetic:	yes

Delivery Specifications

Delivery System: Balloon expandable; self-mounted; available in kit with balloon.

Minimum Guiding Catheter Lumen:	0.064" (6F guide)
Radiopacity of Stent:	low
Deployment Pressure:	3-5 atm
Further Balloon Expansion:	as needed with deployment balloon

Distinctive Features

High radial strength.

FLEXSTENT (GIANTURCO-ROUBIN)

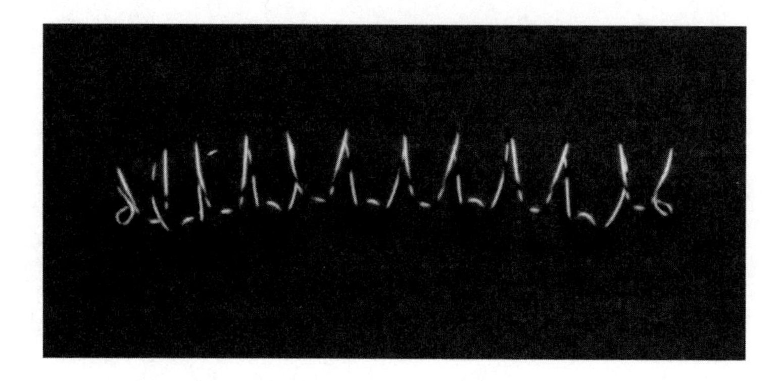

Manufacturer: Cook, Inc.
Description: The original flexible coil

Technical Specifications

Material:	316 L stainless steel
Surface Area After Expansion (%):	10 %
Strut Thickness/Wire Diameter (mm):	0.15 mm
Lengths Available (mm):	12, 20 mm
Shortening After Delivery (%):	none
Diameters Available (mm):	2.0, 2.5, 3.0, 3.5, 4.0 mm
Recoil (%):	15-20%
Profile Before Delivery:	1.78-2.3 mm
Ferromagnetic:	no

Delivery Specifications

Delivery System: Balloon expandable; pre-mounted on a balloon without sheath.

Minimum Guiding Catheter Lumen:	0.077" (2.5, 3.0 mm) 0.086" (3.5, 4.0 mm)
Radiopacity of Stent:	low
Marker Positions:	■////////■
Deployment Pressure:	4-5 atm
Further Balloon Expansion:	as needed being cautious not to overexpand the coils.

Distinctive Features

This is the original "bailout" stent. Has been replaced by the GR II, which provides greater scaffolding, a smoother lumen, and a significantly lower crossing profile.

FREEDOM STENT

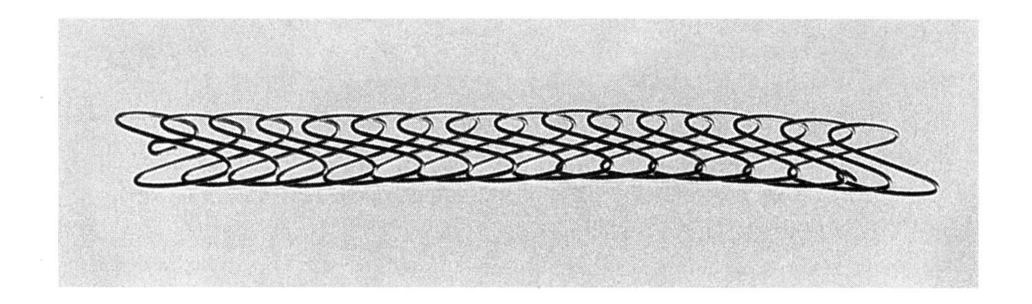

Manufacturer: Global Therapeutics, Inc.
Description: Multiloop design; single wire fishbone

Technical Specifications

Material:	316 LVM stainless steel
Surface Area After Expansion (%):	11%
Strut Thickness/Wire Diameter (mm):	0.175 mm
Lengths Available (mm):	12, 16, 20, 24, 30, 40 mm
Shortening After Delivery (%):	none
Diameters Available (mm):	2.5, 3.0, 3.5, 4.0, 4.5 mm
Recoil (%):	5-7%
Profile Before Delivery:	1.30 mm
Ferromagnetic:	no

Delivery Specifications

Delivery System: Balloon expandable; pre-mounted on a balloon without sheath (available as a bare stent in some markets).

Minimum Guiding Catheter Lumen:	0.065"
Radiopacity of Stent:	medium
Marker Positions:	■#####■
Deployment Pressure:	10-12 atm
Further Balloon Expansion:	as needed

Distinctive Features

Remains flexible and trackable even at longer lengths.

GFX STENT

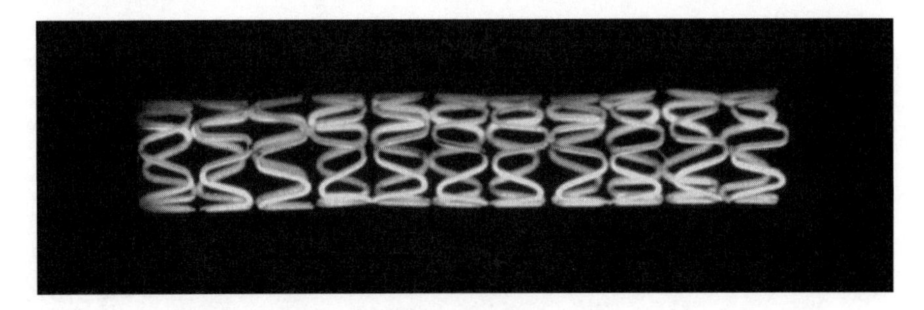

Manufacturer: Arterial Vascular Engineering, Inc
Description: 6 crowns, 2 mm length sinusoidal elements with elliptorectangular struts connected by helical laser fusion technology.

Technical Specifications

Material:	316 L stainless steel
Surface Area after expansion (%):	20%
Strut Thickness/Wire Diameter (mm):	0.125 mm
Lengths Available (mm):	8, 12, 18, 24 mm (GFX-XL: 30, 40 mm)
Shortening After Delivery (%):	negligible
Diameters Available (mm):	2.5, 3.0, 3.5, 4.0 mm
Recoil (%):	4%
Profile Before Delivery:	0.9-0.93 mm
Ferromagnetic:	no

Delivery Specifications

Delivery System: Balloon expandable; pre-mounted on a custom stent delivery system without a sheath. Available as rapid exchange and over the wire.

Minimum Guiding Catheter Lumen:	0.064" (3.0, 3.5 mm) 0.072" (4.0 mm)
Radiopacity of Stent:	moderate
Marker Positions:	■#####■
Deployment Pressure:	9-10 atm
Further Balloon Expansion:	high pressure deployment makes this optional

Distinctive Features

This is an improved iteration of the AVE Micro Stent. 2mm segments have replaced the 3mm segments, there are 6 crowns radially rather than 4, and the round wire has been made elliptical for improved scaffolding. Radiopacity and excellent hoop strength make it good for ostial lesions. The low crossing profile, short lengths, and extreme flexibility and trackability are a good choice for distal lesions and through-stent touch ups. Side branches can be safely approached to perform angioplasty.

GR II STENT

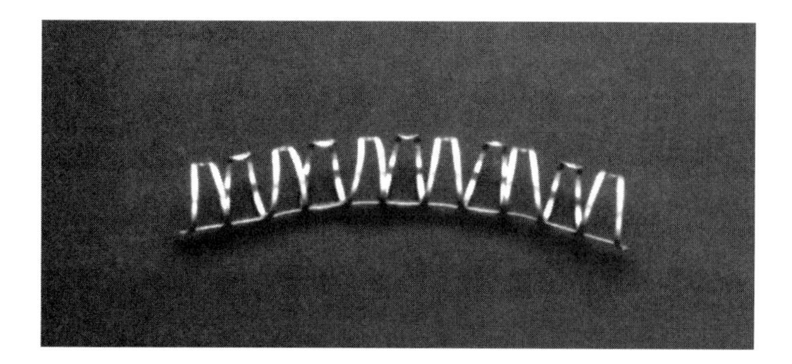

Manufacturer:	Cook, Inc.
Description:	Interdigitating loops of flat wire on a longitudinal spine

Technical Specifications

Material:	316 L stainless steel
Surface Area After Expansion (%):	15-20 %
Strut Thickness/Wire Diameter (mm):	0.075 mm
Lengths Available (mm):	10, 20, 40 mm
Shortening After Delivery (%):	none
Diameters Available (mm):	2.5, 3.0, 3.5, 4.0 mm
Recoil (%):	9-11%
Profile Before Delivery:	1.5-1.7 mm
Ferromagnetic:	no

Delivery Specifications

Delivery System: Balloon expandable; pre-mounted on a minimally compliant balloon without sheath.

Minimum Guiding Catheter Lumen:	0.06" (2.5, 3.0 mm) 0.066" (3.5 mm) 0.07" (4.0")
Radiopacity of Stent:	low but with radiopaque gold markers at the ends
Marker Positions:	■/#/#/#/■
Deployment Pressure:	6 atm
Further Balloon Expansion:	12-14 atm as needed

Distinctive Features

Stent diameter should be sized 0.5 mm larger than the artery. Gold markers at ends make for easy stent positioning. Flat wire design provides better scaffolding and a smoother lumen than the FlexStent (GR-I) device. Safe access to cross the coils and perform angioplasty in side branches.

MICRO STENT II

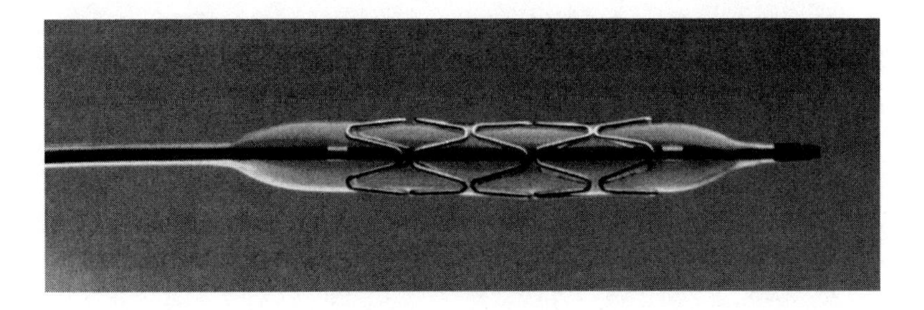

Manufacturer: Arterial Vascular Engineering, Inc
Description: Continuously connected 3 mm sinusoidal elements

Technical Specifications

Material:	316 L stainless steel
Surface Area after expansion (%):	14.5%
Strut Thickness/Wire Diameter (mm):	0.2 mm
Lengths Available (mm):	6, 15, 30 mm (in the U.S.) 9, 12, 18, 24, 30, 39 mm (elsewhere)
Shortening After Delivery (%):	2% at 3.5 mm
Diameters Available (mm):	2.5, 3.0, 3.5, 4.0 mm
Recoil (%):	8%
Profile Before Delivery:	1.63 mm
Ferromagnetic:	no

Delivery Specifications

Delivery System: Balloon expandable; pre-mounted on a custom stent delivery system without a sheath. Available in rapid exchange and over-the-wire configurations.

Minimum Guiding Catheter Lumen:	0.072"
Radiopacity of Stent:	moderate
Marker Positions:	■///////■
Deployment Pressure:	9-12 atm
Further Balloon Expansion:	high pressure deployment makes this optional

Distinctive Features

Good radiopacity and hoop strength make it good for ostial lesions. Low crossing profile and short lengths are good for distal through-stent touch ups. Side branches can be safely approached to perform angioplasty.

MULTI-LINK STENT

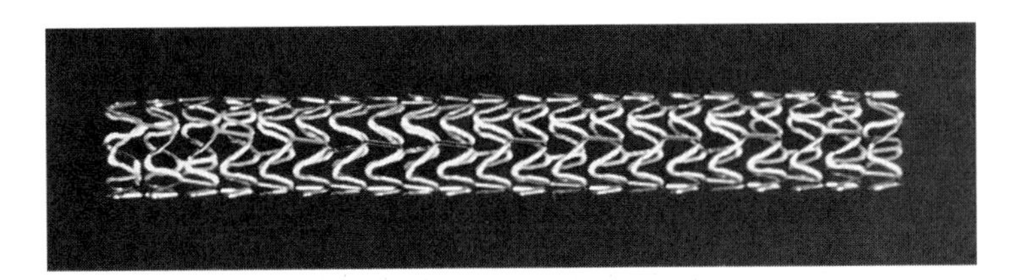

Manufacturer: Guidant/ACS, Inc.
Description: Multiple linked rings

Technical Specifications

Material:	316 L stainless steel
Surface Area After Expansion (%):	<15%
Strut Thickness/Wire Diameter (mm):	0.056 mm
Lengths Available (mm):	15, 25, 35 mm
Shortening After Delivery (%):	< 5%
Diameters Available (mm):	USA: 3.0, 3.5, 3.75mm (high-pressure system) International: 3.0, 3.5, 4.0 (all systems)
Recoil (%):	< 6%
Profile Before Delivery:	1.35-1.38 mm (rapid exchange)
Ferromagnetic:	no

Delivery Specifications

Delivery System: Balloon expandable; pre-mounted on a balloon without protective sheath. Over-the-wire and rapid exchange systems available. A high pressure, low profile delivery system (DUET) and bare stent (SOLO) will be available in some markets this year.

Minimum Guiding Catheter Lumen:	0.064" (all systems)
Radiopacity of Stent:	low-to-moderate
Marker Positions:	■######■
Deployment Pressure:	10 atm (high-pressure systems) 6-7 atm (standard systems)
Further Balloon Expansion:	not recommended on original version but indicated as necessary on high-pressure systems

Distinctive Features

Excellent combination of high radial strength and flexibility. Computer-aided finite element analysis led to design of rings and links with fewer intersection points applying more metal to stress points. Animal modeling suggests that this will result in less intimal reaction and possibly less restenosis. Side branches may be safely accessed for angioplasty as maximum aperture is 3.9mm diameter.

NIR STENT

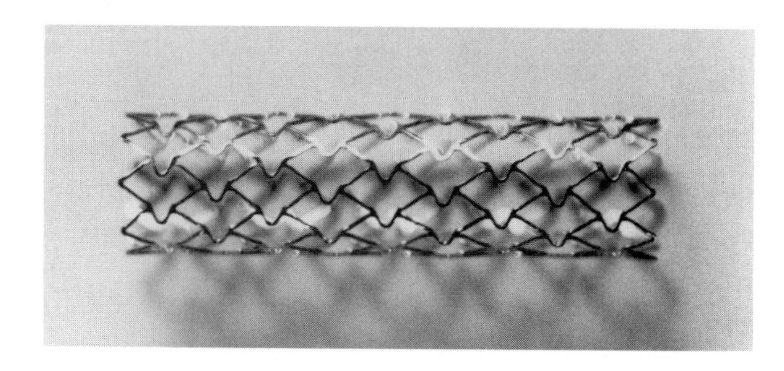

Manufacturer: Boston Scientific/SciMed, Inc.
Description: Expandable uniform cellular mesh

Technical Specifications

Material:	316 LVM stainless steel
Surface Area After Expansion (%):	19% at 3 mm, 14% at 5 mm
Strut Thickness (mm):	0.075 and 0.1 mm
Lengths Available (mm):	9, 16, 25, 32 mm
Shortening After Delivery (%):	< 5% up to 5mm
Diameters Available (mm):	2.0, 2.5, 3.0, 3.5, 4.0, 4.5, 5.0 mm
Recoil (%):	< 5%
Profile Before Delivery:	crimped < 1.0mm
Ferromagnetic:	no

Delivery Specifications

Delivery System: Balloon expandable; pre-mounted on a balloon without sheath or free for hand crimping.

Minimum Guiding Catheter Lumen:	0.064"
Radiopacity of Stent:	low
Marker Positions:	proximal and distal markers on balloon
Deployment Pressure:	7-14 atm
Further Balloon Expansion:	as needed

Distinctive Features

Very low crossing profile and high flexibility make this stent suitable for distal lesions through tortuous segments. High hoop strength and resistance to radial compression are good for ostial lesions.

PALMAZ-SCHATZ (PS153) STENT

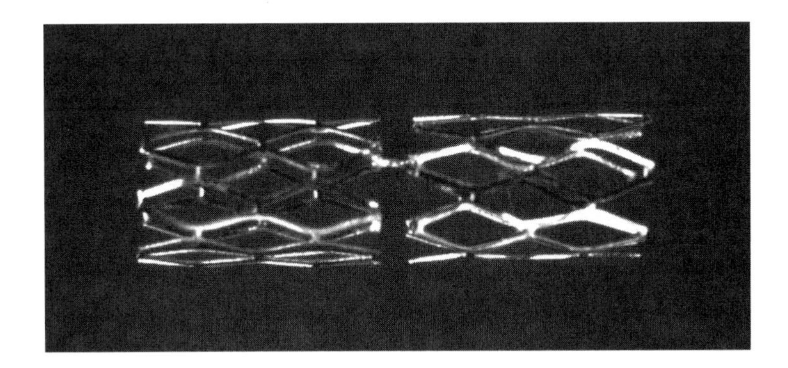

Manufacturer:	Cordis/Johnson & Johnson
Description:	Slotted tube with central articulation

Technical Specifications

Material:	316 L stainless steel
Surface Area After Expansion (%):	< 20%
Strut Thickness/Wire Diameter (mm):	0.0625 mm
Lengths Available (mm):	15 mm
Shortening After Delivery (%):	2.5-15%
Diameters Available (mm):	3.0, 3.5, 4.0, 4.5 mm
Recoil (%):	5-7%
Profile Before Delivery:	1.65 mm
Ferromagnetic:	no

Delivery Specifications

Delivery System: Balloon expandable; pre-mounted on a compliant balloon with sheath. Free stent is available in some markets.

Minimum Guiding Catheter Lumen:	0.084" (0.062" for bare stent)
Radiopacity of Stent:	low
Marker Positions:	■######■....■
Deployment Pressure:	4-6 atm
Further Balloon Expansion:	yes

Distinctive Features

This is the original slotted tube design with proven reduction in restenosis rates compared to angioplasty.

PARAGON (ACT ONE) STENT

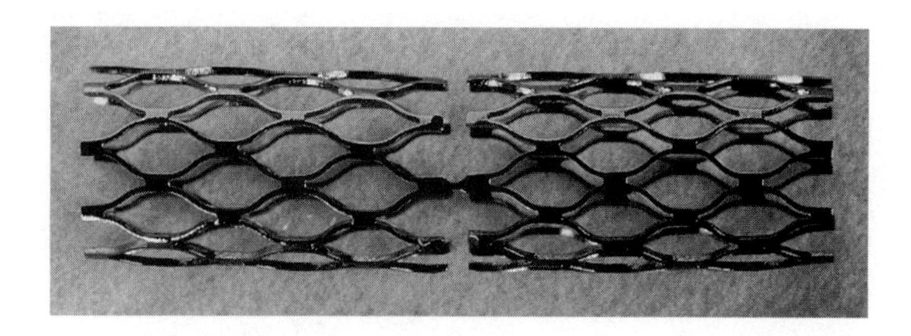

Manufacturer: Progressive Angioplasty Systems, Inc.
Description: Non-articulated slotted tube

Technical Specifications

Material:	Martensitic Nitinol (nickle-titanium)
Surface Area After Expansion (%):	26% at 3 mm size
Strut Thickness/Wire Diameter (mm):	0.15 mm
Lengths Available (mm):	9, 16, 26, 36 mm
Shortening After Delivery (%):	3%
Diameters Available (mm):	3-4 mm
Recoil (%):	5-10%
Profile Before Delivery:	1.3 mm
Ferromagnetic:	no

Delivery Specifications

Delivery System: Balloon expandable; pre-mounted on a balloon without sheath. Over-the-wire and monorail delivery balloons available.

Minimum Guiding Catheter Lumen:	0.062"
Radiopacity of Stent:	moderate
Marker Positions:	■#####■
Deployment Pressure:	8-16 atm
Further Balloon Expansion:	recommended

Distinctive Features

Superb flexibility with a low crossing profile make it a good choice for distal lesions. Good radiopacity helps with ostial lesions. Proton beam irradiation transmutes the stent to the beta emitter vanadium, allowing for a beta emitting stent.

RADIUS STENT

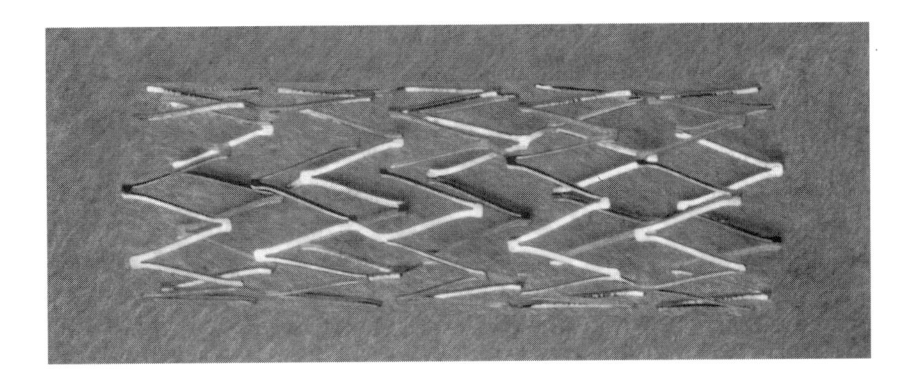

Manufacturer: Boston Scientific/SciMed, Inc
Description: Multiple segment slotted tube

Technical Specifications

Material:	Nitinol
Surface Area After Expansion (%):	22%
Strut Thickness/Wire Diameter (mm):	0.11 mm
Lengths Available (mm):	14, 20, 31 mm
Shortening After Delivery (%):	< 3%
Diameters Available (mm):	3.0, 3.5, 4.0 mm (treats vessels 2.75-4.25 mm)
Recoil (%):	0%
Profile Before Delivery:	1.53 mm
Ferromagnetic:	no

Delivery Specifications

Delivery System: Self-expanding; unique wire pull-back sheath delivery system.

Minimum Guiding Catheter Lumen:	0.072"
Radiopacity of Stent:	moderate
Marker Positions:	■#####■(stent covers to outside edge of marker bands)
Deployment Pressure:	Stent will not expand beyond its unconstrained diameter; therefore, a device with an unconstrained final diameter 0.5-1.0 mm larger than the reference diameter is selected.
Further Balloon Expansion:	as needed

Distinctive Features

Excellent flexibility and low profile provides good trackability.

SPIRAL (Palmaz-Schatz) STENT

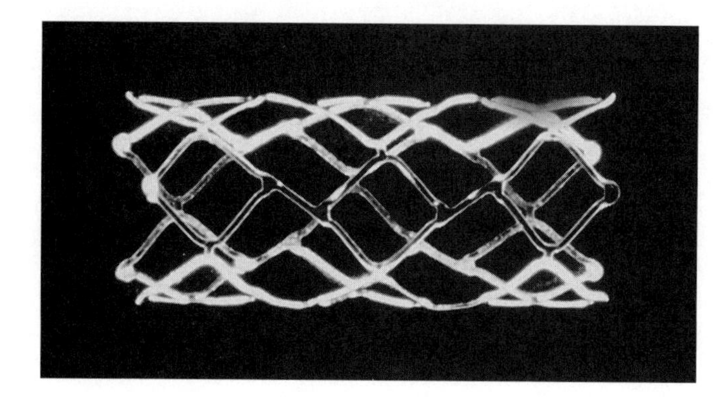

Manufacturer: Cordis/Johnson & Johnson
Description: Slotted tube; 12 row spiral with spiral articulation

Technical Specifications

Material:	316 L stainless steel
Surface Area After Expansion (%):	< 20%
Strut Thickness/Wire Diameter (mm):	0.1 mm
Lengths Available (mm):	8, 9, 14, 18 mm
Shortening After Delivery (%):	2.5-15%
Diameters Available (mm):	3.0, 3.5, 4.0, 4.5, 5.0 mm
Recoil (%):	5-7%
Profile Before Delivery:	1.65 mm
Ferromagnetic:	no

Delivery Specifications

Delivery System: Balloon expandable; pre-mounted on a compliant balloon with sheath. Free stent is available in some markets.

Minimum Guiding Catheter Lumen:	0.084" (0.062" for bare stent)
Radiopacity of Stent:	low
Marker Positions:	on delivery balloon
Deployment Pressure:	depends on the delivery balloon
Further Balloon Expansion:	yes

Distinctive Features

This slotted tube design has a proven reduction in restenosis rates. While the thicker Spiral stent design provides better hoop strength and resistance to radial compression than the original PS-153 design, it is not as flexible in passing tortuous segments. Heparin coating may be an advantage.

SPIRAL (IMPROVED) (Palmaz-Schatz) STENT

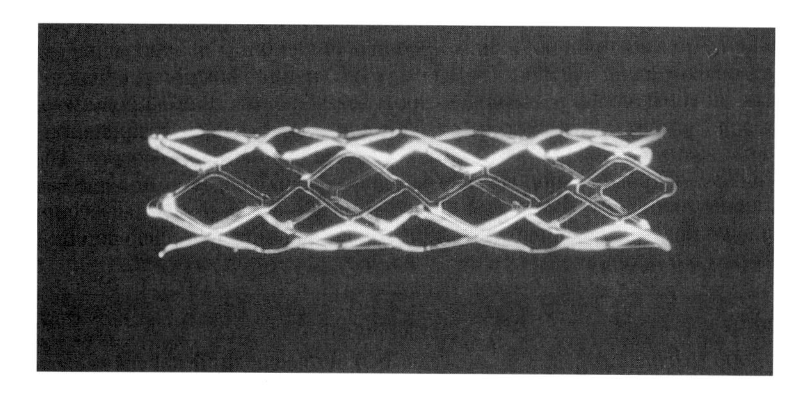

Manufacturer:	Cordis/Johnson & Johnson
Description:	Slotted tube; 10 row spiral with spiral articulation

Technical Specifications

Material:	316 L stainless steel
Surface Area After Expansion (%):	< 20%
Strut Thickness/Wire Diameter (mm):	0.0027"
Lengths Available (mm):	15 mm
Shortening After Delivery (%):	7%
Diameters Available (mm):	3.0, 3.5, 4.0, 4.5, 5.0 mm (mounted on PowerGrip)
Recoil (%):	minimal
Profile Before Delivery:	1.4 mm
Ferromagnetic:	no

Delivery Specifications

Delivery System:	Balloon expandable; pre-mounted on a high-pressure, noncompliant sticky balloon without sheath.

Minimum Guiding Catheter Lumen:	6F
Radiopacity of Stent:	moderate
Marker Positions:	proximal and distal ends
Deployment Pressure:	6 atm
Further Balloon Expansion:	yes, as needed

Distinctive Features

Ease of delivery; increased flexibility compared to regular Spiral stent; no bare area at articulation. High stent retention rates, compatibility with 6F guides, and high-pressure delivery balloon are added features.

TERUMO STENT

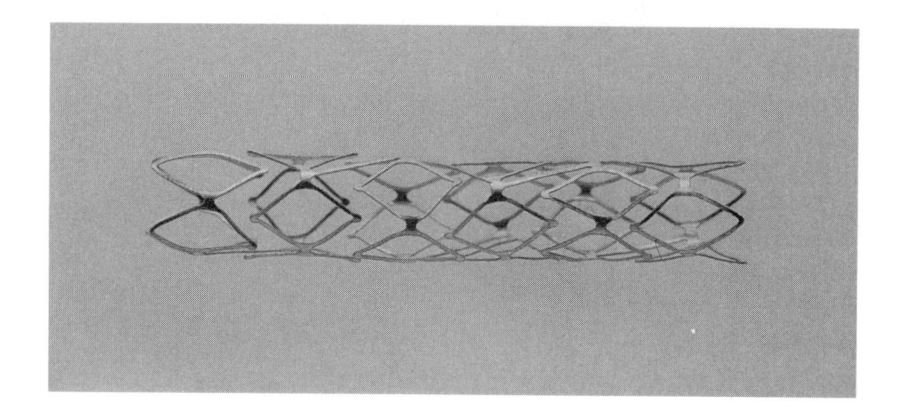

Manufacturer: Terumo Medical Corp.
Description: Four diamonds joined by a single connector

Technical Specifications

Material:	stainless steel
Surface Area After Expansion (%):	18%
Strut Thickness/Wire Diameter (mm):	0.075 mm
Lengths Available (mm):	20 mm
Shortening After Delivery (%):	< 5%
Diameters Available (mm):	3.0, 3.5 mm
Recoil (%):	< 5%
Profile Before Delivery:	not reported
Ferromagnetic:	no

Delivery Specifications

Delivery System: Balloon expandable; only available as a bare stent at this time.

Minimum Guiding Catheter Lumen:	0.065"
Radiopacity of Stent:	low
Marker Positions:	on balloon of choice
Deployment Pressure:	10 atm
Further Balloon Expansion:	as needed

Distinctive Features

Clinical trials started in 1997.

WALLSTENT ("MAGIC WALLSTENT")

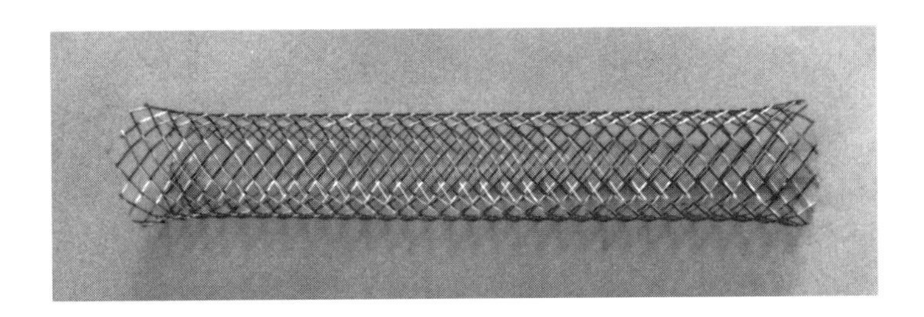

Manufacturer: Schneider (Europe), Inc.
Description: Self-expanding wire braid

Technical Specifications

Material:	Cobalt based alloy; platinum core
Surface Area After Expansion (%):	approximately 14%
Strut Thickness/Wire Diameter (mm):	0.08-0.1 mm
Lengths Available (mm):	15-50 mm (implanted length)
Shortening After Delivery (%):	approximately 20%
Diameters Available (mm):	4.0-6.0 mm
Recoil (%):	no
Profile Before Delivery:	maximum 1.6 mm
Ferromagnetic:	no

Delivery Specifications

Delivery System: Self-expandable after withdrawal of the outer sheath; stent pre-mounted on delivery device

Minimum Guiding Catheter Lumen:	0.064"; inner lumen PTFE coated
Radiopacity of Stent:	moderate
Marker Positions:	ends of stent, end of outer sheath
Deployment Pressure:	no pressure necessary
Further Balloon Expansion:	yes

Distinctive Features

Superb scaffolding; short and long lengths at large diameters make this an excellent choice for vein graft disease or diffuse native vessel disease. Stent protected by outer sheath (no stent loss). Partially released stent can be recaptured and repositioned.

WIKTOR (PRIME AND GX) STENT

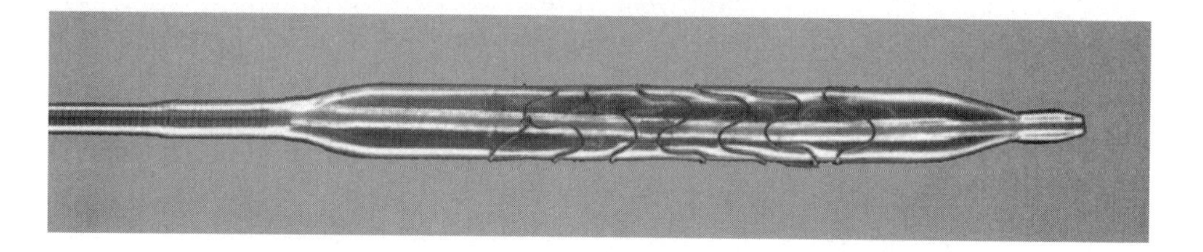

Manufacturer: Medtronic
Description: Single wire sinusoidal helix

Technical Specifications

Material:	Tantalum
Surface Area After Expansion (%):	7-9%
Strut Thickness/Wire Diameter (mm):	0.127 mm
Lengths Available (mm):	16 mm
Shortening After Delivery (%):	4%
Diameters Available (mm):	3.0, 3.5, 4.0, 4.5 mm
Recoil (%):	< 7%
Profile Before Delivery:	1.55-1.77 mm
Ferromagnetic:	no

Delivery Specifications

Delivery System: Balloon expandable; pre-mounted on a balloon without a sheath. Over-the-wire (Prime) and rapid delivery (GX) systems available. Over-the-wire (Wiktor Rival) in clinical trials.

Minimum Guiding Catheter Lumen:	0.079"
Radiopacity of Stent:	high
Marker Positions:	/////■////
Deployment Pressure:	6-8 atm
Further Balloon Expansion:	as needed until stent struts appear to reside just outside vessel lumen

Distinctive Features

Radiopacity and flexibility facilitate precise placement without side branch compromise. This and other coil stents should be avoided at aorto-ostial locations due to their susceptibility to guiding catheter damage. Although radial strength is roughly equivalent (and in some cases superior) to slotted tubular stents, the relatively low metal coverage of this stent makes it a poor selection for calcified or bulky lesions (unless preceded by atherectomy). Complete predilatation of target lesion and moderate proximal disease is essential to allow passage of the stent without risk of altering stent geometry during positioning (sheathless system). Coaxial guide position is essential. Extra-support and stiffer guidewires are often not required and may in fact direct the uncovered stent coils against the vessel wall restricting free passage. Stent should be slightly oversized (10-15%, or 0.5 mm) as compared to the ideal angioplasty balloon in most clinical situations. A well-deployed stent has a characteristic scalloped appearance in which the coils appear to reside slightly outside the arterial lumen. If additional expansion is indicated post-deployment, this should first be attempted with the delivery balloon. High pressure post-dilatation is often not required, and recrossing the freshly deployed stent should be avoided if possible. If higher pressures are indicated clinically, a soft semi-compliant balloon with excellent rewrap characteristics should be used.

WIKTOR-I STENT

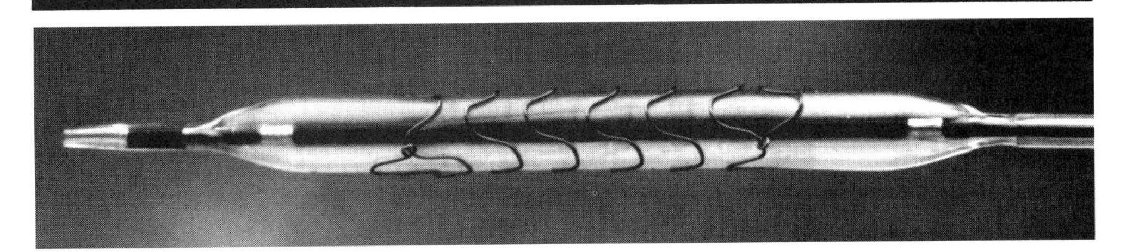

Manufacturer:	Medtronic
Description:	High frequency wave patterns of a single wire sinusoidal helix. Available with or without Hepamed surface (hydrogel with covalently-bound heparin) outside USA.

Technical Specifications

Material:	Tantalum
Surface Area After Expansion (%):	8-9.5%
Strut Thickness/Wire Diameter (mm):	0.127 mm
Lengths Available (mm):	10, 15, 20, 30 mm
Shortening After Delivery (%):	4%
Diameters Available (mm):	2.5, 3.0, 3.5, 4.0 mm
Recoil (%):	< 7%
Profile Before Delivery:	1.27-1.50 mm
Ferromagnetic:	no

Delivery Specifications

Delivery System: Balloon expandable; pre-mounted on a balloon without a sheath. Over-the-wire and rapid delivery systems are available.

Minimum Guiding Catheter Lumen:	0.062" (2.5, 3.0 mm); 0.086" (4.0 mm)
Radiopacity of Stent:	high
Marker Positions:	double markers at stent margins
Deployment Pressure:	8-10 atm
Further Balloon Expansion:	as needed until stent struts appear to reside just outside vessel lumen

Distinctive Features

Radiopacity and flexibility facilitate precise placement without side branch compromise. As such, this stent is especially suitable for tortuous vessels, long lesions, and side branches. This and other coil stents should be avoided at aorto-ostial locations due to their susceptibility to guiding catheter damage. Although radial strength is roughly equivalent (and in some cases superior) to slotted tubular stents, the relatively low metal coverage of this stent makes it a poor selection for calcified or bulky lesions (unless preceded by atherectomy). Complete predilatation of target lesion and moderate proximal disease is essential to allow passage of the stent without risk of altering stent geometry during positioning (sheathless system). Coaxial guide position is essential. Extra-support and stiffer guidewires are often not required and may in fact direct the uncovered stent coils against the vessel wall restricting free passage. Stent should be slightly oversized (10-15%, or 0.5 mm) as compared to the ideal angioplasty balloon in most clinical situations. A well-deployed stent has a characteristic scalloped appearance in which the coils appear to reside slightly outside the arterial lumen. If additional expansion is indicated post-deployment, this should first be attempted with the delivery balloon. High pressure post-dilatation is often not required, and recrossing the freshly deployed stent should be avoided if possible. If higher pressures are indicated clinically, a soft semi-compliant balloon with excellent rewrap characteristics should be used.

XT STENT

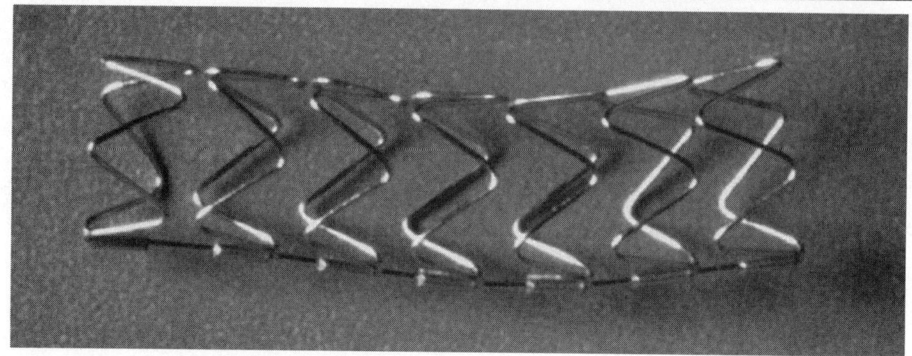

Manufacturer: CR Bard Ireland, Ltd.
Description: Modular zigzag rings on a longitudinal spine

Technical Specifications

Material:	316 LVM stainless steel
Surface Area After Expansion (%):	13-19%
Strut Thickness/Wire Diameter (mm):	0.15 mm
Lengths Available (mm):	bare: 6, 11, 15, 24, 34 mm pre-mounted: 11, 15, 24, 34 mm
Shortening After Delivery (%):	none
Diameters Available (mm):	bare: 2.5, 3.0, 3.5, 4.0 mm pre-mounted: 3.0, 3.5, 4.0 mm
Recoil (%):	5%
Profile Before Delivery:	< 1.28 mm when crimped
Ferromagnetic:	no

Delivery Specifications

Delivery System:	Balloon expandable; free mounted on balloon of choice with a unique loading tool or premounted.
Minimum Guiding Cath. Lumen:	0.062" (bare stent on rapid exchange [RE] catheter or premounted stent on Samba RE delivery catheter); 0.070" (bare stent on over-the-wire [OTW] catheter or premounted stent on Process II OTW catheter)
Radiopacity of Stent:	low overall (but with radiopaque spine markers)
Marker Positions:	one marker per module
Deployment Pressure:	8 atm with Rely balloon material
Further Balloon Expansion:	as needed

Distinctive Features

Excellent flexibility and open design make it a good choice for tortuous segments with side branches. The spine tends to self orient on curves. The excellent radiopacity of the spine allows for accurate positioning of tandem stents on long lesions.

APPENDIX VIII

STENT REFERENCE CHART

The following two pages summarize selected technical and delivery specifications for each of the 26 stents listed in the *Stent Design Compendium (pp. 179-206).* Since most stent designs are in a state of rapid evolution, the reader is referred to the stent manufacturers or the Physicians' Press web site (www.physicianspress.com) for the latest stent specifications.

STENT NAME	COMPANY	MATERIAL	SURFACE AREA (%)	DELIVERY SYSTEM	LENGTHS AVAILABLE
ACCUFLEX	Navius	0.025 mm 316L Stainless Steel	40%	OTW without sheath	8, 16 mm
ANGIOSTENT	Angiodynamics	0.127 mm, 90% platinum, 10% iridium	10-12%	OTW with sheath	15, 25, 35 mm
BE STENT	InStent/ Medtronic	0.11 mm 316 L Stainless Steel	11-18%	Free Stent & RX (outside US)	8, 15, 25 mm
BIOTRONIK/ TENSUM	Biotronik	0.08 mm Tantalum	13%	RX without sheath or Free Stent	9, 14, 19 mm
CARDIOCOIL	InStent/ Medtronic	0.15 mm Nitinol	8-15%	Premounted without sheath	15, 40 mm
CORDIS	Cordis	0.125 mm Tantalum	15%	OTW & RX without sheath	15 mm
CROSSFLEX	Cordis	0.152 mm 316L Stainless Steel	15%	OTW & RX without sheath	15 mm
CROWN	Cordis	0.068 mm 316L Stainless Steel	<20%	RX without sheath	15, 22, 30 mm
ENFORCER	CardioVascular Dynamics	316 L Stainless Steel	10-12%	Free Stent	17, 27 mm
FLEXSTENT (GR I)	Cook	0.15 mm 316L Stainless Steel	10%	OTW	12, 20 mm
FREEDOM	Global Thera-peutics	0.175 mm 316LVM SS	11%	Premounted or Free Stent	12, 16, 20, 24, 30, 40 mm
GFX	Arterial Vascular Engineering	0.125 mm 316L Stainless Steel	20%	OTW & RX without sheath	8, 12, 18, 24 mm
GR II	Cook	0.075 mm316L Stainless Steel	15-20%	OTW without sheath	10, 20, 40 mm
MICRO II	Arterial Vascular Engineering	0.20 mm 316L Stainless Steel	14.5%	OTW & RX without sheath	6, 15, 30 mm (US) 9, 12, 18, 24, 30, 39 mm (elsewhere)
MULTILINK	Guidant/ACS	0.056 mm 316L Stainless Steel	7-15%	OTW & RX with or with-out sheath	15, 25, 35 mm
NIR STENT	SciMed/Boston Scientific	0.075 & 0.1 mm 316LVM SS	14-19%	Premoumted or Free Stent	9, 16, 25, 32 mm
PALMAZ SCHATZ PS153	Cordis	0.063 mm 316L Stainless Steel	<20%	OTW with sheath or Free Stent	15 mm
PALMAZ BILIARY	Cordis	0.138 mm 316L Stainless Steel	<20%	Free Stent	10, 15, 20 mm
PARAGON (ACT-ONE)	Progressive Angioplasty Systems	0.15 mm Nitinol	26%	OTW & RX without sheath	9, 16, 26, 36 mm
RADIUS	Sci Med/Boston Scientific	0.11 mm Nitinol	22%	OTW with sleeve	14, 20, 31 mm
SPIRAL	Cordis	0.1 mm 316L Stainless Steel	<20%	OTW with sheath or Free Stent	8, 9, 14, 18 mm
SPIRAL IMPROVED	Cordis	0.068 mm316L Stainless Steel	<20%	OTW without sheath and Free	15 mm
TERUMO	Terumo	0.075 mm Stainless Steel	18%	Free Stent	20 mm
WALLSTENT (MAGIC)	Schneider Europe	0.08-0.1mm Cobalt based alloy	14-25%	OTW	12 - 50 mm depending on diameter
WIKTOR	Medtronic	0.127mm Tantalum	7-9%	OTW & RX without sheath	i - 10, 15, 20, 30 mm Prime, GX - 16mm
XT	Bard-USCI	0.15mm 316LVM Stainless Steel	13-19%	OTW & RX	bare: 6,11,15,24,34 mm mount: 11,15,24,34mm

Abbreviations: OTW - over the wire; RX - rapid exchange; N/A - not available

STENT NAME	DELIVERY PROFILE	SHORTENING POST DELIVERY %	INFLATION PRESSURES	VISIBILITY ON FLUORO	MINIMUM GUIDING CATHETER	MARKERS
ACCUFLEX	0.12-0.16 mm	0%	3-6 atm	+	0.064"	■#####■
ANGIOSTENT	5 french delivery system	<5%	8-12 atm	++++	0.084"	■#####■; addtl. marker on sheath
BE STENT	<1.0 mm	0%	8 atm	+	6 F	■#####■
BIOTRONIK/ TENSUM	1 mm	7%	8 atm	++++	0.064"	########; stent radiopaque
CARDIOCOIL	1.6 mm	24-32%	self expanding	+++	0.072"	■///////■///
CORDIS	1.50 mm	<10%	8 atm	++++	0.072"	////■////
CROSSFLEX	1.50 mm	N/A	10 atm	++	0.064-0.074"	////■////
CROWN	1.4 mm	7-10%	6 atm	+	6, 7 F	■#####■
ENFORCER	depends on balloon	12%	3-5 atm	+	0.064"	markers on balloon
FLEXSTENT (GR I)	1.78-2.3 mm	0%	4-5 atm	+	0.077 - 0.086"	■////////■
FREEDOM	1.3 mm	0%	10-12 atm	++	0.065"	■#####■
GFX	0.9-0.93 mm	0%	9-10 atm	++	0.064-0.072"	■#####■
GR II	1.5-1.7 mm	0%	6 atm	+++ (gold markers)	0.060- 0.070"	■/#/#/#/■
MICRO II	1.63 mm	2%	9-12 atm	++	0.072"	■///////■
MULTILINK	1.35-1.38 RX 1.7-1.95 OTW	<5%	7 atm OTW 10 atm RX	+	0.064"	■#####■
NIR STENT	<1.0 mm	<5%	7-14 atm	+	0.064"	markers on balloon
PALMAZ SCHATZ PS153	1.65mm	2.5-15%	4-6 atm	+	0.062" bare 0.084"mounted	■ #####■ ...■
PALMAZ BILIARY	depends on balloon	2-15%	delivery balloon	++	0.078"	markers on balloon
PARAGON (ACT-ONE)	1.3 mm	3%	8-16 atm	+++	0.062"	■#####■
RADIUS	1.53 mm	<3%	self expanding	+++	0.072"	■#####■
SPIRAL	1.65 mm	2.5-15%	delivery balloon	++	0.062" bare 0.084"mounted	markers on balloon
SPIRAL IMPROVED	1.4 mm	7%	6 atm	++	6 F	■#####■
TERUMO	depends on balloon	<5%	10 atm	+	0.065"	markers on balloon
WALLSTENT (MAGIC)	1.6 mm	20%	4 atm to allow self expansion	+++	0.064"	ends of stent & end of outer sheath
WIKTOR	1.27-1.77mm	4%	6-10 atm	++++	0.062-0.086"	/////■///// double mark (i)
XT	depends on balloon	0%	8 atm with Rely balloon material	++	0.062-0.070"	one per module

INDEX

About Physicians' Press

– Letter to the Editor –

Adapted from: American Journal of Cardiology (Sept 1, 1997, vol 80)

If you attended the American College of Cardiology meeting in Anaheim last March, and were in a particularly attentive mood when you walked through Publishers Showcase, you may have noticed the following announcement at one of the medical publisher's booths:

Don't Be Fooled!

Before you buy a book from any other medical publisher, ask the sales rep, ***"How current are the literature references?"*** *Don't accept statements such as, "The book is hot-off-the-press," or, "The book is new; of course it's current." Insist on an answer. And if the sales rep says, "Well the references are just a few months old," ask him, "If I determine otherwise, will you return my money and let me keep the book?" (Don't be surprised if you see a bead of sweat start to form on the sales rep's brow when you pose this question.) Just because you're told a book is "new," or you see a shiny "new" sticker on the cover, doesn't mean the information is "current!"* ***Don't buy a book today that has you practicing 1996 medicine. Don't waste your money on out-of-date information.***

And don't be fooled.

This important "public service" announcement comes from Physicians' Press, a unique entry into the medical publishing industry. In addition to being owned and operated by physicians, Physicians' Press stands apart from all other medical publishers in being able to produce completely current publications, with literature references ***less than 2 weeks old*** at the time of book release, compared to 12-18 months old for most other texts! (For example, *The New Manual of Interventional Cardiology* contained literature references from the very same meeting it appeared at — an unprecedented event.) We frequently receive comments such as, "The only books I bother reading are yours, the rest are outdated." Even experts such as Martin B. Leon, MD, one of the world's leading interventional cardiologists, agree: "I remain astounded at how the editors [of *The New Manual of Interventional Cardiology*] have provided fully updated chapters."

Current publications include the Physicians' Press "Interventional Library" (*The New Manual of Interventional Cardiology and Slide Series, The Device Guide, TOUGH CALLS in Interventional Cardiology, Guide To Rotational Atherectomy, Interventional Cardiology: Self-Assessment and Review, The Stenter's Notebook), as well as The Complete Guide To ECGs, and Essentials of Cardiovascular Medicine*, the latter of which has sold more than 200,000 copies. Within the next six months, more than a dozen new titles are due out, including manuals, slides sets, self-assessment & review books, and CD-ROMs on interventional and general cardiology, ECG interpretation, drug therapy & differential diagnosis, and infectious diseases. We have also developed a web site (www.physicianspress.com), which contains interventional cardiology and ECG cases-of-the-week, self-assessment tests, interventional news, quotes & cartoons, and a listing of upcoming meetings and conferences.

Gone are the days when physicians must accept the slow and antiquated methods of medical publishers who produce outdated books and call them "new." Gone are the days when an author has no other choice but to submit a book chapter to a publisher, knowing that some (or much) of the information will be obsolete by the time the book is published.

Whether you're a reader or a writer, we would like to welcome you aboard the "Physicians' Press Express," as we continue to develop the most current, practical, and user-friendly information, and distinguish ourselves as the new gold-standard in medical publishing.

Mark Freed, M.D.
President and Editor-in-Chief

If you have an idea for a publication, or are looking for a publisher, please call us at (248) 645-6443. And don't forget to send us your e-mail address (either by fax to: 248-642-4949, or by e-mail to MFreedMD@flash.net) so we can notify you about new information and services.

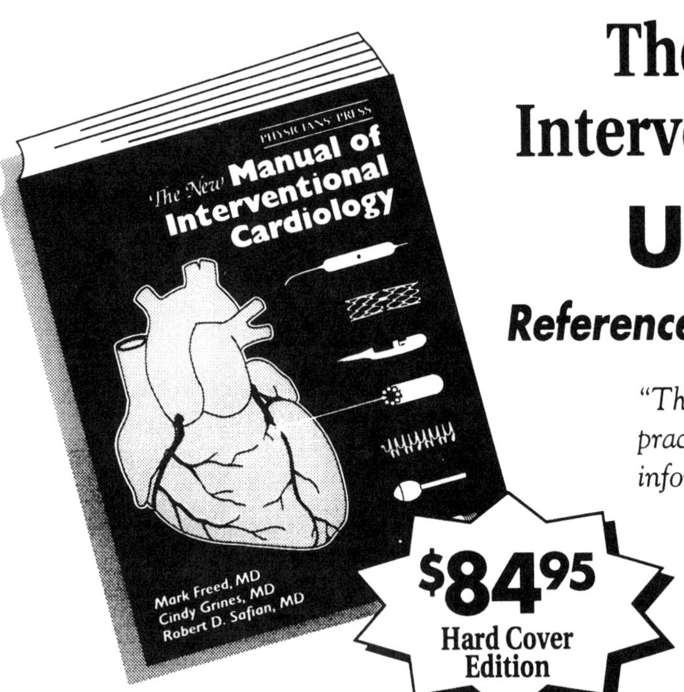

The New Manual of Interventional Cardiology

UPDATED!

References through September 1997

"The most comprehensive body of practical interventional cardiology information I have seen."

Gary Roubin, MD, PhD

"Remarkably comprehensive… I remain astounded at how the editors have provided fully updated chapters… without question, this is a 'must-read'."

Marty Leon, MD

ReoPro vs Placebo for Elective PTCA: The EPILOG TRIAL

30 Day Event	ReoPro	Placebo
Death	0.4**	0.8
Death + MI*	2.6**	8.1
Major Bleeding	1.8	3.1

* CK > 3x normal
** $p<0.001$

Adjunctive ReoPro improves PTCA outcome at 30 days without an increase in bleeding complications.

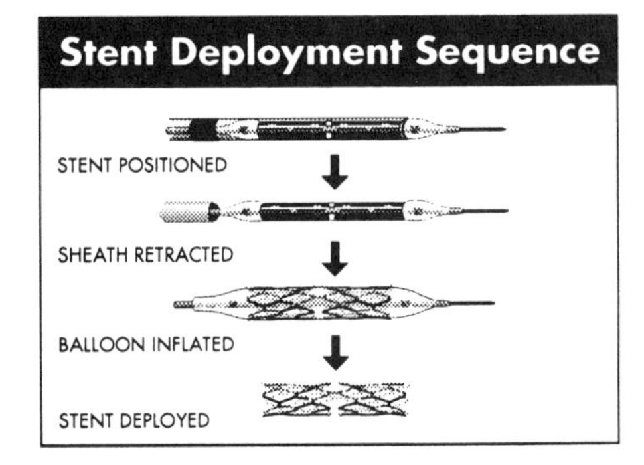

Hundreds of Easy-to-Read Tables, Figures & Algorithms

800 Pages & 40 Chapters In All Including:

- Simple & Complex Angioplasty
- Intervention by Lesion Morphology
- Intraprocedural Complications
- New Devices with Special Emphasis on Stents

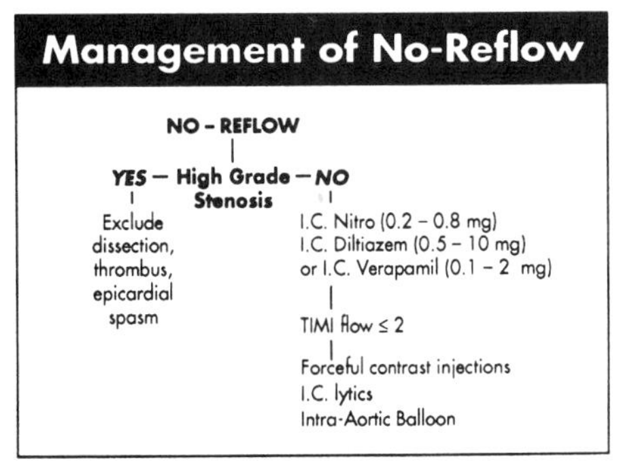

Enjoy The Physicians' Press Advantage:

References less than 2 weeks old at time of publication compared to 12–24 months for other interventional texts!

FAX/MAIL ORDER FORM

ITEM	QUANTITY	TOTAL COST (US Dollars)
______	______	______
______	______	______
______	______	______
______	______	______
______	______	______

5 Ways to Order:

Contact your local medical bookstore or:

By Phone:

(USA) (800) 642-5494

(Outside USA)

(248) 645-6443

By Fax:

Fax order page to:

(248) 642-4949

By Internet:

www.physicianspress.com

By Mail: *Mail to:*

Physicians' Press
555 S. Old Woodward
Suite 1409
Birmingham, Michigan
USA 48009-6679

Sales Tax ______

(Michigan residents add 6%; Canadian residents add 7% GST)

Shipping ______

(Compute shipping charge based on chart below)

TOTAL (U.S. DOLLARS) $ ______

TOTAL PURCHASE	USA *UPS Ground; arrives 3–7 days*	OUTSIDE USA* US Postal Surface *Arrives 6–8 weeks*	US Postal Air *Arrives 10-14 Days*	Express Air *UPS, FEDEX, DHL Arrives 2-5 Days*
$1–35	Add $4	Add $10	Add $20	Add $30
$36–90	Add $7	Add $15	Add $30	Add $60
$91–150	Add $12	Add $20	Add $40	Add $75
$151–400	Add $14	Add $25	Add $50	Add $90
$401–750	Add $16	Add $30	Add $60	Add $120
$751+	Add $20	Add $35	Add $70	Add $150

** If shipping charges exceed those listed in the chart, you will be contacted for approval prior to shipment.*

For shipping outside USA, check one: ☐ Express Air ☐ US Postal Air ☐ US Postal Surface

☐ Check Enclosed *(US Dollars from US Bank)*

☐ Bill Me

☐ Credit Card: ☐ Visa ☐ MasterCard ☐ AMEX

☐ 3-Payment Plan: Orders over $300, bill my credit card each month for 3 consecutive months.

Card No.: ______

Exp. Date: ______

Signature: ______

Name: ______ (PLEASE PRINT)

Address: ______

______

______

Telephone *(important)*: ______

FAX *(important)*: ______

e-mail ______

ORDERING INFORMATION
30 DAY MONEY-BACK GUARANTEE

ELECTROCARDIOGRAPHY

ITEM	DESCRIPTION	PRICE (US Dollars)
1	The Complete Guide to ECGs	$ 49.95
2	The Complete Guide to ECGs Slide Set (100 slides)	69.95
3	The ECG Criteria and ACLS Handbook	12.95

INTERVENTIONAL CARDIOLOGY

ITEM	DESCRIPTION	PRICE (US Dollars)
4	The New Manual of Interventional Cardiology	84.95
5	The New Manual of Interventional Cardiology Slide Series (650 slides)	750.00
6	Tough Calls in Interventional Cardiology	129.95
7	The Device Guide	39.95
8	Guide to Rotational Atherectomy	59.95
9	Interventional Cardiology: Self-Assessment and Review	45.00
10	The Stenter's Notebook	49.95

OTHER PUBLICATIONS

ITEM	DESCRIPTION	PRICE (US Dollars)
11a	Essentials of Cardiovascular Medicine (unabridged)	29.95
11b	Essentials of Cardiovascular Medicine (abridged)	12.95
11c	Essentials of Cardiovascular Medicine (bookset)	39.95
12	After Residency: The Young Physician's Guide to the Universe	19.95

DISCOUNT PACKAGES

ITEM	DESCRIPTION	PRICE (US Dollars)	
13	Interventional Package I: Items 4, 6, & 7	229.95	SAVE $25
14	Interventional Package II: Items 4, 5, 6, & 7	899.95	SAVE $105
15	Interventional Package III: All 6 Interventional Publications & Slides	1009.75	SAVE $150

§ Prices subject to change.

Sales Tax: Michigan residents add 6%; Canadian residents add 7% GST

Shipping & Handling Policy: Books & Slides are shipped immediately upon publication. It is possible to receive 2 or more shipments. **Overnight delivery available – call for charge.**

5 Ways to Order:

Contact your local medical bookstore or:

By Phone:

(USA)
(800) 642-5494
(Outside USA)
(248) 645-6443

By Fax:

Fax order page to:
(248) 642-4949

By Internet:

www.physicianspress.c

By Mail: *Mail to:*

Physicians' Press
555 S. Old Woodwarc
Suite 1409
Birmingham, Michigan
USA 48009-6679

FAX/MAIL ORDER FORM

ITEM	QUANTITY	TOTAL COST (US Dollars)
______	______	______
______	______	______
______	______	______
______	______	______
______	______	______

5 Ways to Order:

Contact your local medical bookstore or:

By Phone:

(USA) (800) 642-5494
(Outside USA)
(248) 645-6443

By Fax:

Fax order page to:
(248) 642-4949

By Internet:

www.physicianspress.com

By Mail: *Mail to:*

Physicians' Press
555 S. Old Woodward
Suite 1409
Birmingham, Michigan
USA 48009-6679

Sales Tax ______
(Michigan residents add 6%; Canadian residents add 7% GST)

Shipping ______
(Compute shipping charge based on chart below)

TOTAL (U.S. DOLLARS) $ ______

TOTAL PURCHASE	USA *UPS Ground; arrives 3–7 days*	OUTSIDE USA* US Postal Surface *Arrives 6–8 weeks*	US Postal Air *Arrives 10-14 Days*	Express Air *UPS, FEDEX, DHL Arrives 2-5 Days*
$1–35	Add $4	Add $10	Add $20	Add $30
$36–90	Add $7	Add $15	Add $30	Add $60
$91–150	Add $12	Add $20	Add $40	Add $75
$151–400	Add $14	Add $25	Add $50	Add $90
$401–750	Add $16	Add $30	Add $60	Add $120
$751+	Add $20	Add $35	Add $70	Add $150

** If shipping charges exceed those listed in the chart, you will be contacted for approval prior to shipment.*

For shipping outside USA, check one: ☐ Express Air ☐ US Postal Air ☐ US Postal Surface

☐ Check Enclosed *(US Dollars from US Bank)*

☐ Bill Me

☐ Credit Card: ☐ Visa ☐ MasterCard ☐ AMEX

☐ 3-Payment Plan: Orders over $300, bill my credit card each month for 3 consecutive months.

Card No.: ______

Exp. Date: ______

Signature: ______

Name: ______ (PLEASE PRINT)

Address: ______

______

______

Telephone *(important)*: ______

FAX *(important)*: ______

e-mail ______